T0177551

# Neuroscience at the Intersection of Mind and Brain

Jack M. Gorman, MD

Co-Founder and President, Critica LLC

CEO and Chief Scientific Officer

Franklin Behavioral Health Consultants

New York, NY

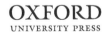

OXFORD
UNIVERSITY PRESS

OXFORD
UNIVERSITY PRESS

Oxford University Press is a department of the University of Oxford. It furthers
the University's objective of excellence in research, scholarship, and education
by publishing worldwide. Oxford is a registered trade mark of Oxford University
Press in the UK and certain other countries.

Published in the United States of America by Oxford University Press
198 Madison Avenue, New York, NY 10016, United States of America.

CIP data is on file at the Library of Congress
ISBN 978–0–19–085012–8

1 3 5 7 9 8 6 4 2

Printed by Webcom, Inc., Canada

# Contents

# Preface

... wide as the gap between brain and mind.
—Helen Mort ("Ablation," Poetry Magazine, December, 2015, p. 249)

This book is about neuroscience and experience and what I believe the mind is. Therefore, it seems appropriate that I begin by explaining a bit about the experiences—personal and scientific—that led me to my fascination with the topic and to write this book. In other words, to lay out what is on my mind.

Although during medical school at Columbia University in New York City I was determined to be a pediatrician, I changed my mind during my pediatric internship and began my residency training in psychiatry at Columbia in 1978. Having myself been in psychotherapy during medical school, I was impressed by the intellectual power and therapeutic possibility of psychoanalysis and started my psychiatry residency with the notion of someday becoming a psychoanalyst myself. At the time, there was no shortage of famous psychoanalysts on the faculty of Columbia's Department of Psychiatry and its affiliated Psychoanalytic Clinic for Training and Research.

But there was also a relatively new breed of prominent psychiatrists on that faculty, led by two giants of the field, Donald Klein and Edward Sacher. Klein was one of a handful of pioneers in the relatively new field of psychopharmacology, the study of the use of medication to treat psychiatric illnesses. He had shown, among other things, that the antidepressant drug imipramine could effectively block spontaneous anxiety attacks in patients with the newly described condition called *panic disorder*. These patients suffer supposedly "out-of-the-blue" panic attacks in which their hearts pound, breathing rates speed up, and they fear imminent death. So dreaded are these attacks that many patients become afraid to be alone, often to the point of becoming homebound, a condition called *agoraphobia*. Psychoanalysis had theories about the generation of these attacks and phobias, but Klein used the methodology of the placebo-controlled clinical trial to demonstrate that, after about four weeks, the drug imipramine, and later other antidepressants as well, resulted in a marked decrease and even elimination of the attacks. The phobic avoidance subsequently subsided and the patient seemed virtually cured.

Sacher, who become chairman of our department before suffering a devastating stroke and ultimately taking his own life, was one of the first to show that patients with depression had elevated levels of the adrenal hormone cortisol in their blood and urine. Cortisol was already known to be a marker of the stress response in animals and to be under the control of another hormone synthesized in the brain. Sacher's work suggested that depression involved a disorder of the cortisol system, placing it in the realm of a "biological" rather than a "psychological" condition.

Sacher and Klein were the powerful professors in our department. The psychoanalysts complained about their "superficial" approach to mental illness, but we residents looked up to them and their colleagues as great scientists, which they were. In my last year of residency, I started not only formal psychoanalytic training but became a research fellow in Klein's group. My first project was studying the autonomic nervous system—the part of the nervous system that controls the heart, lungs, and other vital organs—in patients with panic disorder. I quickly received my first grant from the National Institute of Mental Health (NIMH) to pursue my research under Klein's supervision and was soon thrilled to see my name on published papers in scientific journals. My wife Lauren and I had a new baby at home, and I realized that I couldn't pursue both research and psychoanalytic training. I decided to quit psychoanalysis and devote my life to studying the biology of fear and anxiety and to helping develop drugs for people suffering from anxiety, depression, and other emotional disorders.

Klein was my mentor, an internationally renowned figure who traveled the world giving lectures and consulting to pharmaceutical companies. He insisted on rigorous adherence to the scientific method, to carefully designed studies, and to accepting only what the data we generated could support. He hated psychoanalysis and psychotherapy. Under his tutelage, I became a full-fledged psychopharmacologist, specializing in research that sought to uncover exactly what happens in the brain when a person becomes fearful or chronically anxious. My studies extended to a collaboration with a group that focused on separation anxiety in monkeys, to the use of every newly developed brain imaging technique, and to a devotion to emerging findings in the basic neuroscience laboratories at Columbia and elsewhere.

My career flourished—I continued to receive grant funding from the NIMH and to publish papers. I, too, received invitations to speak around the world, to consult to drug companies, and to be on government grant review panels. I was promoted to full professor, became head of my own lab and research group, and taught students and other doctors how to use medications to treat psychiatric disorders.

But, all the while, I was bothered by the persistent claims that there was another, perhaps better way to treat conditions like panic disorder and depression—*cognitive behavioral psychotherapy* (CBT). Klein himself engaged in some rather ferocious debates with an English physician named Isaac Marks who insisted that drugs only worked while the patient continued to take them, but CBT could induce a more durable response. Unlike psychoanalysis, which the CBT people seemed to dislike even more than the psychopharmacologists, CBT ignored childhood trauma, dreams, the unconscious, and transference in favor of confronting one's irrational fears and behaviors. The treatment lasts only about 12 sessions over three months, not the years that a psychoanalytic treatment takes. Also unlike psychoanalytic psychotherapies, there were actual studies showing that CBT worked.

Klein and other psychopharmacologists dismissed the CBT group's claims by focusing on methodological problems with their study designs. Ever since World War

II, the coin of the realm in biomedical research has been what is called the *double-blind, placebo-controlled, randomized clinical trial* (RCT). The three main elements are that (1) the treatment under investigation is compared to a control treatment, usually either an inert substance (placebo) and/or an already established medication; (2) neither the investigators nor the patients know who is getting the new treatment under investigation and who is getting the placebo or other control treatment; and (3) patients are randomly assigned to receive either investigational treatment or control treatment. All of this is widely felt to reduce the possibilities of investigator bias creeping into the interpretation of the results of the study. The placebos used for medication RCTs are usually sugar pills that look exactly like the drug under investigation. But what is the placebo for a psychotherapy? How do you keep the patient and the therapist "blind" as to whether the patient is getting real CBT or some kind of "placebo" therapy?

And yet the data coming from the CBT studies seemed persuasive to me and I felt hypocritical for ignoring it. I was trained, after all, to accept whatever the data show. So I contacted one of the leading scientists in the CBT world, David Barlow, who was then a professor at the State University of New York in Albany, and challenged him to design a study with me comparing the drug imipramine with CBT for the treatment of panic disorder. To my surprise, Barlow told me he was already discussing this possibility with another psychopharmacologist, Yale University's Scott Woods. Ultimately, we decided to ask another CBT proponent, psychiatrist M. Katherine Shear, then at the University of Pittsburgh, to join us in designing a four-site study. Our goal was to come up with a design that would satisfy both sides of the debate, so that no one could attack the methods and everyone would have to accept the results. We received funding from NIMH to do the study and spent months hammering out the technical issues of how to do it. The study took us several years to complete, but I had no doubt all along that the results would show that the drug imipramine was a superior treatment to both CBT and placebo.

I was wrong. In what we called the *acute phase* of the study—the first six weeks—imipramine, CBT, and the combination of imipramine and CBT were all better than placebo and equally effective with each other. We kept the responders on whatever treatment they had responded to for an additional six months of a maintenance phase and saw the same results. But the surprise came in the follow-up phase after we discontinued the treatments and assessed how the patients were doing during a six-month no-treatment period. To our surprise, the patients who had been on CBT were doing better than those who had been assigned to either imipramine or the combination of drug plus CBT. It was as if taking the drug somehow made things worse in the long run.

Needless to say, I hated these results. We psychopharmacologists tried to find something wrong with the study or the way we had analyzed the results. By the time the study results were published in 2000, in the *Journal of the American Medical Association* (JAMA),[1] drugs like imipramine had been replaced by fluoxetine (brand name: Prozac) and similar new medications of a class called the *selective serotonin*

---

[1] Barlow DH, Gorman JM, Shear MK, Woods SW: Cognitive-behavioral therapy, imipramine, or their combination for panic disorder: a randomized controlled trial. *JAMA* 2000;283:2529–2536.

*reuptake inhibitors* (SSRIs). Some die-hard psychopharmacologists tried to say that if we had used Prozac instead of imipramine, we would have beaten CBT. For a variety of reasons, that is not a very likely prediction, and, indeed, the only choice I had was to accept that CBT was a better treatment for panic disorder than imipramine.

My other work in the laboratory also led to some unpredicted findings, and I came to believe that I had been barking up the wrong tree in my studies. I had been treating psychiatric illnesses as if they were no different from pneumonia or cancer, things that happen to people without any emotional input.[2] Panic disorder, according to this view, was caused by some brain circuits and chemicals going awry, and the solution was to give a medication that fixed the problem. In fact, there is no question that medication makes people better. But I now saw that the thoughts and emotions that patients have are more complicated and that therapies that addressed them seemed more capable of inducing longer lasting cures. Much as I hated to admit it, Marks was right: medication only worked as long as the patient was taking it, whereas CBT seemed to give the patient new sets of skills and behaviors to stay well even after the therapy was finished. Moreover, it was obvious how CBT worked: each component addressed one of the aspects of the disorder directly. Patients with panic disorder hyperventilate, so there was a breathing retraining component. They think they are going to die during an attack, so a cognitive strategy to get them to rethink that irrational idea was pursued. They were afraid to leave the house, so an exposure component in which they took trips of increasing length from their front door was included. By contrast, by 2000, we had to admit that we had absolutely no idea how imipramine, Prozac, or any of our antidepressant drugs actually work. Even one of psychiatry's real miracle drugs, lithium, which is so effective for people with bipolar disorder, has an entirely obscure mechanism of action in the brain.

The second thing that changed the trajectory of my thinking and career began when a surprise candidate was selected as the new director of the NIMH in 1996, Steven Hyman. Hyman was at the time an associate professor at Harvard and not as well known in the psychiatry world as had been previous NIMH directors. He was among a small number of psychiatrists who worked in a basic science laboratory and distinguished himself as a molecular neuroscientist. Up until then, however, most of the NIMH directors had been national figures in psychiatry, usually chairs of a medical school department. Hyman's appointment signaled a welcome recognition that psychiatry and mental health research needed to be placed on a firmer scientific basis than was then so far the case.

I didn't know Hyman well at the time of his appointment, but every time I saw him after he became NIMH director he would say to me "you should be working with Joe LeDoux." Although that name was familiar to me, I really had no idea what LeDoux had done that might be relevant to me. Nevertheless, after Hyman said this to me on several occasions, I finally looked up LeDoux and went to see him.

---

[2] Of course, there are almost no medical illnesses that don't have an emotional or behavioral aspect. But that is another story.

What LeDoux had done—and continues to do—is of staggering innovation and importance. Based at New York University's Center for Neural Science, LeDoux has managed to elucidate some of the most basic aspects of what happens in the brain during the experience of fear. The details of his work will be described later in this book, but basically LeDoux induced a learned fear response in rats and then used a variety of techniques to show that a small region deep in the mammalian brain called the *amygdala* is absolutely essential for the animal to manifest the fear response. He then traced the pathways to and from the amygdala that underlie all of the many manifestations of fear, including freezing and increases in heart rate, respiration, and stress hormone release. Finally, and perhaps most important, he and his group isolated a cascade of genes and proteins necessary for the acquisition, consolidation, extinction, and reinstatement of learned fear. For the first time, the circuitry and molecular biology of an emotion common to rats and humans had been revealed.

In 2000, my colleagues and I published a theoretical paper in the *American Journal of Psychiatry* called "The Neuroanatomical Hypothesis of Panic Disorder, Revised,"[3] in which we speculated that perhaps panic attacks in humans also involved abnormal activation of the amygdala. It is still unclear whether this hypothesis is correct, but it represented for me a first attempt to try to match clinical research observations with what had been discovered in the basic neuroscience laboratory. This effort is known as "translational neuroscience," and it became an important part of my subsequent work.

Together with several other researchers at New York City institutions, including Bruce McEwen of Rockefeller University, John Morrison of Mount Sinai School of Medicine, and David Silbersweig, then of Cornell University's medical school, we obtained a large research grant from the NIMH to pursue the translational neuroscience of fear and anxiety. Among other things, we began applying advanced brain imaging techniques to patients with anxiety disorders to see if we could find traces of the same biology LeDoux and McEwen had found in rats and mice.

One of the things that impressed me as I began this new phase of work was the enormous changes in brain structure and function that could be produced by exposing laboratory animals to both negative experiences, like stress, and positive experiences, like an enriched environment. It was not just that the animals' behaviors could be changed, but also that the projections from neurons that form brain connections with other neurons retracted or sprouted, genes were activated, proteins synthesized, and long-term memories created. We were able to go back and forth between the clinical and basic laboratories, as I will explain in more detail in subsequent chapters, to show the effects of lived experience and learning on how the brain works.

By 2000, my ideas and interests had radically changed. I now believed that psychotherapy was not only effective but could be studied in the same rigorous way as medications; that although genes undoubtedly are important factors for mental illness, experience plays at least as great a role; and that we have much to learn from

[3] Gorman JM, Kent JM, Sullivan GM, Coplan JD: Neuroanatomical hypothesis of panic disorder, revised. *Am J Psychiatry* 2000;157:493–505.

basic neuroscientists. I used my exposure to LeDoux and McEwen to try to forge relationships with other basic scientists and to learn as much neuroscience as I could.

Unfortunately, these efforts came to a grinding halt for me in 2006. A variety of factors forced me to begin a decade of rehabilitation and reflection. The devotion of family and friends got me through my exit from academic psychiatry and enabled me to see many things more clearly than ever before. Not having the pressures of writing grants and papers and managing a large research team freed me to think about science and consider how a new set of personal experiences—however stressful—might give me further insights into the role of experience in changing the brain. I plan in a future book to explain much more about my personal travails, but in this book I want to focus on what I learned about psychiatry, psychology, and neuroscience. I will frequently interject personal experiences and recollections because my story involves the important element of what scientists do when they are confronted with data that do not fit their hypotheses and beliefs and how they change—or fail to change—their thinking and work as a result. As psychiatry and psychology struggle to become more "scientific," the issue of how scientists come to conclusions and how these conclusions are conveyed to the public they serve becomes increasingly critical.

In the first chapter, I will give a brief and admittedly very subjective history of the recent relationships among various schools of thought in the mental health field, including the debate about whether the brain and the mind are the same or different entities and to what extent neuroscience is relevant to both brain and mind. Subsequent chapters will use selected emotions, experiences, or mental disorders to illustrate specific aspects of brain function that are relevant to the ways in which experiences affect brain function and structure. Chapter 2 will engage in the current discussion of just how different our brains are from our nearest genetic neighbors, the chimpanzee and bonobo, and what that can tell us about severe brain disorders like schizophrenia. Is it the ineffable "mind" that makes us a different intellectual creature than our genetic relatives, or something physical about the brain? This is a crucial question to address in the mind versus brain arena. In Chapter 3, I will use the experience of stressful life events as the platform to discuss the genetics and something called *epigenetics* of the brain. Then, in Chapter 4, we will advance from the molecular to the cellular level of brain function and discuss how neurons connect with each other and how, under limited circumstances, new neurons can sometimes be created. Among other things, these processes are very important in understanding some aspects of depression. Before advancing to the next level of brain organization, I will take a brief detour in Chapter 5 to explain the various technologies we use to image living, human brains as we experience the world around us. It is important for the reader to understand that enthusiasm for the power of clinical neuroscience must be tempered by a recognition of the limitations of our technology. Then, in Chapter 6, we will see how these brain imaging techniques are used to visualize connections between different regions of the brain and to determine which connections between different brain regions may be crucial for the experience of fear and the development of anxiety disorders. In Chapter 7, I will review the biology of social affiliation and romantic love, which involve the brain's reward system and the hormone oxytocin. I will then turn in

Chapter 8 to the most speculative chapter of the book: a discussion of whether there is a scientific basis to psychotherapy and psychoanalysis, focusing attention on neural processes called *extinction* and *reconsolidation of memory*. Finally, in the last chapter, I will endeavor to bring all of these biological processes together and trace how a series of adverse experiences, particularly in early life, can change the physical brain in the direction of emotional disturbance and suffering and how drugs and psychotherapy act on those brain changes to promote mental health, resilience, and even, may I dare say, happiness. All along, I will build a case that there is no physical or scientific difference between what we call the mind and what we know to be the brain. Perceived differences between "mind" and "brain" rest, I believe, only in what neuroscience has yet to figure out.

There are, of course, some very technical aspects to all of this, but my hope is to make these accessible to the interested nonscientist without oversimplifying the science or the issues. I expect that there will be many objections to my outlook, both from those who insist that a former psychopharmacologist has no business delving into the world of psychotherapy and those who will be unconvinced that neuroscience is anything more than a way to reduce the human mind to chemicals. Most welcome to me, however, will be comments and criticisms on how I have depicted the science of experience.

# Acknowledgments

This is the fourth book I have worked on with Oxford University Press. Each time, the editors at the Press have proved to be wonderful professionals. For this book, I am indebted to editors Andrea Knobloch and Allison Pratt, whose help and support have been invaluable.

Thanks also to illustrator Catherine DiDesidero who drew several figures in Chapters 6 and 8.

Many scientists, psychiatrists, and therapists profoundly influenced me and helped me through the four decades of my research and clinical career. I want to extend my deepest gratitude to Drs. Joseph LeDoux, Bruce McEwen, Steven Roose, Jeremy Coplan, Leonard Rosenblum, Cindy Aaronson, Jerry Gliklich, Jan Mohlman, Richard Munich, David Barlow, Scott Woods, M. Katherine Shear, Charles Nemeroff, Karen Winer, Aaron Beck, Alan Weiner, Ezra Susser, and Peter Nathan.

I am blessed with several great professionals to whom I also happen to be related. My brother-in-law, Sandy Winer, an eminent attorney, has offered me invaluable personal support in recent years. I have two amazing and brilliant scholars as sons-in-law, Dr. David Moster and Dr. Robert Kohen, who are both inspiring.

My daughters are also my teachers and colleagues. Dr. Rachel Moster, a psychiatrist who specializes in treating people with severe mental illness, has blossomed into a superb clinician and advocate for the disadvantaged. She is everything a physician should be. Dr. Sara Gorman is the co-author of my previous book, *Denying to the Grave* and co-founder with me of Critica LLC, our company devoted to fighting science denial, and my intellectual mentor.

This book deals a lot with the effects of early life experiences. While writing it, I have had the wonderful experience of watching how this works in my granddaughter, Hannah Beth Moster. Of course, as a doting Grandpa I believe she is totally exceptional and I am dazzled by how a new person embraces her environment, learning so many complex things so quickly. I hope it is not too long before she can read this paragraph (she is two years old now) and realize how amazing I think she is.

I have also had adverse life experiences while writing this book, the saddest of all was the passing of my mother, Kate Gorman, who, among other things, taught me to love literature and learning. This book is dedicated to her blessed memory.

When I am finally done with a book, I write down acknowledgments like these to people I admire and want to thank. Each time, as I get to the end of this section, my eyes reflexively fill with tears of gratitude. How lucky am I that I get to finish by thanking my wife, Dr. Lauren Kantor Gorman. I am not by far the only person who is grateful to her: she is a psychiatrist who has devoted decades to helping so many people overcome life's challenges. It certainly helps in writing a book about the brain to be married to the world's best psychiatrist. Her knowledge and insights are palpable throughout this book and everything else I do. Her love is even more apparent.

# 1

# Introduction

The brain is the organ of the mind.
—Eric Kandel

Neuroscience has captured the attention of both the scientific community and the general public. Perhaps beginning around 2000, when the Nobel Prize for Medicine or Physiology was awarded to three neuroscientists, there is a widespread sense that we now have an unprecedented ability to study the intricacies of brain function in order to understand many aspects of human behavior and emotion as well as the basis for psychiatric disorders and their treatments. There have been many presentations to the public using various forms of print and electronic media to explain these important advances.

But among psychiatrists, psychologists, and other mental health professionals, not everyone is so enthusiastic about neuroscience's popularity or its explanatory potential. For some, contemporary neuroscience is another way for those who promote the use of medication as the main method for treating mental illness to argue that their views are uniquely "scientific." Proponents of the idea that medication is the first-line approach for most conditions, often called the *psychopharmacology group*, have long insisted that there is little scientific evidence supporting either the theory or usefulness of any form of psychotherapy. The psychopharmacologists claim to know what drugs do in the brain and can point to many rigorously designed studies that show that these medications work for most psychiatric disorders, including the most common ones: depression and anxiety disorders. In its most extreme form, the psychopharmacologists believe that all mental illnesses are ultimately due to abnormal genes and that adverse life experiences play almost no role in causing them. Ultimately, they insist, those genes will be uncovered, the precise neurobiological mechanisms for emotional problems revealed, and increasingly better medications that target specific brain abnormalities developed. Brain science, the psychopharmacologists assert, is on their side.[1]

---

[1] It will be important as we proceed through this book to bear in mind that there is no formal field called psychopharmacology. Addiction psychiatry, forensic psychiatry, and geriatric psychiatry are among the recognized subspecialties of psychiatry, but psychopharmacology is not one of them. All psychiatrists are qualified to prescribe psychiatric medications. Those who call themselves psychopharmacologists are self-describing their particular interest and not a special credential.

Two brilliant neuroscientists, Daniel Geschwind and Jonathan Flint, wrote a few years ago that:

> Genetic findings are set to illuminate the causes and to challenge the existing nosology of psychiatric conditions, some of which, until recently, were purported to have a non-biological etiology. After decades of false starts, we now have confirmed associations between genetic variants that increase the risk of schizophrenia (SCZ), autism spectrum disorder (ASD), major depression, and bipolar disorder (BPD), and in some cases the underlying gene(s) have been identified. (p. 1489)[2]

This strong statement implies that the inheritance of disease genes will ultimately explain the cause and direct the treatment of most psychiatric disorders. By "non-biological etiology" Geschwind and Flint mean all those messy things that happen to us that make us feel sad, or worried, or scared. Those things, they assert, can now be dismissed in favor of real "biology." It is unsurprising that mental health professionals who specialize in psychotherapy, including those without a medical degree who cannot prescribe medication, object strongly to this characterization. The "psychotherapy" group frequently criticizes neuroscience as "reductionistic," that is, an attempt to describe the complexities of human behavior and emotions by the actions of a handful of brain chemicals and neurons. Contrary to the psychopharmacologists' claim that clinical trial evidence is limited to medication, psychotherapists can point to many very good studies demonstrating that some forms of psychotherapy are at least as good and in many cases better than medications for treating several psychiatric illnesses. But the main contention of the people who characterize neuroscience as reductionistic is that brain science cannot possibly explain how the human mind works. Only psychotherapy, they argue, with its emphasis on understanding our minds can offer more than the superficial remedy that a psychiatric patient gets from taking an antidepressant or antianxiety drug.

It is the main thesis of this book that both camps misunderstand and/or mischaracterize the state of contemporary neuroscience and are missing opportunities to advance our understanding of how mental illnesses develop and how interventions we currently have work, thus limiting opportunities to develop better treatments. Patients suffering from psychiatric problems are put at a great disadvantage by these professional battles. It is time to develop a broad understanding of both the wonderful developments in neuroscience that are directly applicable to human behavior and, just as important, the many things we still do not know or understand. In general, the psychopharmacologists overvalue and the psychotherapists underappreciate the

Many psychiatrists are actually far more comfortable treating patients with psychotherapy than with medication.

[2] Geschwind DH, Flint J: Genetics and genomics of psychiatric disease. *Science* 2015;349:1489–1494.

Neuroscience at the Intersection of Mind and Brain

relevance of both basic and clinical neuroscience to their fields. The aim here is to try to grapple with these issues and to demonstrate what we know and what we need to find out.

## DO SCIENCE AND EXPERIENCE GO TOGETHER?

A focus on the science of experience will help us achieve that goal. Putting the words "science" and "experience" together was, until fairly recently, a controversial notion in psychiatry and psychology. Yet this connection is clearly true for many diseases in physical medicine as well. Let's take an unfortunately all too common example, type 2 diabetes mellitus. Sadly, millions of people around the world are developing diabetes at a pandemic rate. It is known that the biology of type 2 diabetes involves an inability of cells to respond to insulin. This is different from type 1 diabetes, which usually develops in childhood and involves an inability of the pancreas to produce insulin. In the type 2 version there is enough insulin, but cells become resistant to its effects, leading to abnormally high glucose levels in the blood and a host of terrible complications. It is well-known that obesity is a major risk factor for type 2 diabetes, and, in some cases, diabetes can be averted by weight loss. Yet not everyone who gains too much weight develops type 2 diabetes, and there is very likely a genetic predisposition to do so.

So here we have a situation in which some as yet unknown genetic mutation(s) increases the likelihood that a life experience—becoming obese—will cause a biological change: insulin resistance. The details of how these are connected are complex and not entirely worked out, but it is obvious that there are going to be two main ways of attacking this problem: changing people's behavior so they lose weight and developing drugs that overcome the biological abnormality. Dealing with the genetics is not yet an option and probably won't be for many decades at least. This is because it is almost certainly not one but multiple genetic mutations that are involved in type 2 diabetes, each conferring a very small part of the overall genetic risk. The former solution, changing behavior, is a very difficult task—getting people to diet and exercise is notoriously frustrating and often unsuccessful. The latter is tough as well, but drugs that treat type 2 diabetes are very effective and profitable. And for patients with type 2 diabetes, taking a pill to fix the problem may seem much simpler and more desirable than losing weight and running on the treadmill every day. The result is that scientists will focus on developing more and better medications for diabetes. Those medications will be expensive and have adverse side effects, but the risk of untreated diabetes is a far worse situation. The role of the life event—becoming obese—takes on less and less importance in scientific circles until it seems nearly forgotten.

But this runs the risk of deemphasizing the important part that behavior plays in causing type 2 diabetes and of limiting efforts to figure out better ways to help people live healthier lives. Drugs to treat type 2 diabetes work and are absolutely a necessary part of dealing with this enormous problem, but perhaps we should not lose sight of the fact that we know very little about why people eat too much, hate to exercise, and tolerate getting fat. Science should be addressing those issues as well. It is, of course, absolutely not that we should stop trying to develop better and safer medications for diabetes but rather that we should add to that scientific effort more work to figure out why we are so enamored with our totally unhealthy approaches to diet and physical activity.

This tendency to push the importance of life experiences into the background was becoming the case for psychiatry as well. When it comes to mental health, it may seem obvious at first that life's experiences are relevant. We all know that bad news makes us sad and that things we worry about cause anxiety. That, of course, was the view of the early psychoanalysts like Sigmund Freud, who insisted that events occurring from birth through early childhood have permanent influences on our emotions and behaviors as adults (Freud did give passing mention to a "constitutional" predisposition to neuroses that is something like our modern-day notion of genetic risk). Psychoanalysis developed in part as a way to understand long-forgotten early life experiences and then to figure out how those events can have such enduring effects that they adversely affect the lives of adults.

But as medicine became increasingly more scientific following World War II, there was an enormous desire among psychiatrists to follow the trend of using clinical trial methodology to decide which treatments work. When a medication is involved, that means taking a large sample of people with an illness and randomly assigning one group of them to receive the new medication under consideration and the other group to receive either an older medication already known to work for the illness or a placebo pill. This kind of rigorously conducted experiment is highly effective in showing that medications do or do not work for a given illness, but they are very difficult to conduct with psychotherapies like psychoanalysis. In addition to the issue of figuring out what could possibly be the "placebo" condition that mirrors psychoanalysis but doesn't have any effect, psychoanalysis takes years to work; it is impossible to conduct a clinical research trial that lasts that long—three months is a much more practical length of time for a practical, affordable *randomized control trial* (RCT). And so, psychiatrists turned to the possibility that medications might be helpful for mental illnesses as they are for physical medical illnesses. When several medications indeed passed the RCT test in the 1950s, the new field of psychopharmacology was born. Psychiatrists started feeling like "real doctors," buoyed by a scientific foundation for their specialty and a pharmaceutical industry that immediately recognized the enormous profits to be gained from psychiatric drugs. In time, it seemed that antidepressants and antipsychotics were scientific and psychotherapy merely old-fashioned. This is the situation I found when I started my psychiatric residency training in 1978.

Along with the success of psychiatric medications came a tendency to reject not only the practice of psychoanalysis but also everything that psychoanalytic theory had posited. Whether correct or not (and, indeed, I will show in later chapters that the notion is not correct), psychiatric medications were believed to work on physical processes in the brain that were not subject to environmental influences. The earliest antidepressants, for example, increased levels of one or both of two chemical neurotransmitters, serotonin and norepinephrine. Scientists and psychiatrists leaped to the conclusion that people with depression must suffer from a deficiency in these neurotransmitters, caused by some abnormal gene. The antidepressants worked regardless of whether the patient's depression followed on the heels of a personal tragedy or loss or seemed instead to come "out of the blue." Hence, life experience seemed irrelevant to the new pharmacology. Although it is now quite clear that illnesses like depression are not caused by a simple deficiency of any neurotransmitters, we still see instances in which psychopharmacologists recommend switching a patient who has not responded to a drug that affects one neurotransmitter to a different drug that works on a different neurotransmitter in order to take advantage of a different "mechanism of action." In fact, the implied mechanisms of action are entirely elusive at this point.

In the nature versus nurture debate that swept through the mental health field, problems in nature were clearly winning out as the cause of psychiatric illness, at least as far as the psychopharmacologists were concerned. What your relationship was with your parents or any other aspect of your early life environment became irrelevant. Even traumatic experiences occurring during adult life seemed in this view of minor importance. Scientists began extensive and expensive searches for hardwired genetic effects as the cause of mental illness.

## IS NEUROSCIENCE JUST FOR DRUGS?

At the same time, the psychotherapy camp believed that neuroscience existed only to explain the mechanism of action of psychiatric drugs. They recognized immediately that a syndrome as complex and varied as depression probably could not be attributed just to low brain levels of one or two neurotransmitters and therefore tended to demean neuroscience in general. The human mind was seen as distinct from the physical brain, the former an ineffable entity containing the human spirit. Trying to explain mind by referencing brain chemicals and cells seemed simplistic and "reductionistic."

That view, too, turns out to be wrong. In fact, as we will see, modern neuroscience can describe in elegant detail how life's experiences translate into physical changes in our brains and even begin to explain how psychotherapy, including psychoanalysis, might work. "Plasticity" is the term often applied to the ability of the living brain to change itself physically in response to both stimuli and the absence of stimuli. Norman Doidge, a psychoanalyst whom I knew when he was one of our psychiatric residents at Columbia University, writes in his book *The Brain that Changes Itself*:

> Everything your "immaterial" mind imagines leaves material traces. Each thought alters the physical state of your brain synapses at a microscopic level.

Each time you imagine moving your fingers across the keys to play the piano, you alter the tendrils in your living brain.[3]

Neuroscience of the brain, far from being reductionistic, describes an incredibly rich, complex, and elegant human mind. Appreciating this, as I hope this book will influence its readers to do, immediately renders the reductionist idea obsolete.

Although some of the rabid debates between the psychopharmacology and psychotherapy groups that took place when I trained to be a psychiatrist in the late 1970s have simmered down a bit, this battle is ongoing today. To the extent that people who suffer with psychiatric problems deserve the very best possible treatments that modern science can discover and provide, a debate like this places us at a disadvantage. A person with severe depression isn't interested in whose school of thought is right and doesn't want scientists and clinicians wasting time battling it out; he or she wants to get better with whatever is safest and most effective to accomplish that goal. So it is definitely worth our while to explore what is behind this fight and whether it can be resolved in a way that preserves adherence to scientific evidence.

Studying the science of experience is therefore a wonderful pathway to seeing more clearly the complex ways in which brain function determines how we feel and act; how events in our lives affect us; some of the things that go wrong when we develop clinical depression, anxiety, and other mental health disorders; and even how different types of psychotherapy and medications can successfully treat those disorders.

Emphasizing the importance of the neuroscience of life's experiences by no means entails denying the role of genetics in human emotion and behavior. For the most part, the genes we inherit cannot be changed during life. Some diseases that afflict us are purely genetic, like Huntington's disease and sickle cell anemia. In those cases, the patient inherits a disease-producing genetic mutation, and succumbing to the disease is inevitable. There is no question that many psychiatric illnesses, like schizophrenia and bipolar disorder, have strong genetic roots. But it is probably true that most purely genetic diseases are already known and that diseases for which we have not uncovered a discrete mutation, like type 2 diabetes and depression, probably involve the work of many genes and many environmental events. Throughout all of medicine, there is a tendency to say that such diseases are caused by a combination of "genes and the environment." That is, abnormal genes increase the susceptibility we have to adverse environmental influences, as in the type 2 diabetes situation discussed earlier.

The problem we face today, however, is that we do not know what most of the abnormal genes actually are that increase our susceptibility to adverse life experiences. There are many leads for many genes that may be involved in psychiatric illnesses, as Geschwind and Flint point out in the article I cited earlier, but each one of these genes at best explains a very small part of the reason anyone gets an illness like schizophrenia. Coupled with the fact that there is at present little we can do to reverse the effects of most abnormal mutations (although techniques like CRISPR may soon

---

[3] Doidge N: *The Brain that Heals Itself*. New York, Penguin, 2007, p. 213.

change that statement), let alone those caused by multiple mutations, it is clear that finding the hereditary basis of mental illness is still a distance away. It is important to keep looking, and someday these efforts should yield important insights. At the same time, however, this book will show that neuroscience already has some good handles on how the environmental causes of mental illness work to alter normal brain function and that some of these may be amenable to therapies we currently have available. Throughout the book, I will try to make clear what genetic, or "hardwired," influences we know about in order to keep a proper balance. But my primary aim is to delineate the scientific basis for the environmental side of the ledger.

## NEUROSCIENCE COMES OF AGE

In this book, I will not shy away from mentioning a number of personal experiences in my scientific and medical career that influence my views. It is probably already clear that I am somewhat enamored of the work done so far by neuroscientists and the potential for even more major insights into how the human brain works. I will try to temper this with realistic appraisals of the many shortcomings of what is known and with recognition of the overstatements of the implications of some findings that have been advanced. But I hope that, even when I acknowledge that I may be getting a bit carried away with some finding or other—like my enthusiasm for the amygdala as central to the human experience of fear and anxiety—the reader does not lose sight of the big picture: neuroscience has taken us to depths of understanding of brain function that are both marvelous and challenging.

How did neuroscience reach the point that we now have so much useful information about emotion, behavior, and mental illness? There have been and are many great neuroscientists at work, but because Eric Kandel was a prominent and highly visible member of the Department of Psychiatry at Columbia University in which I worked for more than two decades, his seminal contributions feel to me especially critical in making neuroscience the advanced and promising field it is today.

When I took my required medical school neuroanatomy course in the late 1970s, what we were taught about neuroscience resembled the New York City subway map— a complex web of nerve tracts connecting different parts of the brain to different parts of the body. Much to the chagrin of my classmates and myself, we were expected to memorize every aspect of that map. One brain region supposedly controlled speech, another vision, and yet another hearing. Damage one of the nerve tracts from the brain and you would immobilize the left leg; lesion another and sensation to the right cheek would be lost; severing a third would result in the loss of the ability to move the diaphragm during breathing. The message we received was that the brain is a hardwired organ that "controls" the functions of the rest of the body.

Scientific breakthroughs often involve a genius confronting an apparent paradox and asking a simple but radical question. Einstein, for example, asked how it could be that nothing goes faster than the speed of light if the light emanating from a flashlight held by a man on a train must be going at the speed of light plus the speed of the train. Thus was born one of the twentieth-century's two greatest revolutions in physics, the theory of relativity. Although I don't know for sure that this is what went on in Kandel's mind, I can imagine him thinking "if everything in the brain is set in stone, so to speak, like those neural pathways we teach in neuroanatomy class, then how do we ever learn a new fact or lay down a new memory? Something in the brain *must undergo change* in order for these things to happen." In this thought I am sure he had many forbears, including the great scientist Donald Hobbs, who probably first advanced the idea that when a specific set of neurons are together involved in a learning process they undergo chemical changes that strengthen the connections among them. But Kandel's work is not only brilliant, it opened our eyes to the fundamental ways in which brains change as they experience.

Starting with a primitive organism, the invertebrate sea slug called *Aplysia*; eventually advancing to flies, worms, mice, and rats; and using ever more sophisticated methods, from placing microelectrodes to record from single neurons to knocking out genes in living mice, Kandel and his group of extremely talented scientists discovered the basic ways in which gene activation in the brain makes new proteins and new synaptic connections every time we learn something new and remember it. This information, which Kandel and his Columbia University neuroscience team are still hard at work gathering, showed in the most advanced way yet that the brain is a plastic organ, one that changes as we experience our worlds and confront new things. These insights do not replace our earlier understanding of brain tracts to peripheral organ. It is true that lesioning a specific part of the brain or a specific nerve tract can result in a very specific deficit, like the inability to move one arm or to speak coherently. Sadly, a severed spinal cord cannot be repaired, and paralysis is never reversed. Rather, these new insights into the brain's plasticity formed the basis for our understanding that the brain is capable of ongoing change and greatly expanded our appreciation for the complexities of brain function down to the level of cells and molecules.[4]

The implications for psychiatry of this new work are tremendous: life's experiences, including undergoing psychotherapy, must affect the brain on the molecular and cellular levels that Kandel's work had elucidated. At the same time, major advances were being made in our ability to image the living, human brain. In most areas of medicine and medical research, it is possible to get access to the tissues involved in normal function and disease. Blood and urine samples tell us directly what is going on in bones, muscles, the liver, and the kidneys. If necessary, we can obtain biopsies of heart, lung, lymph node, or liver tissue. But when it comes to the brain, such access is almost never possible. The brain lives inside something called the *blood–brain barrier*, and, consequently, almost nothing in blood or urine reflects what is going on in the brain. We cannot sample actual brain tissue except in certain relatively uncommon circumstances

---

[4] It is, of course, a bit of unabashed hero worship that I seem to be attributing all of this work to Eric Kandel. I am well aware that not only have many talented scientists worked with him, but that the elucidation of the biology of learning and memory required contributions from many laboratories in many countries over many years. Kandel himself would surely cite colleagues and students like Tom Carew, Jimmie Schwartz, Steve Siegelbaum, Tom Jessel, Richard Axel, and Rene Hen among many others.

involving devastating brain diseases. Hence, it has traditionally been very difficult to understand what happens in the living human brain. Fortunately, throughout the last third of the twentieth century, when Kandel was doing his important molecular and cellular work on brain plasticity in animals, new brain imaging techniques like functional magnetic resonance imaging (fMRI) and positron emission tomography (PET) became increasingly sophisticated, enabling us to see aspects of human brain function for the first time. The coupling of scientific and technological advances that have occurred in the past 50 years revolutionized what we know about the brain and how we think of its capacity for dynamic responses and change.

## DON'T SLIGHT THE MIND

But, as explained earlier, along with this justified enthusiasm for the power of both laboratory and clinical neuroscience came the suspicion that somehow neuroscience was going to "reduce" the intricacies of human abilities and feelings to explanations that rely "simply" on chemicals called neurotransmitters and their receptors in the brain. It is relatively easy to define what the human brain is: an approximately 3-pound organ comprised of several types of cells, including about 86 billion cells[5] called *neurons* and $10^{14}$ (that's a 1 with 14 zeroes after it) connections among them, called *synapses*. Each individual neuron is connected to, on average, thousands of other neurons, some located long distances away in the brain.[6] On a functional level, neurons can send signals to each other at speeds of anywhere from 1 to more than 260 mph and can send 1,000 impulses per second.[7] This makes mapping brain connections a task that only teams of scientists using powerful computing resources can solve.

In contrast, there really is no such clear-cut definition of the "mind." The "mind" some insist, cannot be explained by this new "brain science." People are spiritual beings with huge intellectual capacities and wide-ranging emotions. Brain chemistry, this argument goes, cannot be a sufficient basis to explain all of the mind's wonderful complexity. This way of thinking is clearly stated in an article in the *Christian Worldview Journal* in which the work of a prominent neuroscientist, Michael Merzenich, was reviewed,

> There is no question that contemporary neuroscience has certainly made huge strides in understanding the processes that go into making our brains, personalities, and emotions what they are. But to claim that brain science can define our very *nature*, and that the recent discoveries about brain plasticity have finally laid to rest all philosophical and religious questions about the self, is a *non sequitur* of enormous proportions. It would be like me saying that we can

[5] Herculano-Houzel S: *The Human Advantage: A New Understanding of How Our Brain Became Remarkable.* Cambridge, MA: MIT Press, 2016.

[6] Huang ZJ, Luo L: It takes the world to understand the brain. *Science* 2015;350:42.

[7] http://virtuallabs.stanford.edu/tech/images/ReactionTime.SU-Tech.pdf

understand the nature of the soul from examining the body, or that we can fully define the mind because we know what happens in the brain, or that we can define the nature of love merely because we understand what happens chemically, physiologically, and neurologically when a husband and wife have sex.[8]

And the famous spiritual author and lecturer Deepak Chopra believes the mind is something much grander than the mere organ we know as the brain. He writes in an essay on the difference between brain and mind:

Ultimately, the current brain fetish will reach a dead end, if it hasn't already. Society will return to the concept of the mind, and something startling but obvious will emerge and become accepted. Consciousness is primary, the brain is secondary. This is like saying that music is primary, the radio is secondary. Whatever is primary comes first and holds the essence of life.[9]

Finally, this way of thinking is a very eloquently put by Vivian Gornick in her review of a book of essays by Siri Hustvedt called *A Woman Looking at Men Looking at Women: Essays on Art, Sex, and the Mind.* Gornick writes:

To stand, even for a moment, at the edge of that emotional abyss into which the candidate for suicide stares daily—and to be aware that it is only a matter of time before he or she dives in—is to be in the presence of one of the great mysteries of human existence; one that language, especially the impoverished language of science, cannot demystify.[10]

But what does Gornick mean by "the impoverished language of science?" She seems to be saying that suicide is a complex behavior based on mysterious thoughts and feelings to which scientists have no access. The language of science is "impoverished" according to Gornick because it is the language of brain and not of mind. And she seems to believe that a terrible outcome like suicide is forged by the mind and not the brain.

To writers like Chopra and Gornick, the mind is an ineffable repository of our feelings, ideas, yearnings, and strivings. It has in many people's view a nearly spiritual quality, as if it is separate from any other aspect of the body's physiological function.[11] This is the version articulated by Renee Descartes in the seventeenth century!

---

[8] http://www.colsoncenter.org/the-center/columns/changepoint/19312-neuroscience-and-the-reductionist-temptation. Another great example is to be found at http://articles.latimes.com/2008/jan/20/opinion/op-lehrer20

[9] http://www.oprah.com/spirit/The-Difference-Between-the-Mind-and-the-Brain

[10] Gornick V: Mind-Body Problems. *New York Times Book Review*, December 18, 2016, p. 16.

[11] Some of these contentions are, of course, religious in nature, and, as a religious person myself, I do not mean to dismiss them out of hand. While it is possible to see how the brain works when someone prays and to recognize that contemplating one's religious convictions stimulates specific

In the realm of psychiatric illness and treatment, this argument is sometimes translated into the fear that neuroscience is intent on promoting only medication as the solution for disorders like depression, phobias, substance abuse, and schizophrenia. Psychotherapy and its attempt to understand beliefs, motivations, feelings, and thoughts will get left behind. Neuroscience, it is said, cannot possibly understand or explain psychotherapy. According to George Makari of Weill Cornell Medical College, "Unfortunately . . . there was a sustained effort by academic research leaders in American psychiatry to promote these [psychopharmacology] successes, and to fight the stigmatization of the mentally ill by forgoing the complexities of the biopsychosocial model for a simpler, more authoritative claim: Mental illness is a brain disease. . . .There is, and should continue to be, a rich, solid arena for scientific research and clinical work that does not turn all mental health and illness into the mantra of 'it's the brain, stupid', and falsely oppose 'real' brain ills with 'unreal' mental ones."[12] As will be seen, I completely agree with Makari's concerns that US—indeed international—psychiatry has become too focused on pharmacology to the exclusion of research into the effects of life events and psychotherapy on the course of mental illness. But I will contend that mental illness *is* a brain disease. We need to retire the term "biopsychosocial" with its implication that somehow psychological and social factors are not biological. Everything we experience, learn, see, and do (or don't do) affects the brain, which mediates all of our thoughts, responses, and memories. It is definitely, as Makari points out, far more difficult to figure out how being raised by abusive parents, living in poverty, or losing a loved one affects the brain compared to understanding what a drug does. Nevertheless, the difficulty inherent in understanding how psychological and social factors affect brain biology to produce mental illness should not dissuade us from trying to do so or to simply creating a separate and mysterious category of phenomena called "mind."

In fact, much of the fear that neuroscience will subvert our appreciation for the complexity of the human mind and push medications as a solution to all of life's problems comes from a misunderstanding about how neuroscience works and what it intends to learn. Part of the problem, to be sure, stems from exaggerated claims by neuroscientists and florid descriptions of what neuroscience has learned in the general media. Too much is often made of the usefulness of new technologies like MRI and genetic testing, while extrapolations of things learned from rodents in the laboratory to human behavior are often leaps beyond what the data really allow. It is therefore important to explain not only what neuroscience has learned about brain function but also what we still do not understand. In doing so, it will become clear that, far from an attempt to reduce the human spirit to mere chemistry, neuroscience is slowly but surely elucidating the wonders and complexity of the human mind. This book will help show why we can be comfortable when Kandel and co-author A. J. Hudspeth

brain regions, this of course has no bearing on religious beliefs. It is perfectly possible to study the biology of prayer, for example, without in any way demeaning one's religious faith.

[12] Makari G: Psychiatry's mind-brain problem. *New York Times*, November 11, 2015.

write "What we commonly call the mind is a set of operations carried out by the brain."[13]

That brain that serves as the organ of mind is thus clearly not simply a collection of chemicals connecting nerve cells in order to conduct electrical currents. Rather, the brain is an amazing construction of many kinds of molecules, ion channels, scaffolding proteins, cells, hormones, connecting processes, and transmitters that act out a dynamic and ever-changing drama, one that is scripted both by our genes and our life's experiences. It is the case that all of our actions, feelings, and ideas can ultimately be explained in terms of the way the physical brain works, but once we understand how complex and dynamic our brains are, this will never seem simplistic or reductionist. As I will explain in a later chapter, even our nearest genetic neighbor, the chimpanzee, which shares more than 98% of our genes, cannot muster the mental processes that we take for granted in the regular course of human life. The evolution of the human brain is a remarkable feat of nature. This enormous complexity, however, is also the basis for what can go wrong in our brains and cause us to develop all of the distressing emotions and abnormal behaviors that animals do not manifest but that form the basis of psychiatric disorders. While our brains are clearly capable of doing things no other animal can, it is clearly wrong in my opinion to say we are superior. After all, we are the species whose tremendous brain capacity finds us currently destroying our planet by burning fossil fuels.

## IS PSYCHIATRY STALLED?

Because of our brains' incredible complexity, science has only provided hints so far about what causes mental illness. Some people are discouraged about the lack of progress and characterize psychiatric research as stalled. I can understand their point of view, as two examples will demonstrate.

First, I had occasion to ask a young psychiatrist recently the following question: "if you have a very psychotic patient in the emergency department who is delusional and hallucinating and violent and requires emergency medical treatment, what drug do you generally use?" Her answer was—haloperidol (brand name, Haldol). This is the same drug I used when I worked in the psychiatric emergency room at what was then Columbia Presbyterian Medical Center in New York City more than 30 years ago. The fact is that psychiatrists today use drugs that are really minor variations on those that were first introduced in the 1950s and '60s. The newer medications tend to be better tolerated and in some cases a bit safer, but they work no better in treating depression, anxiety, bipolar disorder, or schizophrenia and have pretty much the same chemical actions in the brain.

[13] Kandel ER, Hudspeth AJ: The Brain and Behavior. In Eric R. Kandel, James H. Schwartz, Tomas M. Jessell, Steven A. Siegelbaum, A. J. Hudspeth, eds. *Principles of Neural Science.* 5th ed. McGraw-Hill, 2013, p. 5.

Second, psychiatry seems to be grasping at straws in trying to identify treatment breakthroughs. In the past few years, scientists have shown that a one-time injection of an anesthetic agent called ketamine can almost immediately relieve a patient's severe depression for several weeks.[14] More recently, some in the field seemed dazzled by two papers reporting that the hallucinogen psilocybin, also known as "mushrooms," dramatically reduced depressive symptoms in patients with cancer.[15] Ketamine blocks the activity of a neurotransmitter called glutamine, while psilocybin stimulates serotonin receptors in the brain. Both can be drugs of abuse. Although I am intrigued by these findings and hope they pan out, I also have reason to curtail my enthusiasm a bit. Neither the ketamine nor psilocybin findings tells us much about the underlying cause of depression, why some people get depressed and others don't, and what exactly is wrong in the brains of patients with depression. We could probably give any number of commonly abused drugs to depressed people, including LSD, alcohol, opioids, and amphetamines and see some decrease in symptoms. If we do get more effective medications, that will indeed be a wonderful development; our primary aim is to help suffering people get better. But the science of mental illness is not necessarily advanced by these findings, and it is rare in the history of medicine that real breakthroughs are accomplished without understanding the underlying physiology of the disease.

But those who are discouraged at the lack of progress in psychiatric research are focusing exclusively on just one area of that research: psychopharmacology. While drug research so far has given us few new agents and no better understanding of what is going on in the brains of people with mental illnesses, there has been tremendous progress in other areas. We have learned that stressful life events and childhood maltreatment are major precursors of most forms of psychiatric illness. We have convincing evidence that several forms of psychotherapy are highly effective in treating many different conditions. And we have detailed information from the basic science laboratory about the ways in which stress and adversity cause molecular and cellular changes in the brain that can endure for prolonged periods of time, even an entire life. Indeed, by understanding how complicated the brain is, we begin to see how psychiatric medications offer a valuable but always relatively blunt tool for helping people. Neuroscience suggests that psychotherapy, by changing the ways our brains respond to the events we experience throughout our lives, does indeed have the potential for providing more durable solutions for many emotional and behavioral problems.

[14] Abdallah CG, Adams TG, Kelmendi B, Esterlis I, Sanacora G, Krystal JH: Ketamine's mechanism of action: a path to rapid-acting antidepressants. *Depress Anxiety* 2016;33:689–697.
[15] Griffiths RR, Johnson MW, Carducci MA, Umbricht A, Richards WA, Richards BD, Cosimano MP, Klinedinst MA: Psilocybin produces substantial and sustained decreases in depression and anxiety in patients with life-threatening cancer: a randomized double-blind trial. *J Psychopharmacol* 2016;30:1181–1197.

# THE RDOC: A PROMISING ADVANCE

A potentially positive step in putting the study of the brain and psychiatric disorders on a firmer scientific basis is the brainchild of the immediate past director of the National Institute of Mental Health (NIMH), Thomas Insel. When I first met Insel, he was a clinical researcher at the NIMH, focusing on obsessive compulsive disorder (OCD). But he eventually abandoned clinical research for basic neurobiology. In a brilliant series of studies that I will return to in Chapter 7, Insel demonstrated on a molecular and cellular level how the brain hormones oxytocin and vasopressin are involved in pair bonding and monogamy in laboratory animals. In 2001, he was appointed director of NIMH, a post he held until 2015. In 2009, he announced a plan for the comprehensive overhaul of the psychiatric diagnostic system based on neurobiological findings, called the Research Domain Criteria (RDoC).

Since 1980, psychiatric diagnoses are generally made using a system developed by the American Psychiatric Association called the *Diagnostic and Statistical Manual* (DSM). Until the third edition of the DSM (known as DSM-III) was published that year, psychiatric diagnosis was an unreliable game, fraught with all kinds of partisan views and divergent schools of thought. We would joke that if you put 50 psychiatrists in a room with a patient the result would be 51 very reasonable diagnoses because the patient's was as good as anyone else's. While this may seem ecumenical, it meant that if one researcher wrote a paper on a treatment for depression, no one could replicate it because there would be no way to know for sure exactly what illness the patients in the study had. In clinical medicine, if one physician refers a patient with diabetes to another, the second physician has a pretty good idea of what the patient has. But, before DSM-III, if I referred a patient with schizophrenia to another psychiatrist, I would either have to describe all the symptoms to my colleague or she would have to do the entire diagnostic workup all over again because there was no agreement on what the term "schizophrenia" actually entailed.

The late Robert Spitzer and his colleagues at Columbia University developed a system that used explicit criteria to make each psychiatric diagnosis and showed that these could be made reliably, such that multiple observers will agree on the same diagnosis for a given patient. This system, which is the basis for DSM-III, was followed by several revisions and is now known as the DSM-5. While there is no question that this approach has helped psychiatry and everyone who deals with patients with psychiatric illness enormously, 35 years later, the system is clearly showing its substantial flaws. Among other things, it puts different illnesses into categories that are largely traditional and often arbitrary. Perhaps most troubling for people like Insel, it bears no relationship whatsoever to what is known about how the brain actually works.[16] As Hyman, now at Harvard University, put it, "the modern DSM system, intended to create a shared language, also creates epistemic blinders that impede progress toward

---

[16] Cuthbert BN, Insel TR: Toward the future of psychiatric diagnosis: the seven pillars of RDoc. *BMC Med* 2013;11:126.

valid diagnoses. Insights that are beginning to emerge from psychology, neuroscience, and genetics suggest possible strategies for moving forward."[17]

There are five domains to the RDoC system that each isolate a system of human emotion, behavior, or cognition, such as emotion, motivation, attention, social affiliation, and sleep. The RDoC does not seem to favor any particular type of treatment but rather calls for including information about genes, molecules, cells, circuits, physiology, behavior, self-report, and various experimental paradigms to generate diagnoses that more clearly match what is going on in the human brain. As Yager and Feinstein point out in their discussion of the RDoC, "Each domain has been variably associated with increasingly well-defined neurocircuits, many of which have been associated with specific psychopathological conditions."[18] Now, for example, instead of a diagnosis of "depression" defined by feeling sad and losing interest in things, we may get a category of disorders that primarily involve abnormally elevated fear, characterized by specific thoughts and behaviors and mirrored by exaggerated activity in the amygdala and decreased input from the prefrontal cortex.

It is too early to know if this new system will prove useful, and, of course, it has been criticized for its emphasis on biology, but I believe it is a clear advance in the way we think about mental illness. Support for it comes, for example, from a recent study by Stanford University researchers in which 420 people with either depression, an anxiety disorder, or no psychiatric illness underwent multiple assessments that included tests of real-world function, cognitive ability, self-reported symptoms, and physiological brain mapping. They found that six separate categories best described these individuals: tension, anxious arousal, general anxiety, anhedonia (the inability to experience pleasure), melancholia, and normative mood.[19] These categories better described these people than the DSM-5 categories of depression or anxiety disorders. A similar approach is being taken in Europe by the STRATIFY study, which uses brain imaging to link patterns of brain function to symptoms that may cut across our current diagnostic categories in psychiatry.

As scientists do more and more sophisticated studies of psychiatric disorders, they often find that there are important basic biological similarities among different DSM-5 categories. In a study of how genes are expressed in 700 brains obtained from deceased people with and without several psychiatric illnesses, common genetic signatures were found linking autism, schizophrenia, and bipolar disorder.[20] Depression, on the other hand, had a distinctive genetic signature in this study. These findings will be refreshing

[17] Hyman SE: The diagnosis of mental disorders: the problem of reification. *Annu Rev Clin Psychol* 2010;6:155–179.
[18] Yager J, Feinstein RE: Potential applications of the National Institute of Mental Health's Research Domain Criteria (RDoC) to clinical psychiatric practice. *J Clin Psychiatry* 2017;78:423–432, p. 424.
[19] Grisanzio KA, Goldstein-Piekarski AN, Wang MY, Rashed Ahmed AP, Samara Z, Williams LM. Transdiagnostic symptom clusters and associations with brain, behavior, and daily function in mood, anxiety, and trauma disorders. *JAMA Psychiatry* December 03, 2017.
[20] Gandal MJ, Haney JR, Parikshank, et al.: Shared molecular neuropathology across major psciatric disorders parallels polygenic overlap. *Science* 2018;359:693–697.

to psychiatrists and psychologists who routinely struggle to figure out whether a patient with psychotic symptoms has schizophrenia or is in the manic phase of bipolar disorder. Genetic neuroscience suggests that there is a biological reason why it is so hard to differentiate these two conditions clinically: they may really not be such different illnesses after all.

I have often said that, long before we knew that heart attacks involve clogging of the coronary arteries and shutting off the oxygen supply to the heart muscle, it was known that the heart is a muscle with four chambers and four valves that beats according to certain physiologically determined rules. By contrast, we have been making psychiatric diagnoses for centuries without knowing much about the way the brain actually looks or works. Now that we have at least some of this information, it is imperative that we use it. Hopefully, that is the direction the RDoC is going.

## TOWARD A NEUROSCIENCE FOR ALL

Typical of the criticism of the RDoC and of similar efforts was a recent op-ed in the *New York Times* by a Columbia University psychiatrist, John Markowitz, titled "There's Such a Thing As Too Much Neuroscience." Markowitz believes that the RDoC shifts the NIMH funding focus to neuroscience, thereby "strangling its clinical research budget."[21] He asks "where does that leave patients whom today's treatments do not help? Can they wait for neuroscience developments that may take decades to appear or prove illusory?" Markowitz also fears that the NIMH has been slow to listen to voices like his. "We have too often been reluctant to voice our protest, for fear of incurring the institute's displeasure and losing whatever opportunities we still have for funding." He concludes with the warning, "Many patients continue to suffer. . . . Some will kill themselves. . . . Patients cannot afford to wait 10 years or 20 years or longer for the results neuroscience promises. Gene therapy, for example, is unlikely to eliminate suicide or to diminish it in the next decade."

And yet Markowitz acknowledges that NIMH has, for years, provided funding for psychotherapy research, producing, as I have pointed out, ample evidence of its efficacy. Right now, the problem is that health insurance companies will not pay for psychotherapy, and, even when they do, there are too few psychotherapists trained in evidence-based psychotherapies who accept health insurance. Developing more psychotherapy evidence is not going to help anyone until health insurance companies agree to pay for it and therapists are trained to deliver it. That is not a research issue; for the NIMH to continue to fund studies for treatments no one has access to is the real waste of money. As Hyman and Mount Sinai's Eric Nestler point out in their reply to Markowitz, "People suffering from severe mental disorders need and deserve more effective treatments, and this goal requires more neuroscience, not less."[22] Until we accept the fact that the brain is the organ of the mind and that its structure and function

---

[21] Markowitz JC: There's such a thing as too much neuroscience. *New York Times*, October 14, 2016.
[22] Nestler EJ, Hyman SE: More neuroscience, not less. *New York Times*, October 21, 2016.

are responsible for both mental health and mental illness, we will be left to tinker with decades-old treatments of varying effectiveness. There is no conspiracy to silence psychotherapy research advocates; rather, there is finally a concerted effort to look at what we already know about how the brain works, apply it to what we observe in human behavior, and then devise new experiments to learn more. Because neuroscience continues to teach us that positive experience can overcome a history of abuse and stress, better psychotherapy is destined to be an important result of that effort.

This book will explain in accessible terms many of the new technologies and findings that have made the neuroscience of human behavior and emotion so exciting and promising. This will include clear and understandable discussions of a number of the fascinating technical aspects of modern neuroscience, including genetics, epigenetics, brain circuitry, neurogenesis, neurohormones, brain imaging, and optogenetics. From this, it will be much easier to understand how life's experiences are translated into biological processes in our brains, how everything we see or feel or learn during our lifetimes stimulates a variety of changes in the brain. I will use this information to explain how psychiatric problems can develop, why we harbor irrational fears and resentments and succumb to harmful influences, and how we develop attachments to other people and to groups of people. Finally, I will explain the relatively simple ways in which psychiatric drugs work and the much more complicated ways in which the various forms of psychotherapy may be affecting physical processes in the brain. By elucidating the science of experience, we will see how neuroscience now lives at the intersection of mind and brain, unifying the two into a complicated, elegant, and researchable whole.

# 2

# Is the Human Brain Unique?

Did a big brain raise us into mountains
—Yosef Komunyakaa[1]

There must be something unique about the human brain. After all, we alone among all the species on earth have a written language, create symphonies, invent machines, build rockets, perform mathematical equations, and cook our food. Our nearest genetic neighbors are the chimpanzee (*Pan troglodytes*) and bonobo (*Pan paniscus*), followed by the gorilla and orangutan. Chimpanzees have about 98% of the same genes as do humans,[2] even though the two species separated from a common evolutionary ancestor about 6 million years ago.[3] Chimpanzees, like all animals that are the subjects of Animal or National Geographic Channel documentaries, are frequently described as "these magnificent creatures." Indeed, they are capable of doing many remarkable things, including using—and teaching their offspring how to use—tools, cooperating in large social groups, and demonstrating emotions. As we will see and to some extent dispute, there are some scientists who believe we have actually made too much of the difference in intellectual power between humans and chimpanzees.

It was once fashionable to call the thing that differentiates us from animals the "soul." Nowadays, it has become the "mind." It is clear that animals learn from experience just as humans do, and we will have occasion many times throughout this book to consider studies that document how experience changes the structure and function of these animals' brains. Neuroscientists rely a great deal on animal models to understand how the human brain functions, making it disingenuous to claim at the same time that there are no similarities between rat, monkey, and human brains. If, however, the contention that the mind and the brain are the same thing is true, then it is absolutely necessary that we figure out the biological basis for why humans can write novels and make bombs. Furthermore, understanding these phenomena might give us insights into where to look for the causes of the brain diseases that are unique to humans.

---

[1] From "Nighttime," a poem by Yosef Komunyakaa, published in *Poetry*, November 2017;211(2):112.
[2] Cyranoski D: Almost human. *Nature* 2002;418:910–912.
[3] Patterson N, Richter DJ, Gnerre S, Lander ES, Reich D: Genetic evidence for complex speciation of humans and chimpanzees. *Nature* 2006;441:1103–1108.

Several possibilities have been considered for what differentiates our brains from those of the great apes. Here, we will consider the three that are most often mentioned in the scientific literature:

1. *Structural*: Is the human brain larger, larger in proportion to total body size, or organized differently? Does it have more neurons?
2. *Genetic*: Are the few genes that are not the same between humans and apes responsible for the differences?
3. *Gene expression*: As we will discuss in this chapter and in Chapter 3 on epigenetics, not all genes are actually expressed or expressed at the same rate at the same time. Do differences in the amount of protein generated by genes in the brain account for the differences?


## IS HUMAN BEHAVIOR REALLY DIFFERENT?

A few years ago, some colleagues of mine (including Rachel, one of my daughters) and I published a paper in which we proposed "the reason other species are immune from mental illness is because they do not have the organ of the body necessary to sustain such disorders, namely a fully-developed prefrontal cortex."[4] We further suggested that it is specifically an increase in the number of genes that are expressed in the prefrontal cortex that is responsible for both our unique abilities and defects. The contention, however, that we are all that unique is not universally accepted.

Once, while giving a lecture to the Emory University Medical School's Department of Psychiatry, I asserted that we are the only species with a sense of the future and therefore the only species capable of worrying about it. The chairman of the department at the time, the great psychiatrist and neuroscientist Charles Nemeroff, interrupted me and asked a member of the audience who is an expert on animal cognition if my assertion is actually true. He answered that he agreed with my claim, and I breathed a sigh of relief and continued the lecture. But I think that if he hadn't also been caught by surprise by the question, he might have been less agreeable.

I have wondered since if perhaps the man in the audience was the renowned ethologist and biologist, Frans de Waal, who is a professor at Emory. I may be flattering myself to think that so eminent a scientist as de Waal would have taken the time to attend my lecture in another school and department of the University, but questions of exactly what intellectual feats animals are capable of are his specialty. It has long been de Waal's contention that the only reason we think we are special is because we are the ones making the judgments. Squirrels, de Waal points out in one of his books, *Are We Smart Enough to Know How Smart Animals Are?*,[5] squirrels can remember where they

---

[4] Berkowitz RL, Coplan JD, Reddy DP, Gorman JM: The human dimension: how the prefrontal cortex modulates the subcortical fear response. *Rev Neurosci* 2007;18:191–207, p. 195.
[5] de Waal F: *Are We Smart Enough to Know How Smart Animals Are?* New York, WW Norton, 2016.

hid hundreds of acorns, and bats, by using systems of echolocation that are far superior to anything of which we are capable.

In the thirteenth century, Albertus Magnus wrote what for more than 700 years was pretty much felt to be the state of animal intelligence:

> Some of them [animals] participate in acts of foresight with no premeditation of future events but rather out of natural instinct. When they gather up food they are not conjecturing a future lack of time, but do so out of greediness over food which is present.[6]

For the next seven centuries, scientists and philosophers believed that animals are incapable of social cooperation and altruism; unlike humans, the argument goes, animals, including chimpanzees, do only what is directly to their individual advantages. In the nineteenth century, Darwin challenged the notion that there is such a qualitative difference between animal and human behavior. He described the differences as purely quantitative and on a continuum. According to Darwin, we merely do cognitive and intellectual things to a greater extent than other species, but we are not special any more than a cheetah that runs faster than a lion is a superior species on the basis of speed.

Today, biologists and zoologists seem intent on proving that many of the things we believed to be uniquely human are instead also present in other animals. As a science writer put it, "It seems that hardly a week goes by without a new report about animals performing marvelous feats we once thought only humans could do. Crows make tools, chimpanzees seem to mourn their dead, and rats supposedly empathize with one another's pain" (p. 1036).[7] de Waal has coined the term "anthropodenial" to connote the automatic resistance we have to accepting that animals and humans have similar traits. In a provocative editorial in the *New York Times*, he wrote that "this is why science nowadays often starts from the opposite end, assuming continuity between humans and animals, while shifting the burden of proof to those who insist on differences. Anyone who asks me to believe that a tickled ape, who almost chokes on his hoarse giggles, is in a different state of mind than a tickled human child has his work cut out for him."[8] For de Waal, "Apes are special in that they seek logical connections based on how they believe the world works."[9] On the other hand, he asserts that "Human reflection is chronically overrated."[10]

One by one, cognitive abilities once thought exclusively human are found in chimpanzees and bonobos as well. Imagine, for instance, a group of two- and

---

[6] Magnus A: *On Animals: A Medieval Summa Zoologica*, translated of *De animalibus* by Kenneth F. Kitchell, Jr. and Irven Michael Resnick. Baltimore: Johns Hopkins University Press, 1999. With thanks to my daughter, Sara Gorman, for calling this quotation to my attention.

[7] Balter M: "Killjoys" challenge claims of clever animals. *Science* 2012;335:1036–1037.

[8] de Waal F: What I learned from tickling apes. *New York Times*, April 8, 2016.

[9] de Waal F: *Are We Smart Enough?*, p. 55.

[10] Ibid., p. 58.

three-year-old children in an audience. On stage, an actor hides an apple under the cushion of a couch and walks off stage. Another actor comes on stage and moves the apple to a hiding place behind a bookshelf. Then the first actor returns and says, "I am going to get my apple and eat it now." The children in the audience will expect him to look behind the bookshelf, where they know the apple has been moved. Until about four years of age, children are unable to grasp the fact that other people have minds of their own and that the first actor can't possibly know the apple has been moved. At around four, however, the children know immediately that the first actor will go to the couch, and they will yell to him from the audience to go to the bookshelf instead. This ability to understand that other minds have their own thoughts and experiences is formally known as *theory of mind* (ToM). The scientific literature has long held that only humans are capable of this kind of sophisticated mind-reading. A scientist declared in a 2011 review of ToM that "ToM develops fully only in human beings; the presence of a rudimentary ToM in some nonhuman primates and other animals is arguable although they can show very complex social behavior."[11]

Except it turns out that this assumption is wrong. In 2016, scientists, using a new infrared eye-tracking technology, showed for the first time that chimpanzees, bonobos, and orangutans do have ToM.[12] As de Waal points out over and over again, it seems that, if we try hard enough, we find evidence of sophisticated mentation in apes that we once ascribed possible only for humans. Chimpanzees manifest a range of human-like social activities, including seeming to risk their own safety on behalf of other chimpanzees and sharing food. The degree to which these activities are motivated by actual altruism is a subject much debated among specialists.[13] It has been shown that monkeys, dolphins, and apes are capable of introspection and reflection on their own memories, a feat that cognitive scientists call *metacognition*.[14] The chimpanzee in Figure 2.1 surely looks deep in thought!

If we underestimate the abilities of other animals, we may also fail to recognize that they, too, suffer from mental illness. There is, for instance, the heartbreaking story of the baby elephant mourning the death of its mother, killed by poachers.[15] Similar mourning behavior is reported among many species, challenging the idea that only humans experience depression. Monkeys display sad-appearing faces, and veterinarians prescribe antidepressants to dogs that seem depressed.[16] Dogs can also

[11] Korkmaz B: Theory of mind and neurodevelopmental disorders of childhood. *Pediatr Res* 2011;69:101R–108R.

[12] Morell V: Mind-reading great apes. *Science* 2016;354:1520.; Krupenye C, Kano F, Hirata S, Call J, Tomasello: Great apes anticipate that other individuals will act according to false beliefs. *Science* 2016;354:110–114.

[13] Tennie C, Jansen K, Call J: The nature of prosociality in chimpanzees. *Nat Commun* 2016;7:13195.

[14] Miyamoto K, Osada T, Setsuie R, Takeda M, Tamura K, Adachi Y, Miyashita Y: Causal neural network of metamemory for retrospection in primates. *Science* 2017;355:188–193.

[15] http://www.dailymail.co.uk/news/article-2879816/Heartbreaking-moment-orphaned-baby-elephant-mourns-death-mother-killed-poachers-poisoned-spear.html

[16] http://news.nationalgeographic.com/news/2012/10/121004-animals-depression-health-science/

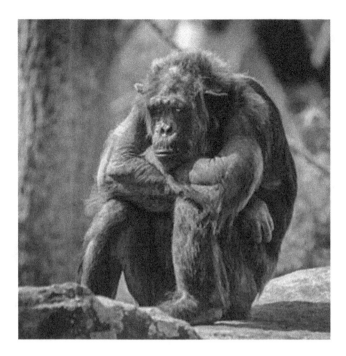

**Figure 2.1** What is going on in this chimpanzee's mind? We will never know, but whatever it is appears to be profound.

Image in public domain, https://cdn.pixabay.com/photo/2015/10/09/06/46/chimpanzee-978809_960_720.jpg

develop compulsive licking and scratching behavior in response to stress or boredom that resembles obsessive compulsive disorder (OCD) in humans. Chimpanzees demonstrate many of the signs and symptoms of posttraumatic disorder when subjected to traumatic stresses.[17] Who knows what emotions these depressed and obsessional animals are experiencing? For all we know, they may actually be feeling sad or irrationally believe that germs are covering their bodies. Could the chimpanzee in captivity in Figure 2.2 be suffering from depression that would meet the criteria of the *Diagnostic and Statistical Manual of Mental Disorders* (DSM-5)?

And it may not even be the case that only humans worry about the future. Nicholas Mulcahy and Joseph Call showed that bonobos and orangutans save tools for later use, anticipating that they will need them in the future.[18] In their paper, they challenged the whole notion that future planning is a uniquely human ability. They note that the animals "executed a response (tool transport) that had not been reinforced during training . . . that produced no consequences or reduced any present needs but

---

[17] Ferdowsian HR, Durham DL, Kimwele C, Kranedonk G, Otall E, Akugizibwe T, Mulcahy JB, Ajarova L, Johnson CM: Signs of mood and anxiety disorders in chimpanzees. *PLOS One* 2011;6:e19855.

[18] Mulcahy NJ, Call J: Apes save tools for future use. *Science* 2006;312:1040.

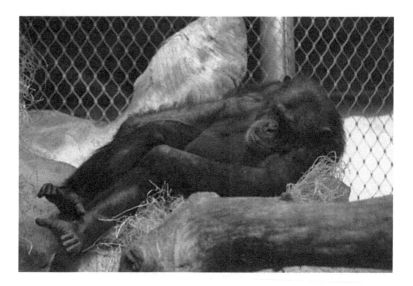

**Figure 2.2** This chimpanzee in captivity certainly appears sad. Perhaps he is suffering from a major depressive episode.

Image in public domain, https://cdn.pixabay.com/photo/2015/09/26/23/25/monkey-959978__340.jpg

was crucial to meet future ones . . . [O]ur results suggest that future planning is not a uniquely human ability" (pp. 1039–1040). If apes and perhaps other animals can plan for the future, then is it possible that they can worry about it as well? Once again, there is no way for us to know for sure.

For our purposes here, it would in some ways be easier if in fact there were no differences between human and animal brains. Perhaps human cognitive and intellectual abilities are not special but merely on a continuum of attributes. Then the whole issue of what is the mind would seemingly go away; we aren't generally concerned about the minds of animals because we can never know for sure what is going on in them. If the chimpanzee and bonobo brains are no different from ours, we could then perhaps justify only dealing with brains on a physiological level.

But this just doesn't feel right; we want to agree that chimpanzees, bonobos, gorillas, and orangutans are our remarkably talented primate cousins, but from a cognitive and intellectual perspective they aren't the same as humans. Some scientists insist that although nonhuman animals do use tools and solve problems, they cannot apply those talents over the wide range of tasks that humans can.[19] Not everyone is willing to agree with Darwin that we differ from chimpanzee only by degree.[20] Dissenters to Darwin's point of view contend that humans can solve many more different kinds of problems and use a much broader range of tools than can apes. Ethologist like de Waal are perhaps

[19] Balter M: How human intelligence evolved—is it science or 'paleofantasy'? *Science* 2008;319:1028.
[20] Penn DC, Holyoak KJ, Povinelli DJ: Darwin's mistake: explaining the discontinuity between human and nonhuman minds. *Behav Brain Sci* 2008;31:109–178.

right to wax with great enthusiasm every time their life-long careful observations reveal a new cognitive skill in a chimpanzee. But, as an observer of human development, most recently that of my first grandchild, Hannah Beth Moster, it is difficult for me not to appreciate the uniqueness of humans. It takes enormous experimental effort, cleverly designed methods, and years of observation to see things in chimpanzees that human children pick up on their own in the first few months and years of life. As early as six months, a human infant can actually recognize what the word "apple" stands for, and, by two years of age, a toddler begins speaking in full sentences with very little special training other than listening to what adults are saying. It isn't because monkeys and apes lack the vocal apparatus to make speech. Recent studies show that baboons, for example, produce five vowel-like sounds that are comparable to human speech.[21] In the domains humans care about—language, self-awareness, impulse control, planning, and the like—apes demonstrate a level of cognitive sophistication that is roughly equivalent to a three-year-old child.

Even scientists who spend their lives among apes, as do Dorothy Cheney and Robert Seyfarth of the University of Pennsylvania, notice these differences. This husband-wife team clearly understands the advanced social and cognitive abilities of apes, yet they also acknowledge their profound differences from humans. "Although there are tantalizing hints that some monkey calls function like words," a science writer who spent time with Cheney and Seyfarth explains, "the vocal repertoires of monkeys and apes are still very limited, especially when compared with our own ability to learn to produce new sounds. Cheney and Seyfarth say very little progress has been made in understanding this limitation, and why monkeys don't seem to learn phonetically" (p. 25).[22]

For all their seeming ability to demonstrate caring and empathy, no other creature but humans cries for emotional reasons. Is that evidence of superiority? Hardly. But it is evidence of difference, and to dismiss this seems just as foolish as failing to appreciate an animal's accomplishments. Six million years after the two species' lineages diverted, humans live everywhere on earth; some of us are systematically destroying the few habitats in Africa where chimpanzees still live while others of us are struggling to protect them from extinction. The reverse, of course, is not the case.

I think I understand what is going on here. As Paul Bloom points out in his recent book *Against Empathy*, we most easily empathize with individuals who are closest to ourselves.[23] That is, if we understand that "empathy" means the process of identifying with another individual's experiences, we do that most readily when the person has characteristics similar to ours. Bloom believes that empathy is actually a source of racism because people of one race, he asserts, naturally empathize best with people

[21] Boe L-J, Berthommier F, Legou T, Captier G, Kemp C, Sawallis TR, Becker Y, Rey A, Fagot J: Evidence of a vocalic proto-system in the baboon (*Papio papio*) suggests pre-hominin speech precursors. *PLOS One* January 11, 2017

[22] Cole B: Field notes: how Dorothy Cheney and Robert Seyfarth's life among primates is influencing the next generation of scientists. *Omnia*, Spring/Summer 2016, 18–25.

[23] Bloom P: *Against Empathy: The Case for Rational Compassion*. New York, HarperCollins, 2016.

of their own race. "Empathy is biased, pushing in the direction of parochialism and racism" (p. 9), he writes. Although the idea that we should dispense with empathy because it promotes racism is not without controversy (and I do not personally agree with it), it seems obvious that, when talking about other species, Bloom's ideas must be correct: it is certainly easier for us to empathize with fellow humans than with animals. I think this is what Frans de Waal is getting at when he writes, "At the same time, we feel threatened by primates. We laugh hysterically at apes in movies and sitcoms, not because they are inherently funny—there are much funnier-looking animals, such as giraffes and ostriches—but because we like to keep our fellow primates at arm's length."[24]

Those who want humans to treat animals with more dignity and respect and less abuse and exploitation therefore naturally find it advantageous to encourage us to think of animals as having as many human characteristics as possible so that we more easily empathize with them. I think the sense is that if we empathize with chimpanzees, we will be less likely to want to lock them up in cages in zoos because that is not something we would want for ourselves. Thus, emphasizing all the ways that apes and other species have human characteristics is in the service of promoting animal welfare. If animals can plan for the future and feel sad just like we do, then we will be less likely to abuse them.

Does pointing out the differences between chimpanzees and humans therefore encourage us to treat them cruelly? I do understand this conundrum. As someone who has participated in animal research (although I have never personally handled them for any experiments), I have taken great interest in the gradual acknowledgment over the past few decades of our shameful treatment of them and the need for serious reform. Animals do feel both physical and emotional pain, and some of the things scientists have done to them are clearly wrong.

I remember learning about the work of the University of Wisconsin psychologist Harry Harlow in college. Harlow reared infant monkeys in isolation, showing that maternal deprivation led to severe emotional and behavioral abnormalities that lasted throughout the animals' lives. Never did any professor or textbook back then mention the fact that these experiments were incredibly cruel and by today's standards totally unacceptable. I confess that it never occurred to me at the time to question whether Harlow's work was unethical either; it was taught to us as groundbreaking, and I accepted that judgment. That attitude now feels shameful to me and makes me wonder if it represented a failure of empathy. In some ways, I suppose it did; had I thought of those poor infant monkeys as I do about human babies I might not have glossed over the cruelty.

It is extremely important, then, to assert that locating differences between humans and animals is not a justification for exploiting animals in the laboratory, zoos, or in any context. Because humans can write poems and chimpanzees cannot (or at least do not) does not mean we have the right to lock them up in tiny cages for life. But

[24] de Waal F: *Are We Smart Enough?*, p. 11.

it does not seem tenable to deny that humans have capabilities that no other species has, some of which are decidedly negative. And given that there are some potential advantages for understanding the basis for those differences—and without disagreeing with de Waal or anyone else who is able to show that animals have more human-like abilities and emotions than previously known—I do want to try to make some distinctions. And for our purposes here, the most important distinctions have undesirable connotations: humans seem more prone to devastating disorders of emotion and behavior than any other species.

While it is true that we do not know the full extent to which animals are self-aware because they cannot describe to us what they are thinking or how they feel, there are some behaviors and brain diseases they do not seem to have. Among them are schizophrenia, suicide, and anorexia nervosa. Here is a fictionalized but entirely typical case of schizophrenia.

## A CASE OF SCHIZOPHRENIA: AN EXCLUSIVELY HUMAN DISORDER

Richard was seemingly normal when he joined the army at age 19. Basic training was a bit harder for him than for other recruits—he had trouble following the rules and seemed a bit "odd" to others in his cohort. His bed was never made quite right, and his weapon not quite correctly assembled. But he got through training and was assigned to a unit based in the United States that specializes in communications. Here, things started going downhill. Richard appeared distracted and forgetful to others. He wandered off without permission and began to drink heavily when off duty. He made few friends and seemed easily offended. Often, he made a big deal out of comments that were plainly innocuous but seemed to him critical or even threatening. He got into several fights and ultimately was given an early discharge. Once out of the army, he was fired from one job after another, unable to even hold down work delivering take-out food. He returned to living in his parents' home, smoking marijuana daily, shaving and showering only occasionally, and spending most of his time playing video games or watching television.

Then, one night, he disappears from home and is found three blocks away banging on a stranger's door, demanding to be let in. Alarmed, the homeowners call the police. When the police arrive, Richard appears disheveled, his shirt unbuttoned, his hair uncombed, his shoelaces untied. The police officers try to talk to him, but he curses, calls them "pigs," and yells that he will kill them if they come closer. Ultimately, the officers are able to subdue Richard and bring him to a local emergency department. There, a psychiatrist is called who is able to elicit that the patient is hearing voices telling him that his parents are about to kill him and he must seek refuge elsewhere to be saved. He thinks they have inserted a tracking device into his head and know where he is. He believes the psychiatrist is in on the plan to kill him.

The psychiatrist diagnoses an acute psychotic state and orders an injection of an antipsychotic medication. After a few such injections over the next several hours in the emergency room, Richard's mind starts to clear a bit and he is willing to consider that perhaps he is mistaken about his parents' intentions. He remains suspicious, however, and insists that he would be better off living in the street than returning home. Richard is admitted to the psychiatry ward of the hospital, where, after a few days of medication and therapy, he no longer believes his parents are trying to kill him or that there is a tracking device in his head.

Richard is discharged after a week in the hospital. The mental health care team taking care of him wants to keep him a bit longer to make sure he is stable and on the right dose of medication, but, as is usually the case, Richard's insurance company refuses to allow the admission to be extended. Sadly, once back home, Richard soon stops taking his medication and relapses. Over the next several months, he has to be admitted to the hospital two more times, once after assaulting his father in a violent rage. Although he is ultimately placed on a stable medication regimen and no longer has hallucinations and persecutory delusions, he is never again able to hold a job or maintain friendships. He seems chronically unmotivated and talks as little as possible. Today, Richard spends most of his time in bed or watching television, seemingly content.

This is a classical description of the evolution of one of the most devastating of all diseases, schizophrenia. Medication and therapy can lead to better outcomes than Richard's, but it is not a curable condition and frequently has a devastating downhill course.

Schizophrenia is a devastating disease that probably has its roots during fetal brain development, but usually only first comes to clinical attention between late adolescence and early adulthood. The diagnosis is typically made when a set of what are called "psychotic" or "positive" symptoms persist in the patient over the course of at least six months. These symptoms include auditory hallucinations (hearing voices), delusions (fixed and incorrect ideas such as the patient believing he is the target of an organized conspiracy), thought disorder (speech that makes little or no sense to the listener), and grossly bizarre and disorganized behavior (such as hoarding garbage or a catatonic state). Although these are not the only symptoms of schizophrenia, they are the ones that usually result in the patient being taken to an emergency department or psychiatrist's office because they are obvious and sometimes threatening to observers.

There are no reports that psychosis ever occurs among any other animal species in the wild.[25] It is an illness that seems to attack the highest forms of human thought and cognition, disrupting logical processes and speech. If we agree that these examples of higher order cognition are uniquely human abilities, then it makes sense that only humans can develop an abnormality that affects them. If we then think about what part of the brain these faculties are most tied to, we immediately turn our attention to the prefrontal cortex (PFC), the part of the brain that, as we will see, most differentiates us from our nearest genetic neighbors. As Bret Stetka put it in his article in *Scientific American*, "with complicated, highly social human thought—and the

---

[25] Stetka B: Why don't animals get schizophrenia (and how come we do)? *SciAm* March 24, 2015. https://www.scientificamerican.com/article/why-don-t-animals-get-schizophrenia-and-how-come-we-do/

complicated genetics at the root of higher cognition—perhaps there's just more that can go wrong: complex function begets complex malfunction."[26] We will come back to schizophrenia when we discuss differences in gene expression patterns between humans and apes later in this chapter.

Another example of a unique human behavior is suicide. This assertion may meet with some disagreement because animals are known to self-mutilate under adverse conditions, and, as Katherine Gammon points out, "Self-destruction in the natural world is fairly common."[27] But as Gammon also explains, "It's more likely that animals will inadvertently terminate their own lives when depressed or lonely." Although suicide is not a common phenomenon among humans, it is the tenth leading cause of death in the United States, far more frequent than anything observed among animals. Although most people who take their lives suffer with depression at the time of their deaths, depression alone is an insufficient explanation because the vast majority of depressed people do not attempt suicide. Rather, suicide often follows what feels like devastating disappointments, personal catastrophes, and total loss of hope. Many survivors of suicide attempts describe thinking "I am better off dead," "my family will be better off if I am no longer around," or "my situation is hopeless." Once again, we are dealing with complex cognitions that only humans appear condemned to maintain.

Finally, I have picked anorexia nervosa as an example of a uniquely human disorder. Once again, we know that depressed animals will stop eating. But that is not what happens to patients with anorexia nervosa. The main problem for people with anorexia nervosa is distorted body image—the belief that they are fat. This drives the patient to starve herself, and, even when she becomes dangerously thin, she still sees herself as obese. No amount of objective evidence dissuades her—not seeing herself emaciated in the mirror or her critically low weight on a scale. Despite feeling hungry, the patient gets a triumphant rush when she avoids eating and experiences anger and despondency when she is forced to eat. No animal species voluntarily starves itself in its natural environment because of such an overwhelming cognitive error.

I considered adding Alzheimer's disease to this list, but that is problematic. It is true that dementia is not observed among elderly great apes, at least not anywhere near the rate it is among humans, and some studies suggest that the chimpanzee brain does not shrink with age the way the human brain does.[28] Furthermore, a key protein system involved in the risk for Alzheimer's disease in humans—called apoE—is not

---

[26] Ibid.

[27] Gammon K: Can animals commit suicide? *Live Science* March 29, 2012. http://www.livescience.com/33805-animals-commit-suicide.html. Note that the phrase "commit suicide" is considered inappropriate by most mental health advocates as it implies that suicide is a criminal behavior rather than a consequence of mental illness.

[28] Sherwood CC, Gordon AD, Allen JS, Phillips KAS, Erwin JM, Hof PR, Hopkins WD: Aging of the cerebral cortex differs between humans and chimpanzees. *Proc Natl Acad Sci USA* 2011;108:13029–13034.

found in any other primate.[29] However, all of this is possibly simply due to the fact that humans live much longer than apes, about twice as long in fact. So, the unique aspect of being human may not be the capacity to develop dementia but rather the things we have figured out to do in order to increase our lifespan, like improved sanitation, antibiotics, and vaccines. Apes perhaps would develop Alzheimer's disease if they lived long enough, but they will never figure out how to purify a water supply or invent penicillin. Frans de Waal can argue that such activities simply do not interest chimpanzees, and perhaps he is correct, but it clearly marks a major difference between how species regard health and mortality.

One could probably mention many other brain ailments that are unique to humans, but the point is that we have paid a hefty price for the rapid evolution of our advanced cognitive capacities. The same brain that appreciates Shakespeare and develops antibiotics also suffers from unprovoked fears and self-denigration. Perhaps we are not special, but we are surely different in many ways that involve emotion, intellect, and behavior. We will not be able to obliterate the "mind" issue by claiming that humans and chimpanzees are simply versions of each other. The task, then, is to figure out exactly what aspect of brain biology is responsible for this state of affairs.

## DOES THE HUMAN BRAIN LOOK DIFFERENT?

We will first consider the possibility that there is something about the brain's physical structure that differentiates us from chimpanzees and bonobos. It is commonly stated that it is the expansion of the outer layer of our brains, called the *cerebral cortex*, comprising 80% of the human brain, that accounts for *Homo sapiens'* unique cognitive abilities. As the eminent neuroscientists Daniel Geschwind and Pasko Rakic put it:

> Since the time of Darwin's *The Origin of Species* about 200 years ago, there has been little disagreement among scientists that the brain, and more specifically its covering, cerebral cortex, is the organ that enables human extraordinary cognitive capacity that includes abstract thinking, language, and other higher cognitive functions.[30]

Innumerable studies have looked at differences in the weights of the entire brains of various species. The human brain weighs about three pounds, about three times heavier than a chimpanzee brain even though we are about the same body size (see Figure 2.3). But we, of course, don't have the biggest brains: dolphins' brains are about the same size, and elephants and whales have much bigger brains. So, brain size alone cannot be the distinguishing feature. Nor is it the ratio of brain size to body mass,

[29] Finch CE, Sapolsky RM: The evolution of Alzheimer disease, the reproductive schedule, and apoE isoforms. *Neurobiol Aging* 1999;20:407–428.
[30] Geschwind DH, Rakic P: Cortical evolution: judge the brain by its cover. *Neuron* 2013;80:633–647, p. 633.

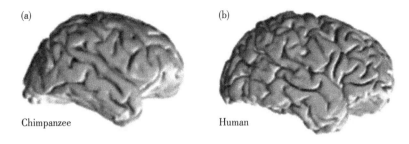

(a)  Chimpanzee          (b)  Human

**Figure 2.3** The human brain is about three times bigger than the chimpanzee brain but still smaller than the brains of elephants and whales.
National Chimpanzee Brain Resource supported by NIH—National Institute of Neurological Disorders and Stroke, http://www.chimpanzeebrain.org/chimpanzee-brain-facts/

the so-called *encephalization quotient*. The human brain constitutes about 2–2.5% of total body mass. Unique? Not really: a species of electric fish from Africa that uses weak electrical pulses to find prey and communicate with other electric fish has a brain about 3% of body size.[31]

Some studies have looked at specific parts of the brain, most notably the prefrontal cortex because it is the part of the brain most involved in thought and reflection. But, here again, even though it is true that humans have an exceptionally large prefrontal cortex, it isn't the largest or out of scale compared to other animals. Studies that have compared the pattern of peaks and valleys on the surface of the brain, called *sulci* and *gyri*, looking for differences in pattern, shape, and depth have similarly not yielded the key to what makes humans different.

It may be that the spacing of neurons is different in the brains of humans and apes. For example, in the prefrontal cortex, where neurons are arranged in minicolumns, spacing may be greater in the human brain.[32] What difference would this make? Perhaps greater spacing would allow for the axons and dendrites that project from neurons to make more connections.[33] Once again, however, exceptions to the rule make the spacing hypothesis difficult to sustain.

Then there are studies that examine the cellular components of the brain. The *neuron* is one of the three main cell types in the mammalian brain, the others being (1) the *glial cells* or *glia*, which in turn are divided into three subtypes: astrocytes, oligodendroglia, and microglia; and (2) the *endothelial cells* that line the small blood vessels of the brain and regulate what can traverse the *blood–brain barrier*, the system that carefully separates the brain from the circulating blood.

---

[31] Sukhum KV, Freiler MK, Wang R, Carlson BA: The costs of a big brain: extreme encephalization results in higher energetic demand and reduced hypoxia tolerance in weakly electric African fishes. *Proc Biol Sci* 2016;283:20162157.

[32] Semeneferi K, Teffer K, Buxhoevden BP, et al.: Spatial organization of neurons in the frontal pole sets humans apart from great apes. *Cereb Cortex* 2011;21:1485–1497.

[33] Miller G: New clues about what makes the human brain special. *Science* 2010;3301167.

We will have much occasion as we proceed to discuss the structure of neurons and occasionally to mention the other types of cells, but for now it is sufficient to note that it is the neurons that store memories and conduct information. Do human brains have more or larger neurons than chimpanzees and other apes? Are there more neurons in the human prefrontal cortex, or is the ratio of neurons to other cells different? One intriguing possible difference between ape and human brains at the cellular level occurs during fetal development, when the area of the cortex known as the subventricular zone undergoes greater expansion in humans than in other primates. The cells in the fetal subventricular zone divide rapidly, and this appears to explain the greater expansion of cortical regions that are needed for our advanced associative and executive functions.[34] But, in general, our neurons look pretty much the same as neurons in the brains of mice, rats, and monkeys.

There is one possible exception to this litany of negative answers, and that comes from the remarkable work of neuroscientist Suzana Herculano-Houzel of the Federal University of Rio de Janeiro.[35] She noticed that papers and textbooks all put the number of neurons in the human brain at 100 billion, but no one seemed to know where that number comes from. Primates in general pack more neurons into a given brain space than do other species, making distances for neural transmission relatively short and efficient. But how do humans compare to our primate cousins?

In order to find out how many neurons there really are in a brain, Herculano-Houzel developed a very clever new technique for counting them and applied it to brains from many species, including chimpanzees and humans. Her story of how she got brains from all these species makes for very interesting reading. It turns out that there are 86 billion neurons in the human brain, and Herculano-Houzel emphasizes that we not treat the mythical 14 million that don't exist as a rounding error; that is a bit more than the total number of neurons in a baboon's brain.

Most important, humans have far more neurons than chimpanzees or any other primate in the frontal cortex, giving us the largest ratio of frontal cortex to total brain mass among primates. Humans, according to Herculano-Houzel's work, have 16 billion neurons in the frontal cortex; chimpanzee have only 6 billion. This phenomenon of frontal cortical expansion appears to be the defining characteristic of human brain development. Our number of neurons is still proportional to body size among primates—we don't have more than expected. In fact, gorillas and orangutans, with their larger body mass, have *fewer* neurons than predicted. "The human cerebral cortex is therefore not outstanding in its neuronal composition," she writes. "It has just the mass that a primate cortex with its number of neurons would be expected to have."[36] We are not special in the sense of the ratio of neurons in the prefrontal cortex to body mass, Herculano-Houzel tells us, but our cognitive abilities are best understood as a

---

[34] McKenzie M, Fishell G: Human brains teach us a surprising lesson. *Science* 2016;3543:38–39.

[35] Herculano-Houzel S: *The Human Advantage: A New Understanding of How Our Brain Became Remarkable.* Cambridge, MA, MIT Press, 2016.

[36] Ibid., p. 81.

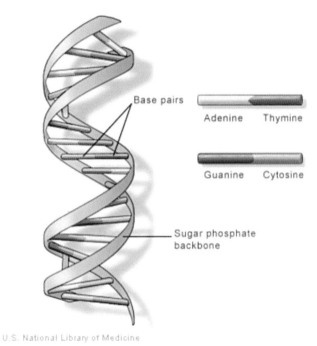

Base pairs

Adenine    Thymine

Guanine    Cytosine

Sugar phosphate
backbone

**Figure 2.4** The hereditary molecule, DNA, is shown here in its familiar double helix shape. The "rungs" of the ladder comprise four bases that are joined by hydrogen bonds. The sides of the ladder are composed of sugar (deoxyribose) and phosphate molecules.

From the National Library of Medicine, https://ghr.nlm.nih.gov/primer/illustrations/dnastructure.jpg

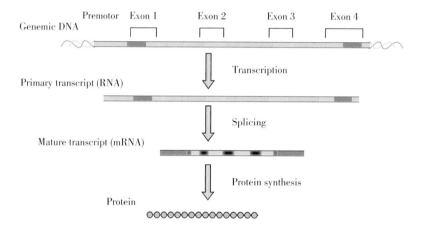

**Figure 2.5** How a gene works. Genes are located along a strand of DNA. The sequence of the four bases (G, C, T, A) within a gene determines what messenger RNA (mRNA) and protein are made from each gene. Each gene has many parts. The exons are the regions of a gene that are actually transcribed to messenger RNA (mRNA). In between them are the introns (not shown in this figure), which are essentially silent. The promoter region is a part of the gene that regulates how and when the gene will be transcribed or expressed. The RNA that is first transcribed from a gene undergoes a splicing process in which some bases are clipped out. The final RNA copy is then translated into a protein.

From the National Center for Biotechnology Information, National Library of Medicine, https://www.ncbi. nlm.nih.gov/probe/docs/applexpression/

function of the greater absolute number of neurons in our frontal cortex. Her conclusion is that

> Our single largest advantage over other animals is most easily ascribed to the sheer number of neurons available in the cerebral cortex, and in the prefrontal cortex in particular, to process information in complex, flexible ways that can predict future outcomes and act as required, particularly in way that intelligently maximizes future possibilities.[37]

Interestingly, all these neurons put a big energy demand on us: the human brain that is only about 2% of total body mass nevertheless uses about 25% of total body energy, about 500 kilocalories a day. In a fascinating set of speculations, Herculano-Houzel proposes that the only way to get all those calories in a day is to have a big mouth and cook our food, which makes its energy more easily available. Thus, she proposes, rats can't have so many neurons as we do because their mouths are too small to eat enough food, and gorillas, chimpanzees, and bonobos cannot because they eat their food raw.

We have then the first possible reason that humans have different cognitive abilities—more neurons in the part of the brain that is needed for doing things only we can do. This explanation favors Darwin's notion that we are quantitatively but not qualitatively different from other primates: writing a poem is simply a more advanced example of the kind of thinking chimpanzees can do, not an entirely unique phenomenon. Let us see, however, if there might be other differences.

## ARE THERE GENES THAT MAKE OUR BRAINS DIFFERENT?

About 2% of human genes are different from chimpanzee genes. If humans have about 20,000 total genes, this would still leave about 400 candidates to explain differences between species. Of course, many of these between-species differences have little to do with the brain or cognitive abilities. Genes on the Y chromosome, the sex chromosome that only males have, are markedly different between humans and chimpanzees for example.[38] Other genetic differences must be present to account for the chimpanzees far greater strength and furrier bodies and our bipedal stance. But there are probably still enough genes that differ between the species to make looking for ones that affect brain function of interest.

It is important to digress a moment here and remind readers what a "gene" is. You might want to bookmark the next several pages as the information here on some of the basic aspects of genetics will crop up throughout the rest of this book. The

---

[37] Ibid., p. 143.

[38] Huges JF, Skaletsky H, Pynitkova T, et al.: Chimpanzee and human Y chromosomes are remarkably divergent in structure and gene content. *Nature* 2010;463:536–539.

double helix, the structure of the genetic molecule deoxyribonucleic acid (DNA), first described in 1953 by Frances Crick, James Watson, and Maurice Wilkins with the crucial but sadly until recently unacknowledged contribution of Rosalind Franklin, is familiar to everyone. The double helix is composed of two strands of DNA wound around each other. Most of the DNA is found inside the nucleus of cells, including neurons. As Figure 2.4 shows, DNA belongs to class of molecules called *nucleic acids* that are composed of four bases or nucleotides that are aligned along each strand in various combinations. The four varieties are commonly referred to as A, C, G, and T (standing for adenine, cytosine, guanine, and thymine). A base on one strand is linked to a base on the complementary strand of DNA, A with T and C with G, by a sugar molecule, called *deoxyribose*, and a phosphate molecule. The structure looks like a twisted ladder, with the bases as the rungs and the sugar and phosphate molecules forming the sides. There are about 3 billion total bases in any person's DNA.

Genes are aligned along the DNA strands, and the main function of a gene (although not the only function of genes) is to provide the information for making proteins, the molecules that do the body's work. Only one of the twisted complementary strands

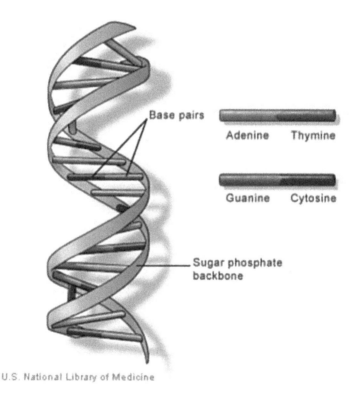

**Figure 2.4** The hereditary molecule, DNA, is shown here in its familiar double helix shape. The "rungs" of the ladder comprise four bases that are joined by hydrogen bonds. The sides of the ladder are composed of sugar (deoxyribose) and phosphate molecules.

From the National Library of Medicine, https://ghr.nlm.nih.gov/primer/illustrations/dnastructure.jpg

is usually functional, and, along that strand, the sequence of bases determines the exact function of each gene and where one gene stops and another gene starts. A gene must first be *transcribed* by an enzyme into a corresponding strand of messenger RNA (mRNA), and the mRNA molecule then moves out of the nucleus, where it is then *translated* into a protein. When we say that a gene "codes" for a protein, we generally mean that the gene is transcribed to an mRNA that is then translated into a protein because not all RNA molecules are translated into proteins. I always remember that transcription precedes translation because the letter "c" precedes the letter "l" in the English alphabet. Figure 2.5 depicts this general process of transcription to translation, with an additional step in which a newly transcribed RNA molecule is spliced. One of the interesting things is that the RNA that is transcribed from DNA can itself be worked on by enzymes and broken up and recombined in various ways before it is translated to protein. This slicing process means that each gene can actually be associated with more than one protein, depending on how its RNA gets broken and recombined after transcription.

It is also important to note that most of our DNA is not associated with proteins at all. First, within a gene, there are "coding" regions called *exons* that are transcribed into RNA and "noncoding" regions, called *introns*, that are skipped over by the transcribing or polymerase enzyme. And then, in between genes, there are long stretches of DNA that don't contain genes at all. In fact, most of our DNA falls within these stretches.

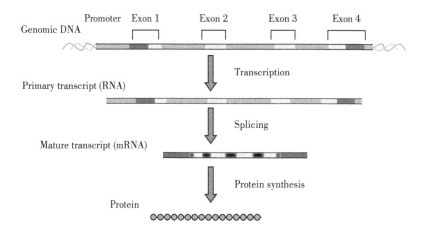

**Figure 2.5** How a gene works. Genes are located along a strand of DNA. The sequence of the four bases (G, C, T, A) within a gene determines what messenger RNA (mRNA) and protein are made from each gene. Each gene has many parts. The exons are the regions of a gene that are actually transcribed to messenger RNA (mRNA). In between them are the introns (not shown in this figure), which are essentially silent. The promoter region is a part of the gene that regulates how and when the gene will be transcribed or expressed. The RNA that is first transcribed from a gene undergoes a splicing process in which some bases are clipped out. The final RNA copy is then translated into a protein.

From the National Center for Biotechnology Information, National Library of Medicine, https://www.ncbi. nlm.nih.gov/probe/docs/applexpression/

Some of that DNA is transcribed into RNA molecules that, instead of being translated into proteins, function as regulators that bind to coding sections of the DNA and determine when and to what degree they are actively transcribed. There are multiple other ways that gene activity is regulated, and we will turn to some of them later in this chapter and in future chapters in this book.

We inherit all of our genes from our parents. We get one set of 23 chromosomes from our mothers and the other set of 23 chromosomes from our fathers. The structure of those genes is basically invariant throughout our lives, and 99% of our DNA is the same among all humans. This means that the sequence of nucleotide bases that contain the information for making proteins largely does not change once the fetus is formed. Moreover, the sequence of nucleotide base pairs in our genes is pretty much the same from one person to the next (although bear in mind that 1% of the 3 billion bases we each have in our DNA still equals a fairly large potential basis for differences among us). During fetal life, when cells rapidly divide, changes or mutations in the DNA base sequence can occur each time the cells divide as the fetus gets larger. Once we are born, most of the cells in our bodies are still capable of dividing, and therefore mutations can still occur although such mutations become much less frequent. The fact that most cells in the body can continue to divide explains why broken bones or torn skin heal—the cells divide by a process called *mitosis* and heal the wound. It is also how we make new blood cells and immune cells throughout life as stem cells in our bone marrow divide and mature into the red blood cells that carry oxygen and the white blood cells that fight infection. Each time a cell divides, it is possible for an error to occur in the way the DNA is processed so that a mutation arises. Some cancer cells have mutations that cause the cell to divide out of control, for example. Ultraviolet radiation from sunlight can cause a mutation and give us skin cancer; cigarette smoke can induce mutations that cause lung and other cancers. Most mutations, however, are silent, and so it is important to emphasize again that, for the most part, the genes we inherit are the ones we live with for our entire lives.

There is an exception to one aspect of the process just described, and this applies to the neurons in the central nervous system. The nervous system is divided into two parts, the peripheral and the central nervous systems. The peripheral nervous system is composed of the nerves that go to and from the spinal cord and innervate all parts of our body. They bring signals to muscles to allow us to move, breathe, and digest our food and keep our hearts beating, and they transport the signals from our skin and other organs that allow us to feel pain and other sensations. The other part of our nervous system, the central nervous system (CNS), comprises the brain and the spinal cord.

Now if you get a really deep cut on a finger and sever a peripheral nerve, the two ends can grow back together because the nerve cells will divide and bridge the gap. But if you transect the spinal cord, it cannot ever be repaired; with a few exceptions, which we will discuss in Chapter 4, the neurons in the CNS cannot divide. They are sometimes referred to as "post-mitotic," meaning that they have entered a stage of life beyond the point where cell division, or mitosis, is still possible.

This means that as far as neurons in the CNS—the brain and spinal cord—go, there is virtually no chance for mutations to occur during life. In the nuclei of neurons in the brains of mammals like us, the genes that we are born with cannot, therefore, change during life. The other cells in the brain (glial cells and endothelial cells), by the way, are capable of continuous mitosis throughout life and therefore can sustain occasional mutations just like cells elsewhere in the body. Incidentally, this is the reason why brain tumors almost never involve neurons but rather are composed of other brain cell types. The worst brain tumor, called *glioblastoma multiforme* (GBM), which is almost invariably fatal, is made of glial cells that divide out of control.

Let's summarize where we are at this point in understanding how genetics might (or might not) explain why the human brain is unique. Throughout the rest of the book, the most important things to remember as we pursue both the possible differences between human and chimpanzee brains in this chapter and the ways in which experience changes our brains are:

1. For the most part, the genes we inherit from our parents stay exactly the same throughout our lives.
2. We share about 98% of our DNA with chimpanzees and about 99% with each other, so the opportunity for differences at the level of the sequence of bases is restricted.
3. The sequence of base pairs (nucleotides) in a gene determines what proteins are made, but genes are subject to all kinds of regulatory influences, and the mRNA that genes produce by transcription is also altered by splicing. Hence, although the sequence of bases on a gene is invariant throughout life, the way that gene actually works changes on a second-by-second basis.
4. Neurons, unlike other types of cells in the brain and throughout the rest of the body, do not divide during the life of any mammal, with a few exceptions that will be discussed in a separate chapter. Hence, for our purposes, it is fair to state that mutations in the base sequence of DNA in neurons in the brain cannot occur.

As we mentioned earlier, the lineages that resulted in our species, *Homo sapiens*, and that resulted in chimpanzees, *Pan troglodytes*, and bonobos, *Pan paniscus*, separated from each other about 6 million years ago. That means we have had 6 million years for evolution to change the structure of those approximately 400 genes we have that chimpanzees don't, and perhaps some of them code for proteins that are at the root of the reason that humans and chimpanzees have different cognitive abilities and emotional repertoires. When scientists sequenced the DNA in human chromosome 21 and the corresponding chimpanzee chromosome 22, they found that only in only 1.44% was one nucleotide (that is, an A, G, T, or C) substituted for another nucleotide.[39] There were 68,000 instances in which a nucleotide was added or deleted for one or the other chromosome, which is really a very small number compared to the

[39] Fuykyama WH, Hattori M, Taylor TD, et al.: DNA sequence and comparative analysis of chimpanzee chromosome 22. *Nature* 2004;429:382–388.

millions of nucleotides in a single chromosome and the fact that most such insertions and deletions have no consequences. Although these changes in DNA sequences did result in changes to the corresponding proteins they code for, most of these changes don't represent much in the way of functional significance. Thus, it doesn't look as if structural differences in the sequence of base pairs in genes between humans and chimpanzees can explain much about why the two species are different.

While it was necessary to go through all of this basic genetic information in order to understand many of the concepts in this book, the bottom line for the topic at hand is that, so far, very little in the way of structural genetic differences has been found that accounts for the big differences between us and chimpanzees in cognitive abilities. There does not seem to be a single gene for written language or mathematical prowess or getting schizophrenia. How nice it would be if the reason humans get schizophrenia and chimpanzees don't is because of a mutation in a single gene that we have and chimps don't. If such a gene existed, we would probably have found it by now. For complex diseases like schizophrenia, however, the evidence now suggests that the genetic contribution comes from mutations in many different genes, each one responsible for only a very small part of the risk for getting the disease. In order to get schizophrenia, according to the multiple gene model, it is necessary to have mutations in several different genes, but exactly what those combinations are is still a mystery.

Before we leave the subject of structural gene differences between humans and chimpanzees, however, I will mention a few instances in which, as it turns out, there is some evidence that variations in the base sequences of a small number of genes account for at least a few of the important differences in the brains of humans and apes. For example, a gene with the designation *ARHGAP11B*, that first appeared in humans after we diverged from chimpanzees (but before we separated from Neanderthals), increases cell division in the brain and folding of the cerebral cortex.[40] When this gene is inserted into the DNA of a developing mouse, the normally smooth surface of the mouse brain develops human-like folds that increase its overall surface area. Neither the ARHGAP11B gene nor its protein product are found in the chimpanzee brain.

It further turns out that the evolutionary predecessor of the ARHGAP11B gene is a gene not surprisingly called *ARHGAP11A*. Scientists at the Max Planck Institute in Dresden, Germany, were surprised to find out that the change from the "A" to the "B" version involves only a single point mutation, the substitution of a G (guanine) nucleotide base for a C (cytosine) nucleotide base.[41] Remember that human DNA has about 3 billion base pairs and that single substitutions of one base for another are both common and generally without functional significance. But this change completely alters the length of the mRNA that is transcribed from the gene and the protein that is

[40] Florio M, Albert M, Taverna E, et al.: Human specific gene *ARHGAP11B* promotes basal progenitor amplification and neocortex expansion. *Science* 2015;347:1465–1470.

[41] Florio M, Namba T, Paabo S, Hiller M, Huttner WB: A single splice site mutation in human-specific AFHGAP11B causes basal progenitor amplification. *Sci Adv*, December 7 2016. doi:10.1126/sciadv.1601941

subsequently translated. Hence, one very tiny change in a single gene seems to play an important role in the expansion of the human cortex.

If you remember the work of Herculano-Houzel described earlier in this chapter, you realize that the ARHGAP11B gene may be of critical significance. Herculano-Houzel contends that the important difference between humans and other primates is the greater number of neurons we have in our frontal cortex. The mutation that produced the uniquely human ARHGAP11B gene seems to be involved in that expansion of the human frontal cortex and therefore may be an important structural DNA reason behind our species' particular abilities.

In another example of possibly significant differences in the physical compositions of genes between humans and chimpanzees, scientists at Duke University focused attention on a region of DNA called *human-accelerated regulatory enhancer* (HARE$_5$).[42] The Duke team recognized that the genes in this region, which are important in brain development, are slightly different between humans and chimpanzees—a difference of only about 16 changes in nucleotide base sequence. But when the DNA from humans and chimpanzees is incorporated into mouse embryos, a striking difference occurred. The human HARE$_5$ sequence, but not the chimpanzee sequence, caused the mice to develop bigger brains by stimulating neural stem cells to divide more actively than is ordinarily the case.

But a mystery of this finding is that the genes in the HARE$_5$ region do not actually code for proteins. So how do they effect this neural stem cell division enhancement? The answer seems to rest in the way genes are actually expressed. Genevieve Konopka, a neuroscientist who works at the University of Texas, Southwestern Medical Center, studies the "genetics of humananess." In a 2009 paper, she and her colleagues wrote:

> As suggested by King and Wilson over 30 years ago, and reaffirmed by the sequencing of both the human and chimpanzee genomes, the phenotypic differences exhibited by humans and chimpanzees cannot be explained by differences in DNA sequence alone, and are likely due to differences in gene expression and regulation. (p. 217)[43]

Finally, a variation in a gene called *FOX2P* may be the reason humans can form words.

I felt obligated to acknowledge the few findings in which structural differences in genes seem to have an impact on differentiating the human and chimpanzee brains, particularly with respect to the size and number of neurons in that all-important prefrontal cortex. It has only been a few years since both the human and chimpanzee genomes were completely sequenced and therefore that this kind of comparison

[42] Boyd JL, Skove SL, Rouanet JP, Pilaz LJ, Bepler T, Gordan R, Wray GA, Silver DL: Human-chimpanzee differences in a FZD8 enhancer alter cell-cycle dynamics in the developing neocortex. *Curr BiolCurr Biol* 2015;25:772–779.
[43] Konopka G, Bomar JM, Winden K, et al.: Human-specific transcriptional regulation of CNS development genes by FOXP2. *Nature* 2009;462:213–217.

became possible on a large scale, so it is absolutely possible that more such structural differences important to brain development will be discovered in the future. Nevertheless, there is an emerging sense that the differences between human and great ape brains lies less in differences in gene structure and more in differences in how genes are expressed. We turn now, then, to these differences.

## DOES THE DIFFERENCE REST IN HOW GENES ARE EXPRESSED?

I alluded to the fact that there are portions within genes called introns and long stretches of DNA on chromosomes between genes that do not ultimately code for any particular proteins. But these noncoding regions of DNA are sometimes transcribed into mRNAs that, rather than being transcribed into protein, bind to regulatory sections on genes. This introduces the topic of gene regulation and expression, which will be extremely important throughout this book, especially in the next chapter on epigenetics and its role in determining the effects of stressful life events.

Almost all cells in the body, regardless of which organ they are in, contain the same DNA coding information. The genes that code for the proteins that make thyroid hormone are present in the cells of the liver, for example, and the genes that code for the enzymes the liver makes to digest the food we eat are present in neurons in the brain. But the liver doesn't make thyroid hormone and the brain doesn't make digestive enzymes (there are actually several exceptions to that statement about the brain and digestive enzymes, but they aren't important right now). The reason is that the thyroid hormone genes are turned off in the liver; they are not transcribed, and so no mRNA is made from them and there is consequently no protein production. Similarly, most of the genes coding for digestive enzymes are turned off in the brain.

Some genes are only turned on some of the time. The gene that codes for the enzyme that digests lactose in milk—lactase—is only activated when we actually drink milk. And then, in most people, it is permanently turned off when we are out of infancy. The genes in the brain structure called the *hypothalamus* that initiate the production of female sex hormones—estrogen and progesterone—are silent until a girl reaches menarche and then turn off again when a woman reaches menopause. In the brain, the expression of about 90% of genes is regulated in different regions and across time.[44]

Every gene has one or more regulatory elements that control whether the gene is transcribed and, when it is, to what degree. The system of gene expression regulation is complex and occurs at every level, from the transcription of a stretch of DNA into mRNA to the size and structure of proteins. Genes have stretches of DNA that are called *regulatory elements* or *promoters* and *inducers*. Other proteins and small

---

[44] Kang HJ, Kawasawa YI, Cheng F, et al.: Spatio-temporal transcriptome of the human brain. *Nature* 2010;478:483–489.

RNA molecules bind to them and start or stop a gene from being transcribed.[45] Furthermore, as will be discussed in Chapter 3 when we discuss epigenetics, the way DNA is folded and surrounded by a type of protein called *histones* also affords another opportunity for gene expression regulation. There's more. Messenger RNA molecules and proteins can be spliced, combined with each other, and altered in a variety of ways once they are made, sometimes making them more or less active or even inactive. And the final product, the protein, can also be cut into several different proteins with different functions. When the genetic code was first revealed, we were taught the mantra "one gene, one protein," meaning that each protein could be traced back to the gene that coded for it. Now we know things are far more complicated. "One gene, many proteins" is actually the case. Our 20,000 genes result in far more than 20,000 proteins—probably somewhere between 250,000 and 1 million—and these proteins are present at different times of the day, month, year, and lifetime.

All of this means that even though we have embedded in that sequence of nucleotide base pairs on our genes that we are born with all the DNA instructions for making proteins we will ever have, whether those instructions are followed and to what degree varies enormously. Is it possible that there are significant differences in gene expression in the prefrontal cortex between humans and apes? Could it be that even though we have almost all the same genes, more of them in the human brain are actually turned on than in the chimpanzee brain? Or, if we want to be careful about using the word "more" when comparing us to them, how about the possibility that different genes in the brains are expressed at different rates between the two species?

Indeed, many recent studies have demonstrated that this is the case. The human brain appears to have more active genes in the brain than those of any other species. This may be because the regulatory regions of those genes are more active, thus increasing the chances that a coding gene will produce more protein.[46] I first became interested in this possibility in 2002, when I read a paper from a research group that included the first author, Wolfgang Enard, who worked at the time at the Max Planck Institute for Evolutionary Anthropology, located in Leipzig, Germany. In this paper (which stimulated my daughter Rachel and I to write a paper we called "The Human Dimension"),[47] Enard and colleagues from multiple institutions in the United States and Europe compared patterns of gene expression in white blood cells (leukocytes), liver, and brain among multiple species including humans, chimpanzees, orangutans, a type of rhesus monkey called the macaque (*Macaca mulatta*), and three species of mice.[48] When looking at liver and blood cells, levels of gene transcription to mRNA

[45] Bose DA, Donahue G, Reinberg D, Shiekhattar R, Bonasio R, Berger SL: RNA binding to CBP stimulates histone acetylation and transcription. *Cell* 2017;168:135–149.

[46] Reilly SK, Yin J, Ayoub AE, Emera D, Leng J, Cotney J, Sarro R, Rakic P, Noonan JP: Evolutionary changes in promoter and enhancer activity during human corticogenesis. *Science* 2015;347:1155–1159.

[47] Berkowitz et al., The human dimension, p. 195.

[48] Enard W, Khaltovich P, Klose J, et al.: Intra- and interspecific variation in primate gene expression patterns. *Science* 2002;296:340–343.

and translation to protein were similar between humans and chimpanzees, both of whom had levels that were significantly greater compared to the macaque. "In stark contrast," the authors reported, "the expression pattern in the chimpanzee brain cortex is more similar to that of the macaques than to that of humans. This is due to a 5.5-fold acceleration of the rate of change in gene expression levels on the lineage leading to humans" (p. 341). A similar finding was reported a year later.[49] More recently, an exhaustive analysis of gene expression in multiple brain regions from humans and several species of apes and monkeys who all died of natural causes found "global, regional, and cell-type-specific species expression differences in protein-coding and non-coding genes (p. 1032)."[50] These findings are all very exciting to me because they offer a solution to the conundrum of such big differences in cognitive ability between apes and humans given such small differences in the actual structure of our genes.

An example of how differences in gene expression between human and nonhuman primates might work in both health and disease may help solve a mystery of human evolution. Schizophrenia, the illness we discussed earlier that appears almost entirely limited to humans, should not persist in the population at the fixed rate of about 1% as epidemiological studies consistently show it does. It is a disorder that is almost 70% inherited but does not seem to confer any reproductive advantage.[51] In fact, people with schizophrenia are less likely to have children than the healthy population: so, why do the genes for schizophrenia persist in human populations? A gene or genes that are responsible for a disease that actually decreases the likelihood that it or they will be passed on to subsequent generations should eventually disappear.

Recall the case of Richard, the unfortunate young man with schizophrenia I described earlier in this chapter. Richard winds up living an isolated, lonely life with little social interaction. He never has a romantic relationship, gets married, or fathers children. Whatever genes he has that contributed to his getting schizophrenia should die when he does. Hence, it should only be possible for schizophrenia to maintain itself as a human genetic disease if the genes that are partially responsible for it also have some beneficial and necessary function. If that were the case, then many if not most people must get these genes that increase the risk for schizophrenia because they are also necessary for a beneficial function but, perhaps because those individuals are not exposed to adverse early life environments, they don't get schizophrenia. Such people only realize the beneficial effect of the genes, reproduce, and pass the schizophrenia-susceptibility genes down to the next generation.

[49] Caceres M, Lachuer J, Zapala MA, et al.: Elevated gene expression levels distinguish human from non-human primate brains. *Proc Natl Acad Sci* 2003;100:13030–13035.

[50] Sousa AMM, Zhu Y, Raghanti MA, et al.: Molecular and cellular reorganization of neural circuits in the human lineage. *Science* 2017;358:10271032.

[51] Srinivasan S, Bettella F, Mattingsdal M, Wang Y, Witoelar A, Schork AJ, Thompson WK, Zuber V, et al.: Genetic markers of human evolution are enriched in schizophrenia. *Biol Psychiatry* 2016;80:284–292.

Ke Xu and colleagues at the Icahn School of Medicine at Mount Sinai in New York City studied genes in the human accelerated regions (HARs), already mentioned.[52] These genes are conserved in chimpanzees and humans through evolution, but the DNA sequences are a bit different between species, and these small differences seem to make a significant difference in brain development. But, again, there is a problem in how we understand this effect because, as I mentioned earlier, the genes in the HARs do not themselves code for proteins. Instead, they seem to be involved in regulating the activity of other genes in the frontal cortex. It is these differences in activity that may, according to the Mount Sinai group, have something to do with why humans but not chimpanzees can succumb to schizophrenia. On the one hand, the genes in the HARs of humans seem both linked to normal brain development, particularly of the brain's main inhibitory neurotransmitter, called γ-*aminobutyric acid* (GABA), and on the other hand, to schizophrenia. In other words, HAR genes that are involved in regulating the activity of other genes serve both beneficial functions and, when bearing relatively small additional changes, in increasing the chance a person will develop schizophrenia. The conclusion is that, in order for the human brain to advance beyond that of the chimpanzee, changes in the regulation of gene expression occurred throughout evolution that were both necessary but could go awry and cause disease.[53]

Another fascinating example of the role played by differences in gene regulation and expression involves speech. Why can't monkeys and apes speak? It was recently shown conclusively that the reason has nothing to do with vocal anatomy.[54] Other primates have vocal cords, pharynxes, tongues, and lips that should be more than adequate to produce speech. The reason they can't talk and we can must therefore reside in the brain. Only one gene so far has been implicated in human speech, called *fox2p*, and it codes for a protein called FOX2P. The human and chimpanzee versions of this gene are almost identical, but there is a very small difference and that difference results in the human protein having two different amino acids in its structure. Is that enough to make a difference? Genevieve Konopka and colleagues performed an exhaustive series of studies on how the FOX2P protein functions in human and chimpanzee brains and showed that these two different amino acids substantially alter the way the protein regulates the expression of other genes in the brain involved in language and speech and even changes in which region of the brain these downstream genes are expressed.[55] Moreover, since FOX2P has also been implicated in disorders of speech and language like autism and dyslexia, we have another example of how small genetic changes leading to more profound gene expression changes can explain both a unique human characteristic and a disorder involving that characteristic.

[52] Xu K, Schadt EE, Pollard KS, Roussos P, Dudley JT: Genomic and network patterns of schizophrenia genetic variation in human evolutionary accelerated regions. *Mol Biol Evol* 2015;32:1148–1160.

[53] Dean B: Is schizophrenia the price of human central nervous system complexity? *Aust NZ J Psychiatry* 2009;43:13–24.

[54] Boe L-J et al.: Evidence of a vocalic proto-system in the baboon.

[55] Konopka G, Bomar JM, Winden K, et al.: Human-specific transcriptional regulation of CNS development genes by FOXP2. *Nature* 2009;462:213–217.

# NOT BETTER, THEN, BUT DIFFERENT

We have, then, three lines of evidence that there are indeed important differences in brain structure and function between humans and their nearest genetic neighbors, the chimpanzee and the bonobo. First, humans have more neurons in the frontal cortex, the part of the brain that has evolved to serve introspection, reason, and creativity. Second, a physical difference in at least one gene is responsible for this expansion in the size of the frontal cortex. Finally, and I am convinced ultimately most importantly, humans express more genes in the frontal cortex.

Does this make us better than other animals? I believe the way around this issue is simply to say that we are not better, but different. Is being able to write a poem evidence of better function than being able to climb a tree and grab fruit? Is having the capacity to pollute the air an indication that we are more advanced than species that do not succumb to schizophrenia, suicide, or anorexia in the wild? These questions seem to me largely philosophical, which does not mean that they are uninteresting. Rather, I believe that by making two stipulations we can move beyond such questions of species-specific cognitive "superiority": first, that we are not superior cognitively or intellectually but rather different, and, second, that differences between us and other species are not in any way a justification to abuse them.

If we agree to these two points, then we notice that we have an important set of leads about where to look for both the benefits and drawbacks of having a human brain. These most likely reside in the way genes in neurons are expressed in the human prefrontal cortex. Although I will not go so far as to say that this is where the human "mind" is located, I will assert here that the particular ways in which prefrontal cortical neurons work are crucial to understanding how the human brain translates our experiences into ideas, memories, emotions, and behaviors. I cannot fully side with scientists like de Waals who seem to want us to believe that chimpanzees and humans are really not that different at all, even though to do so would make it easier for me to dismiss the "mind" as distinct from the brain. Rather, I believe that exploring the interspecies differences as we have in this chapter, using the curious illness of schizophrenia as an example of those differences, tells us a great deal about where to look for the intersection of brain and mind—specifically in the enhanced level of gene expression within neurons in the human prefrontal cortex. In the next chapter, we will delve a bit more into the basic science of how the expression levels of genes in those prefrontal neurons change every time we have a new experience.

# 3

## Life Events Shape Us
### *The Role of Epigenetic Regulation of Gene Expression*

It has memory's ear that can hear without having to hear.
—"The Mind Is a Wonderful Thing," Marianne Moore

Science tries to simplify our world by developing as many straightforward concepts, rules, and causes as possible. It is not uncommon, for instance, for physicists to yearn for a "theory of everything" as they attempt to unify the two great pillars of twentiethcentury physics, quantum mechanics and relativity. It isn't that physicists think these are simple things that can be boiled down to a few short equations. Yet they still hope to take an enormous amount of data—some conflicting—and develop something that helps them unify the information in a coherent way.

Biologists are no different, but the events of our lives are very messy things with which to have to deal. It is satisfying for a biologist to be able to say, "cigarette smoking causes cancer" or "insulin resistance causes type 2 diabetes" because those statements are clear and immediately point to avenues of prevention, treatment, and further research. But behind both of these "cause and effect" or "causal" statements is something much harder to quantify: the behaviors that are involved in these illnesses and the events in our lives that motivate those behaviors. Why do some people smoke and others don't? Is there are a gene involved that makes some people crave nicotine? Is cigarette smoking a way to deal with stress, anxiety, and depression? Do people smoke because they are influenced by advertisements and what their parents did when they were growing up? Or maybe the reasons some people smoke are a combination of these and other factors, all varying in degree of importance from one person to the next.

Similarly, while it is true that type 2 diabetes mellitus, sometimes referred to as "adult-onset" diabetes, involves an inability of cells to respond properly to insulin secreted by the pancreas—so-called insulin resistance—we also know that obesity is a major risk factor for it.[1] Obesity, of course, involves a behavior: eating too much, particularly too much sugar-containing foods. And, once again, we have a similar question

---

[1] Type one diabetes mellitus, sometimes called juvenile diabetes, involves the inability of the pancreas to produce insulin rather than an inability of cells in the body to respond to insulin. Type one diabetes is probably caused by antibodies that attack the pancreas and destroy insulin-producing cells, although why that happens is not entirely clear.

as we did with cigarette smoking and lung cancer: why do some people get obese and develop diabetes and others do not? Do traumatic events in early childhood create a propensity to overeat as adults? Is overeating also a response to stress and anxiety? Do overeating and obesity run in families and have a genetic basis? Here as well, the answer is most likely a combination of these and many other factors.

Given the fact that no two people have the same experiences throughout life, there are as many potential stressful life events as there are people. Science does not like such broad phenomena—it always seeks to try to put things into useable categories or even to discount something that doesn't fit into a theory based on other evidence. Nevertheless, one might think that psychiatry and psychology would have no choice but to accept and deal with all this diversity of life experiences. After all, when a person seeks help from a therapist, isn't figuring out what experiences a person has had among the most important parts of the therapy? It is thus surprising that, in fact, psychiatry and psychology have had a curious and often contentious relationship with life's experiences.

Although Freud did talk about "constitutional" differences among people—presumably traits we are born with and endure throughout life—his psychoanalytic theory and its subsequent modifications are mostly involved with understanding how the things that happen to us after we are born shape our unconscious minds and overt behaviors and emotions. Freud and later psychoanalytic theorists described a now controversial version of what normal development should look like and then explained how deviations from that pattern could cause neuroses. Our early life interactions with parents and siblings are of great importance for psychoanalysts in understanding why some people become neurotic, depressed, or anxious when they are older, and much of a psychoanalytic treatment is spent trying to put together a picture of what those interactions were and how some of them went awry. One of Freud's earliest ideas was that sexual abuse of young girls was repressed and then manifested later as "hysterical" paralysis. Although Freud later came to believe, probably wrongly, that the stories he had been told by his young female patients who could not move their arms or some other body parts were fantasies that never occurred, his later ideas still explain deviations from a notion of ideal early life experiences as the causes of adult emotional disorders.

Nowadays, it is fashionable in many intellectual circles to belittle Freud's and other psychoanalyst's ideas. The "Oedipus complex," for example, seems kind of ridiculous to many, including me: do little boys really want to have sex with their mothers and kill their rival fathers? Watching four-year-old boys play, it is hard to believe that such a thing is on their minds. For Freud, the successful resolution of the Oedipus complex involves a healthy switch from seeing the father as a rival to identifying with him. An abusive, weak, or absent father can impair this transition and lead to a situation in which the desire to kill the father and marry the mother becomes repressed and causes maladaptive feelings and behaviors in adulthood. There is also a version of this for girls, but it is clear that Freud felt more comfortable trying to figure out the early development of boys. Not only is there no evidence that any of this is really true, it is difficult to imagine how such evidence could ever be reliably collected. But that does not mean we are forced to dismiss other aspects of Freud's ideas. We will see if the basic idea—that early life experiences have long-lived effects of our emotions and behaviors—can be validated by scientific investigation.

## DOWNPLAYING LIFE EVENTS

This is, of course, a very abbreviated description of a very complicated theory, and psychoanalysts will be justified in criticizing the brevity of it as dismissive. But the important point for now is not so much trying to explain all the details of the Oedipus complex but to note that it, like many of Freud's theories, had throughout most of the twentieth century little in the way of supporting empirical evidence and increasingly seemed both absurd and even nefarious to many people. Not least of such people were those who were in the forefront of developing medications for psychiatric illness in the 1950s and 1960s and who developed a new psychiatric diagnostic system, referred to as *Diagnostic and Statistical Manual* (DSM-III), that was first published in 1980. As we discussed in the first two chapters of this book, these scientists and psychiatrists were determined to make psychiatry more "scientific," and they were generally appalled at the lack of experimental evidence demonstrating either that any psychoanalytic theories were true or that psychoanalytic treatments actually worked. The DSM-III was supposed to be, among other things, neutral about what caused psychiatric illness (with one important exception we will soon get to). Rather, its aim was simply to describe the "phenomenology" of the illnesses, what could actually be observed by a professional assessing a patient. People with depression feel sad, lose interest in things, can't sleep, don't eat, and the like; people with schizophrenia hear voices that aren't there, believe things that can't possibly be true, exhibit bizarre behaviors, speak without making sense, and so forth; people with alcoholism drink too much and because of it don't go to work, exhibit dangerous behaviors, have withdrawal symptoms if they stop drinking suddenly, and so forth. This is basically how the DSM system, even now in its fifth iteration (DSM-5), describes mental illness—as categories composed of symptom groups, the potential causes of which are, for the most part, not discussed. Because the empiricists believed there was no proof that adverse life events caused psychiatric illness, it was given no place in their new diagnostic system. Having a father die when you were six or a mother call you fat and ugly when you were nine was given no place in DSM-III.

There were other reasons for psychiatry to shun the role of life experiences in causing illness besides the belief that there is no proof of their causal effect. A black mark in the history of psychology and psychiatry was something called the "schizophrenogenic mother." As John Neill explains, at some time in the 1940s, a general notion developed among psychiatrists and psychologists that schizophrenia is the result of an aberrant relationship between a child and his or her mother.[2] This poor mother could not do anything right: if she was overprotective, that caused schizophrenia, but if, on the

---

[2] Neill J: Whatever became of the schizophrenogenic mother? *Am J Psychother* 1990;44:499–505.

other hand, she was rejecting, that also caused schizophrenia. There was never any evidence supporting this idea, and I don't recall ever hearing about a "schizophrenogenic father." The National Alliance for Mental Illness (NAMI), a wonderful nationwide support and advocacy organization, grew in part from parents of people with severe mental illness disputing the idea that they were solely responsible for their children's illnesses.

Blaming maternal behavior for schizophrenia without a shred of evidence was obviously a huge mistake that turned many people off to the whole notion that early life experiences play a role in the genesis of mental illness. And so, by around 1970, the importance of stressful life events in psychiatry seemed about to be overturned by a new view that psychiatric illness is the result of inborn or inherited abnormalities. Some early findings that in fact schizophrenia and other psychiatric illnesses are much more common among siblings and children of people who have these conditions than those who do not helped solidify this new approach to causation. "May the schizophrenogenic mother rest in peace," Neill wrote in 1990 (p. 504), and the search for the genetic mutations underlying mental illness was on. Even today, distinguished neuroscientists hold out hope that psychiatric illness will ultimately prove to be largely a consequence of genetic abnormalities. In an impassioned review article in the prestigious journal *Science*, for example, Daniel Geschwind and Jonathan Flint assert that "Genetic findings are set to illuminate the causes and to challenge the existing nosology of psychiatric conditions, some of which until recently were purported to have a non-biological etiology" (p. 1489).[3]

## THE EXCEPTION: PTSD

There was an important exception to the absence of all mention of causes in the DSM-III, the condition called posttraumatic stress disorder (PTSD). It was clear to the DSM-III framers from epidemiological evidence and their own observations that some people who sustained unusually horrid traumatic experiences did in fact develop a specific set of symptoms as a result. The idea was that anyone who survives a car crash in which there are fatalities, is tortured or raped, or witnesses comrades being killed during a combat mission, regardless of his or her prior psychiatric history or psychological make-up, is at heightened risk to develop a psychiatric disorder. In that sense, a *life trauma* is the direct *cause* of the illness. PTSD itself is characterized by a pattern of reliving the traumatic experience in one's mind, avoiding situations associated with the traumatic event, changes in mood and cognition, and experiencing disturbances in sleep, arousal, and control of the autonomic nervous system.

By now, we know quite a bit about PTSD, and it has captured the popular imagination. Whereas the original DSM-III committee thought of the traumas that qualified as causes of PTSD as severe, unusual, and life-threatening, it was quickly realized that not all of them are sadly so unusual. Rape, for example, causes PTSD and so does child

---

[3]  Geschwind DH, Flint J: Genetics and genomics of psychiatric disease. *Science* 2015;349:1489–1494.

abuse and even being a patient in the intensive care unit. How severe the trauma must be also turned out to be less clear: lawsuits in which someone who had been insulted or humiliated and claimed to have developed a function-impairing case of PTSD became all too common. If your boss criticizes you in front of your co-workers during a meeting you will likely feel embarrassed, even devastated, but is that a trauma sufficient to cause PTSD?

Even more complications arose as researchers began to seriously investigate the consequences of severe life trauma in the decades after DSM-III. They were surprised to find that, in some studies, PTSD is not the most common psychiatric illness that follows on the heels of experiencing a traumatic life event.[4] Depression and anxiety disorders are more common consequences in some cases. Furthermore, people with a history of psychiatric illnesses or even just a family history of psychiatric illnesses are more likely to develop PTSD after a traumatic event than those without such histories. Finally, the level of support from family, friends, clergy, and caregiving institutions modifies the likelihood of getting PTSD. After the 9/11 terrorist attacks, we expected to see a huge upsurge in PTSD cases. Even watching televised images of the planes crashing into the World Trade Center seemed capable of producing PTSD. But the rates were surprisingly lower than anticipated, and we think that was because of the outpouring of support people received following the attacks. Unlike rape victims, who are often ignored and even made to feel guilty, people who witnessed the 9/11 disaster were almost immediately embraced and provided with a variety of services and public recognition.

PTSD, then, is not simply a response to a terrible trauma but a psychiatric illness that is most likely to occur in someone with preexisting risk factors and a lack of strong social supports who experiences a severe traumatic event. At the same time, people exposed to traumatic events are likely to develop a wide variety of psychiatric symptoms and syndromes including but not limited to PTSD, such as depression, panic attacks, phobias, and substance abuse. Whereas in DSM-III in 1980 PTSD was included as one of the anxiety disorders, in DSM-5 in 2013 it is in a new category of "trauma- and stressor-related disorders,"[5] which includes a variety of outcomes for a person who has experienced a traumatic or stressful life event.

## DIFFERENT WAYS TO UNDERSTAND HOW TRAUMA WORKS

Let's look at the ways in which three different schools of thought might look at the effects of a traumatic life experience. Consider Andy, who has just bought a home for the first time. He is very proud of this acquisition, which is the result of his and his

[4] Bryant RA, O'Donnell ML, Creamer M, McFarlane AC, Clark CR, Silove D: The psychiatric sequelae of traumatic injury. *Am J Psychiatry* 2010;167:312–320.

[5] American Psychiatric Association: *Diagnostic and Statistical Manual of Mental Disorders*. 5th ed. (DSM-5). Arlington, VA, 2013.

wife's improved economic circumstances, but he is also nervous about handling all the new demands that home ownership seems to make.

One day, Andy is looking around his new basement and notices that some drains outside of the windows are clogged with leaves. He carefully positions a ladder to easily reach one of these windows, props the window open with a wood panel, and reaches outside to clear the leaves from the drain. Everything is going fine until he accidentally knocks the wood prop with his elbow, dislodging it. The window slams down on the back of his head, banging his nose into the concrete slab windowsill. Andy is thrown off the ladder to the basement floor; he is dazed and there is blood everywhere pouring from his nose. He screams for his wife who rushes him to the local emergency department, where a CAT scan of his head shows no damage. The gash in his nose requires multiple stitches by a plastic surgeon. The pain is substantial. Andy lies on the gurney in the emergency department wondering to himself why all of this happened.[6]

Fortunately, Andy makes a complete recovery—there is only a tiny scar on his nose and no other signs of an injury. A few weeks, later he contemplates returning to his basement to continue clearing the drains, but as he thinks about this he becomes noticeably tremulous and senses his heart racing. It isn't quite as severe as a full-blown panic attack, but bad enough to make him avoid going into the basement at all. He starts to think of himself as a klutz and wonders if he should have bought a house at all. Little by little, he begins to worry that the house is too expensive, that he will never be able to pay for the mortgage, and that he is really a complete failure. He imagines his wife leaving him for a more successful man. Andy is now depressed and anxious around the clock.

Let's first consider what a psychopharmacologist, a specialist in treating psychiatric disorders with medication, would say about Andy's situation. He meets all the criteria for both a major depressive episode and for generalized anxiety disorder (GAD). It turns out that Andy has always been a relatively anxious person and has had two other episodes of depression in his life. The causes of these disorders at this point is unimportant to the psychopharmacologist; an antidepressant is prescribed that increases the levels of an important chemical in the brain, the neurotransmitter serotonin. Four weeks later, Andy feels much better, although he is bothered by some adverse side effects of the drug. He stays on the drug for six more months, during which time he is able to clean all the drains outside the basement windows.

Next, we consider the point of view of a therapist who specializes in cognitive behavioral therapy (CBT). The therapist sees that Andy is burdening himself with guilty and catastrophic thoughts. Andy blames himself for what was obviously a freak accident and then generalizes what happened to every situation in his life. Not only does he think it was his fault that the wooden prop got knocked aside and that this makes him a klutz, but that he is similarly deficient in every other activity of life. The CBT therapist learns that Andy has always tended to be hard on himself and to feeling

---

[6] A version of this story actually happened to me.

excessively guilty. Over the course of the next three months, the CBT therapist works with Andy to help him identify these maladaptive thoughts and to examine them by introducing rational assessments and logical counterarguments. The therapist also has him gradually undertake tasks that he is avoiding. The therapy is successful, and Andy's depression and anxiety remit. He does not need any further treatment, but he does clean out those drains.

Finally, how would a psychoanalytic therapist see things? In taking his history, the analyst learns that Andy's father was extremely handy at all kinds of home repairs. He was also an angry and remote man who often criticized Andy and belittled him. Unconsciously, buying the house feels to Andy like an act of defiance against his father, whom Andy had internalized as a harsh and critical voice telling him he was no good at mechanical chores. This defiance aroused fears of reprisal in Andy's unconscious. Andy's unconscious seeks a solution to this anxiety-provoking conflict between wanting to defy his father and fearing him, and knocking the wooden prop away provides one. Andy has neurotically resolved the conflict by withdrawing from the battle with his father and essentially adopting his father's harsh appraisal of him. Over the course of several years, Andy works out his fear of his father and his tendency to see himself as inadequate. Slowly, he gains confidence in himself and not only cleans the drains but fixes many other things in the house, becoming quite a handyman.

These three scenarios obviously differ substantially in approach, including the length of time it takes for Andy to feel better. We will defer the discussion about which approach is "better" or "best" for now; all three approaches are successful in relieving Andy's depression and anxiety and improving his self-image. The important thing to note is that only the psychoanalyst uses Andy's life experiences preceding his traumatic injury as a critical part of the treatment. Although both the psychoanalyst and the CBT therapist note that Andy has a history of depression and worry, these do not alter the treatment approach. Andy's past, on the other hand, is the preoccupation of the psychoanalytic treatment.

Regardless of which approach we prefer for treating Andy, our research tells us that his past is indeed highly relevant to the way he handles the drain incident. Someone who has a history of anxiety and depression is more likely to experience psychiatric symptoms after a traumatic injury. Today, it is no longer disputed that early life experiences have profound effects on brain function, behavior, and the propensity to develop psychiatric illnesses. Early life experiences can have both positive and negative effects on us. A brain imaging study recently showed, for example, that children aged three to five years who are often read to at home more readily activate a region in the brain that is critical for the development of literacy skills when they listen to stories.[7] Thus, there is a direct relationship between a positive early life experience and a pattern of brain function that may explain why being read to as a child leads to a life-long love of reading and improved reading skills.

[7] Hutton JS, Horowitz-Kraus T, Mendelsohn AL, DeWitt T, Holland SK, et al.: Home reading environment and brain activation in preschool children listening to stories. *Pediatrics* 2015;136:466–478.

On the other side of the life experience spectrum, we now know that early traumatic and stressful life experiences are involved in almost every psychiatric illness. Victims of child abuse and other severe forms of early life adversity are more likely to develop a wide range of problems as adults, including depression, anxiety disorders, eating disorders, and substance abuse.[8] Bipolar disorder (formerly called manic-depressive disorder) is diagnosed in people who have extreme mood swings and suffer from periods of extreme depression that alternate with periods of exhilaration called *mania*. The condition almost always requires medications like lithium, which work well to prevent both the ups and the downs; consequently, it is often thought to be a purely "biological" disorder. Nevertheless, studies show that patients with bipolar disorder have higher rates of experiencing stressful life events before the first signs of the illness appear than do people without bipolar disorder.[9]

Even schizophrenia, which is among the most "genetic" of psychiatric illnesses, is associated with a high rate of environmental exposures and adverse life experiences. My colleague at Columbia University, Ezra Susser, for example, showed that exposure to malnutrition during fetal life increases the risk for developing schizophrenia many years after birth.[10] He and others also showed that when a pregnant woman contracts certain viral infections, like influenza, her offspring have increased risk of developing schizophrenia.[11] Growing up in poverty is also associated with an increased risk for schizophrenia. Adults with psychotic illnesses like schizophrenia are more likely to have experienced severe physical abuse before the age of 12.[12] In fact, a person who experiences a childhood trauma is more than seven times more likely to develop a psychotic illness than his or her own sibling who did not experience a childhood trauma.[13]

The recognition that traumatic events are related to a variety of psychiatric symptoms and syndromes, not just PTSD, obviously reopens the whole issue of if and how what we experience during life plays a causal role in producing psychiatric illness. The idea that a single inherited genetic mutation is the exclusive cause of depression, schizophrenia, or any other psychiatric disorder seems now less likely. These conditions suddenly appear more like cigarette smokers who develop lung cancer and

[8]  Heim C, Shugart M, Craighead WE, Nemeroff CB: Neurobiological and psychiatric consequences of child abuse and neglect. *Dev Psychobiol* 2010;52:671–690.

[9]  Pan L, Goldstein TR, Rooks BT, et al.: The relationship between stressful life events and axis I diagnoses among adolescent offspring of probands with bipolar and non-bipolar psychiatric disorder and healthy controls: the Pittsburgh Bipolar Offspring Study (BIOS). *J Clin Psychiatry* 2017; Epub ahead of print

[10]  Susser E, Neugebauer R, Hoek HSW, Brown AS, Lin S, Labovitz D, Gorman JM: Schizophrenia after prenatal famine. Further evidence. *Arch Gen Psychiatry* 1998;53:25–31.

[11]  Brown AS: Prenatal infection as a risk factor for schizophrenia. *Schizophr Bull* 2006;32:200–203.

[12]  Fisher HL, Jones, PB, Fearon P, et al.: The varying impact of type, timing and frequency of exposure to childhood adversity on its association with adult psychotic disorder. *Psychol Med* 2010;40:1967–1978.

[13]  Barrigon ML, Diaz FJ, Gurpegui M, et al.: Childhood trauma as a risk factor for psychosis: a sib-pair study. *J Psychiatric Research* 2015;70:130–136.

obese people who develop diabetes: all caused by the complex intertwining of multiple factors that include genetics, behavior, and experience.

At first glance, the resurgence of interest in the role of experience in mood, emotion, and behavior might seem to support the idea of a mysterious "mind" that operates above and beyond what we can explain by examining the physical brain. The opponents of the purely psychopharmacological view were correct in asserting that a genetically determined tendency to have too much of this or that neurotransmitter in the brain could not possibly explain why some people get depressed after breaking up with a girlfriend, others start to smoke and consume too much alcohol, and still others—the majority—move on to finding a new girlfriend. The view that neuroscience limits the richness of human experience gains justifiable impetus if things are constructed so narrowly.

But this notion that neuroscience is just about reducing humans to neurotransmitters is itself a reductionistic view of neuroscience. While psychiatry and psychology began to reconsider the importance of life experiences—this time without, we hope, maligning mothers—basic neuroscientists started to show that experiences have some very complex but often predictable effects on the brain at many levels, from the molecular (how genes are expressed), to the cellular (how neurons extend and retract projections called *dendrites*), to the system and structural (how regions of the brain are connected to each other). For the remainder of this chapter, we will focus mostly on the molecular level and, in particular, on the field of epigenetics, which helps determine how genes are expressed. But first, it is important to describe some of the laboratory work that shows how experience changes the brain, and, to do this, I will highlight two laboratories, those of Michael Meaney at McGill University and Leonard Rosenblum and Jeremy Coplan at SUNY Brooklyn.

## HOW YOUR MOTHER TREATS YOU CHANGES YOUR BRAIN

As this will be the first time in this book that I discuss research involving rats, I want to make a few introductory comments about animal research in the behavioral sciences. First, laboratory rats are not like those that we associate with filth and disease. They are bred in and for laboratory use, are quite friendly, and are very smart. I have studied this form of work, called *preclinical* or *basic neuroscience*, and collaborated with many scientists who do it, but I never actually performed experiments on rats or any other animals myself. That does not, however, remove the burden on me of considering the ethics of animal research. I have thought about this a great deal and, in the end, remain comfortable with laboratory research involving animals when they are treated in accordance with the strict animal welfare and ethics regulations that now exist and when that work is done in the service of learning things of importance to furthering human health.

Another aspect about animal research that must be mentioned is that, although I am proud to be an involved father and grandfather myself and take the paternal role seriously, when discussing rodents and most other species, the only player of importance is the mother; rat fathers are not involved in caring for their offspring, and, therefore, everything we can say about the role of early nurturance in a rat's life involves only its relationship with mom. In Chapter 7, we will see a fascinating exception to this rule that only mothers count in rearing young nonhuman animals, but that is indeed a rare exception.

Rat mothers are very attentive to their offspring but show remarkable individual differences in just how attentive. Michael Meaney and his colleagues noticed, for example, that some rat mothers lick and groom (LG behavior) their infants more than others and, on that basis, separated them into two groups, high LG (lick and groom their infants a lot) and low LG (lick and groom less). When the offspring of high LG mothers become adults, they are less fearful than offspring of low LG mothers. Moreover, the high LG offspring have lower activity of a hormonal system that is activated by stress and danger, called the *hypothalamic-pituitary-adrenal* (HPA) axis (see Figure 3.1), throughout their adult lives. Humans have this hormone system,

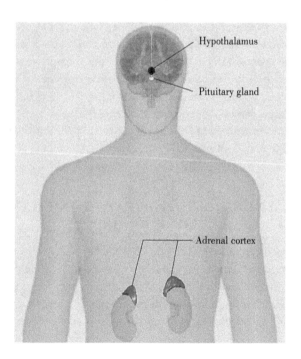

**Figure 3.1** The hypothalamic-pituitary-adrenal (HPA) axis. The hypothalamus releases corticotropin releasing hormone (CRH), which causes the release of corticotropin by the pituitary gland, which in turn causes the release of cortisol by the adrenal gland. Cortisol circulates back up to the brain where it inhibits further release of CRH and corticotropin in what is called a negative feedback loop.

From BodyParts3D/Anatomography, https://upload.wikimedia.org/wikipedia/commons/thumb/c/c5/HPA-axis_-_anterior_view_%28with_text%29.svg/562px-HPA-axis_-_anterior_view_%28with_text%29.svg.png too; it starts with the release of a hormone called *corticotropin releasing hormone* (CRH) in two different places in the brain. The first is the hippocampus, a brain region that is critical for learning and memory. The second is the hypothalamus, a structure that is critical for the control of appetite, sleep, and many other vital biological functions.

CRH is released in the hippocampus whenever an animal is stressed and plays an important role throughout the brain in sustaining fear and anxiety. CRH released by the hypothalamus leads directly to the release of a hormone called *corticotropin* (or ACTH) by the pituitary gland, which in turns leads to the release of the hormone *cortisol* by the adrenal gland, which is located just above the kidneys. When stressful events in rats and humans activate the HPA axis, there is an increased release of all three hormones: CRH, corticotropin, and cortisol. But the less fearful adult rats whose mothers were especially nurturing when they were pups show less HPA activation when confronted with a stressor. Perhaps most remarkably, female rat pups reared by high LG mothers themselves become high LG mothers, whereas offspring of low LG mothers become low LG mothers when adults. The children of high LG daughters—the grandchildren of the first generation—now also show reduced fear and HPA axis responses throughout their lives. Thus, nurturing style not only affects offspring throughout life but is also passed on to a third generation.[14]

Of course, these differences could all be accounted for by a difference in the structure, or nucleotide base sequence, of a gene. Perhaps there is a gene that controls nurturing behavior, fearfulness, and HPA axis activity. Then the offspring of low LG and of high LG mothers might inherit two different versions of that gene, which would explain all the differences. Different versions of the same gene are called *alleles* and involve a structural difference; that is, an inherited difference in one or more nucleotide bases.

To show that they are not a product of inborn genetic (allelic) variation but really the result of the degree of maternal nurturing during infancy, Meaney and his team performed two elegant experiments (Figure 3.2).[15] It is known that briefly separating a rat pup from its mother during the first seven days of life, handling it by humans, and then reuniting it with its mother causes the mother to increase her licking and grooming of the pup. Apparently, the mother smells the scent of human hands on her pup, dislikes it, and vigorously tries to lick it away. Handling pups born to low LG mothers makes the mothers behave as if they were high LG mothers and results in offspring that grow up as if they had been born to high LG mothers—the extra licking and grooming makes them less fearful and have less HPA axis activity throughout their lives. It is, this, an experience that occurs after birth—being vigorously licked—that

[14] Weaver ICG, Cervoni N, Champagne FA, DeAlessio AC, Sharma S, Seckl JR, Dymov S, Szyf M, Meaney MJ: Epigenetic programming by maternal behavior. *Nat Neurosci* 2004;7:847854.
[15] Francis D, Diorio J, Liu D, Meaney MJ: Nongenomic transmission across generations of maternal behavior and stress responses in the rat. *Science* 1999;286:1155–1159.

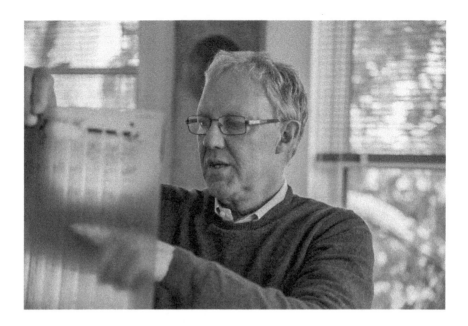

**Figure 3.2** Neuroscientist Michael Meaney of McGill University is among the first to show in laboratory animals that early life experience alters the way genes are expressed in the brain, producing behaviors that are present throughout the animal's life.

Copyright, Jacobs Foundation, https://www.mcgill.ca/newsroom/files/newsroom/channels/image/michaelmeaney.png

alters the infant rat pup's lifelong behavior. Clearly, this result is due entirely to the effect of nurturing rather than to any genetic predisposition.

Next, the Meaney group performed a cross-fostering experiment in which offspring of naturally high LG mother were placed with low LG mothers immediately after birth and vice versa with offspring of low LG mothers. The long-term behavior and HPA axis status turns out to depend entirely on which kind of mother the infant was reared by and not which kind it was born to—a rat born to a low LG mother but reared by a high LG mother shows the same low fearful, low HPA axis activity status as if it had been born to that high LG mother. When the female rats became adults, they themselves are high LG mothers even though their own biological mothers had been low LG. Together, these studies show that the differences in behavior and biochemistry between the two groups of rats is due to the relationship they have with their mothers during infancy, not to a gene. On a molecular level, Meaney and his colleagues showed that the extra licking and grooming provided by high LG mothers changes gene expression in the brains of their infants. We will come back to this and to its implications for humans shortly.

Meaney is not the only scientist who has shown that early life experiences change the life-long behaviors of rodents, but I have always admired his careful, systematic approach to understanding how this works, from behavioral observations down to molecular studies. It is a lovely thing to think of rat mothers taking such good care of their pups, to the point that their offspring are rendered more adaptive and less afraid throughout their lives. To those who say that neuroscience reduces emotion and behavior to mere chemicals, I counter that it takes nothing away from this warm sentiment to know that it is a function of how genes in the brain are working. Understanding the biology of a complex behavior makes it no less compelling.

## ANXIOUS MOMS MAKE ANXIOUS CHILDREN

Research like this from Michael Meaney's lab is convincing that maternal nurturing behavior during infancy can have long-lived effects on the offspring, at least among rodents. With this in mind, I became fascinated by the work of Leonard Rosenblum, who established a laboratory at the State University of New York (SUNY), Downstate, in Brooklyn in 1961, composed of a colony of a type of monkey called the bonnet macaque *(Macaca radiata)*. After training with Harry Harlow at the University of Wisconsin, Len developed a much more subtle, humane, and ecologically realistic method of studying the effects of maternal stress on offspring behavior. Bonnet macaque mothers turn out to be highly nurturing individuals who become anxious whenever they must be separated from their newborn infants to search for food (Figure 3.3). In the Downstate colony, Len randomized mothers of newborn macaques to one of three foraging conditions: in a low foraging demand condition (LFD), food is always presented to the mother directly in front of her. In the high foraging demand condition (HFD), the mother must always dig through wood chips to find her food. Finally, in the variable foraging demand (VFD) condition, the food is sometimes put in front of mother and sometimes she needs to root through the wood chips or perform a task to obtain it, so that she is never certain how much work she must do to

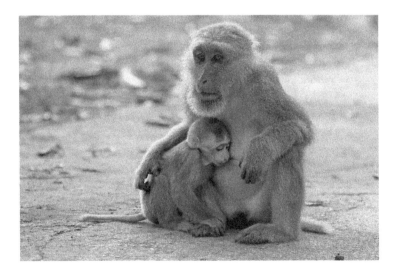

**Figure 3.3** Bonnet macaque mothers are very attentive to and nurturing of their babies. Shutterstock.

secure her daily food ration. The LFD and HFD conditions are, therefore, predictable, whereas the VFD condition is not.[16]

The infants do not seem to care whether their mothers are in the LFD, HFD, or VFD conditions. They can watch their mothers as they root around for food, and they gain weight at the same rate regardless of foraging condition. The mothers do not seem to mind either the LFD or HFD conditions; knowing the conditions under which food is available seems important to them. But they become markedly anxious with the uncertainty of the VFD condition. This condition does not mimic the way animals are fed in laboratories and zoos, which is usually on a regular schedule with food easily available, as in the LFD condition. Nor does it resemble what animals confront in the wild, where they know they must work to get their meals, as in the HFD condition. The introduction of uncertainty to the amount of work needed to secure food with the VFD condition is disorienting for the mother macaques.

The differences in foraging demand conditions begin when the infants are about 17 weeks old and last 12 weeks, at which time the infants are weaned from their mothers. Then all the animals are raised in identical fashion and live their lives together in the colony. To the casual observer, the monkeys raised under the LFD, HFD, and VFD conditions seem to behave identically and normally. They certainly do not resemble the monkeys mentioned in Chapter 2 who were raised by Harry Harlow in complete isolation from their mothers.

But Len and his colleagues made some more penetrating observations: the offspring of mothers who were exposed to the uncertainty of the VFD condition show lower levels of social play and exploration than those whose mothers had been exposed to the two predictable foraging conditions. Any time novelty is introduced into the colony, such as a new toy or a new monkey, the monkeys raised during infancy under the VFD condition become fearful and withdrawn. They do not interact with the new toy or monkey and become visibly distressed. Most important, this situation continues throughout the animals' lifetime, even though the whole foraging condition occupied only a 12-week period of their lives, and they were never physically separated from their mothers.

This effect on life-long behavior that results from varying the mother's experience during her offspring's infancy is clearly not the result of anything inherited. The mothers are all from the same species and are randomized to the three different foraging conditions, so that nothing can account for the differences in offspring behavior other than the foraging conditions experienced by their mothers. In some way, the anxiety provoked in the mother by unpredictable foraging demand seems to result in a form of emotional deprivation of the infant that causes permanent changes in its behavior.

I was fascinated by this work and asked Len Rosenblum if I could meet with him and hear more about it. I first visited his lab at Downstate in the late 1980s and met one of the SUNY Downstate Department of Psychiatry's chief residents, Jeremy Coplan,

---

[16] Rosenblum LA, Paully GS: The effects of varying environmental demands on maternal and infant behavior. *Child Dev* 1984;55:305–314.

who had volunteered to work with Len in his lab. Jeremy struck me immediately as one of the brightest residents I had ever met, and I invited him to do a research fellowship with me at Columbia University after he graduated from his residency. I also asked him whether it would be possible to obtain any biological specimens from the monkeys. I was interested to learn whether the concentrations of the hormones in the HPA axis differed between adult monkeys reared in the VFD condition from those reared in the LFD and HFD conditions.

This began a more than two-decade-long collaboration between Len, Jeremy, and myself that remains one of the most satisfying experiences of my research career. Jeremy performed spinal taps, also called lumbar punctures, on the offspring of the foraging experiment, who were now young adult monkeys, and obtained samples of cerebrospinal fluid (CSF), the fluid that bathes the brain. Obtaining CSF samples may give us a better picture of what is happening in the brain than samples in blood do because the blood–brain barrier prevents many of the neurotransmitters and hormones that are active in the brain from getting into the peripheral circulation. Charles Nemeroff, then at Emory University and an expert on the HPA axis response to stress, measured the levels of CRH, the hormone released by the brain that controls the rest of the HPA axis and is known to increase during acute stress and to be elevated in some human patients with depression. We hypothesized that CRH levels would be higher in VFD than HFD and LFD animals, and we turned out to be correct.[17]

Essentially, we had replicated Michael Meaney's experiments, only this time in a nonhuman primate instead of a rodent. Adult bonnet macaque monkeys whose mothers were exposed to a VFD condition years earlier maintained a biological signature of their early life experience in the form of elevated CRH levels in their spinal fluid. Jeremy, Len, and I, along with many other colleagues, went on to perform several studies examining the long-term effects of VFD rearing. We obtained a grant from the National Institute of Mental Health (NIMH) to transport the monkeys from Brooklyn to Mount Sinai Hospital, where I moved from Columbia in 2002, and we put them into the magnetic resonance imaging (MRI) suite (at night only, when there were no humans having MRI scans). We employed several variations on standard MRI scanning that will be described in more detail in Chapter 5 and found changes in the VFD-reared adult monkeys compared to the LFD-reared animals in brain chemistry using magnetic resonance spectroscopy (MRS)[18] and in the strength of connections

[17] Coplan JD, Andres MW, Rosenblum LA, Owens MJ, Friedman S, Gorman JM, Nemeroff CB: Persistent elevation of cerebrospinal fluid concentrations of corticotropin-releasing factor in adult nonhuman primates exposed to early-life stressors: Implications for the pathophysiology of mood and anxiety disorders. *Proc Natl Acad Sci USA* 1996;93:1619–1623.; Coplan JD, Smith El, Altemus M, Scharf BA, Owens MJ, Nemeroff CB, Gorman JM, Rosenblum LA: Variable foraging demand rearing: sustained elevation in cisternal cerebrospinal fluid corticotropin-releasing factor concentrations in adult primates. *Biol Psychiatry* 2001;50:200–204.

[18] Matthew SJ, Shungu DC, Mao X, Smith El, Perera GM, Kegeles LS, Perera T, Lisanby SH, Rosenblum LA, Gorman JM, Coplan JD: A magnetic resonance spectroscopic imaging study of adult nonhuman primates exposed to early-life stressors. *Biol Psychiatry* 2003;54:727–735.

between regions in the brain using diffusion tensor imaging (DTI).[19] We also found that the VFD animals had enlargement of a structure in the brain tied closely with fear and anxiety, the amygdala.[20]

I want to stress again that although I have highlighted the work of two labs, Michael Meaney's and that of Leonard Rosenblum and Jeremy Coplan, the finding that early life adversity changes behavior and biology for a lifetime is now well-established in the neuroscience laboratory. We can now return to Michael Meaney's laboratory for a glimpse at how this process works at the molecular level of DNA.

## CHANGING THE WAY GENES ARE EXPRESSED

We inherit one-half of our genes from our mothers and one-half from our fathers. Those genes, as we explained in Chapter 3, are strands of DNA that contain the genetic code, a sequence of instructions that is written in four letters, G, C, T, and A, each corresponding to one of four types of molecules called *nucleotide bases*. That sequence of bases does not change, with a few exceptions, during our lifetimes. So, for the most part, the genes we are born with are the genes we will always have.

But if that were the end of the story then we would have trouble explaining several important biological facts. First, humans only have about 20,000 genes, but we have millions of proteins. Second, some proteins are present at different times of the day and month and even at completely different times in our lives. Third, the genetic code is the same in every cell in our bodies, but liver cells don't make thyroid hormone, skin cells don't pump and beat, and bone cells cannot remember names. Each type of cell looks different and makes different proteins. Fourth, identical or monozygotic twins are never exactly identical even though they share all the same genes.

The reason for all this diversity rests with gene expression: some genes are never expressed, some expressed at different times, and some to different degrees at different times. *Epigenetics* is the process behind gene regulation, determining how genes are switched on and off without changing the underlying sequence of nucleotide bases, the genetic code.

To understand how epigenetic control of gene expression works, it is important to realize that the familiar DNA double helix is not exactly how things look inside a neuron's or any other cell's nucleus. First, the double helix is wound around proteins called *histones*, forming something that looks like pearls on a string. Then the DNA-histone complex assembles itself into structures with various 3-D shapes, called

---

[19] Coplan JD, Abdallah CG, Tang CY, Matthew ASJ, Martinez J, Hof PR, Smith EL, Dwork AJ, Perera TD, Pantol G, Carpenter D, Rosenblum LA, Shungu DC, Gelernter J, Kaffman A, Jackowski A, Kaufman J, Gorman JM: The role of early life stress in development of the anterior limb of the internal capsule in nonhuman primates. *Neuroscience Neurosci Lett* 2010;480:93–96.

[20] Coplan JD, Fathy HM, Jackowski Ap, Tang CY, Perera TD, Mathew SJ, Martinez J, Abdallah Cg, Dwork AJ, Pantol G, Carpenter D, Gorman JM, Nemeroff CB, Owens MJ, Kaffman A, Kaufman J: Early life stress and macaque amygdala hypertrophy: preliminary evidence for a role for the serotonin transporter gene. *Front Behav Neurosci* 2014;8:342.

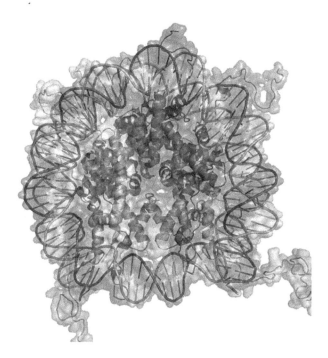

**Figure 3.4** Chromatin is the complex, shown here, of DNA and the proteins called histones. The double helical DNA wraps around the histone proteins, and then the whole assembly curls around in ball-like structures that sequester the DNA. One function of epigenetic factors is to modify the chromatin structure so that the DNA is more accessible to polymerase enzymes that transcribe it to messenger RNA.

Wikipedia.

*chromatin* (see Figure 3.4). The DNA itself is often not on the surface of the chromatin assembly, but hidden by histones. This makes it difficult for the enzymes called *polymerases,* which transcribe the DNA into messenger RNA (mRNA), to reach the DNA itself. And if the DNA is not transcribed to mRNA, the process that leads to protein formation is blocked.

## HOW EPIGENETIC REGULATION WORKS

There are three main ways that the DNA on genes can be activated, repressed, or silenced without altering the base sequence: *DNA methylation, histone modification,* and *RNA interference.* Although this is not an exhaustive list of all the possible regulatory mechanisms, a description of these three will suffice to explain why gene expression regulation is so important to understanding the effects of life events on brain function.

A methyl group is made of a carbon atom attached to three hydrogen atoms $(CH_3)$. Gene expression regulation by DNA methylation occurs when methyl groups attach to one of the four DNA bases, cytosine (C), on DNA. This is accomplished by enzymes called *methyl transferases,* and it alters the way a gene is read by the polymerase enzymes responsible for transcription to mRNA. Usually, but not always, DNA methylation results in a decrease or even silencing of a gene's activity. Methyl groups tend to be very stably attached to DNA and difficult to dislodge. Therefore, when a cell divides, both copies of DNA that go into the two new (called "daughter") cells will have the same pattern of DNA methylation as the parent cell. If a pregnant animal experiences an event that causes a methyl group to attach to a specific gene, the methyl groups will also attach to the genes in the cells of the developing fetus. This means that the effects on gene expression experienced by a pregnant mother can be "passed" on to her offspring. DNA methylation is already known to be involved in some human disease. For example, in certain forms of cancer, there are too few methyl groups on the DNA of the malignant cells. This is called *hypomethylation,* and because it removes a source of control over gene expression, it results in uncontrolled activity and division of the cancerous cells.

The second main mechanism of gene expression regulation is histone modification. Histone proteins can be modified in several ways, mostly by having methyl or acetyl groups bind to them. An acetyl group is made of two carbon atoms, three hydrogen atoms, and one oxygen atom $(CH_3CO)$. In Figure 3.5, we see acetyl groups binding to

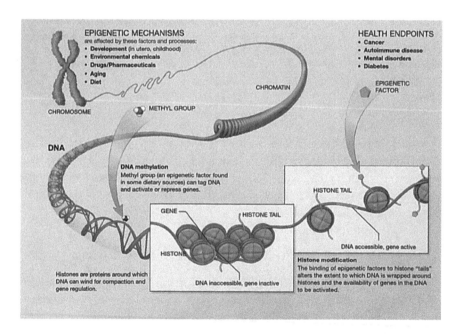

**Figure 3.5** An example of how epigenetics works. DNA is wound around proteins called histones that have tails, to which various epigenetic factors can bind. Methyl and acetyl groups are examples of such epigenetic factors. Here, acetyl groups (the round circles with crosses in the inset) are attaching to histone tails and thereby changing the way the gene can be transcribed and expressed. Also shown is a methyl group attaching directly to DNA.

National Institutes of Health, http://commonfund.nih.gov/epigenomics/figure.aspx

the "tails" of histone proteins. Acetyl groups bind specifically to only one amino acid on the histone protein, lysine. When acetyl groups bind to lysine on histone protein tails, it changes the way the DNA is wound around the histone. This process is also called *chromatin remodeling* because it alters its three-dimensional structure. Among other things, this can result in the DNA itself moving to the surface of the chromatin assembly, making it more easily accessed by the polymerase enzymes, thus increasing transcription. Hence, histone acetylation usually has the opposite effect on gene expression from DNA methylation—it increases gene expression. There are also enzymes called *histone deacetylases* (HDAC), that remove acetyl groups from histones, reversing this process, which therefore slows down gene expression, and drugs that block those enzymes, called *histone deacetylase inhibitors* (or HDAC inhibitors), that keep the acetyl groups bound to histones. This keeps the increase in gene expression caused by histone acetylation going. Acetylation of histones tends to be less stable than DNA methylation, making it easier to dislodge the acetyl group by HDAC enzymes and turn the gene's expression back down. HDAC inhibitors block this process, thus stabilizing chromatin remodeling and maintaining the switched-on gene expression state. A great deal of research is now being conducted to see if drugs based on HDAC inhibitors could be used to increase the expression of genes that are downregulated in certain diseases.

Finally, we have RNA interference. As we discussed in Chapter 2, most of our DNA is transcribed into RNA molecules that never migrate out of the nucleus to engineer protein synthesis. In fact, only about 2% of our DNA actually codes for proteins. The RNA molecules that are never translated into proteins are called *noncoding RNAs* and, the process by which these molecules regulate gene expression is called RNA interference. One type of noncoding RNAs are very small molecules, and these small RNAs bind to mRNA molecules that do code for proteins and alter the way these coding mRNAs are translated into protein. This is called "post-transcriptional" gene expression regulation. Other, longer noncoding RNAs can bind directly to DNA and alter expression.

Many, many things affect epigenetic regulation of gene expression, including drugs, the food we eat, the air we breathe, aging, exercise, and, of course, life's experiences. Epigenetics is one of the most active fields in science now. For someone like me who went to college in the early 1970s, this is exotic stuff. Almost nothing was known back then about gene regulation, and it was thought that there was one gene for every protein. Clearly, the process of gene expression is very complicated—and getting more complicated by the hour.

During cell division, there is a very small chance that, by mistake, a change that has functional significance is made in the DNA base sequence. But we've already noted that neurons in the brain and spinal cord do not divide during our lifetimes the way most other cells do. Therefore, there is almost no chance for them to undergo any changes in DNA base sequence. But gene expression in the brain is vigorously regulated—all kinds of experiences and exposures change levels of gene expression in the brain by DNA methylation, histone modification, RNA silencing, and many other phenomena.

As we have seen, Michael Meaney's high LG mothers have offspring that are less fearful and have less active HPA axes than offspring of low LG mothers. In general, overactivity of any part of the HPA axis is an indicator that an animal or human is in a state of stress or some other uncomfortable mental state like depression. Remember that the HPA axis involves three hormones (see Figure 3.1), increases in any one of which is a sign of stress: CRH, which is released in the brain by two regions, the hypothalamus and the hippocampus; CRH released from the hypothalamus stimulates the release of the second HPA axis hormone, *corticotropin* from the pituitary gland; and corticotropin in turn stimulates the release of *cortisol* from the adrenal gland. Cortisol, a member of a group of compounds called *glucocorticoids*, then travels into the brain and binds to receptors that sense that there is enough cortisol already floating around in the circulation. The effect of cortisol binding to glucocorticoid receptors in the hippocampus and hypothalamus is to turn down the further release of CRH, thus turning down the whole system. Less cortisol is then released by the adrenal gland. This process is called "negative feedback" and is important for many hormonal systems. In the case of CRH it depends on how many glucocorticoid receptors (GR) there are in the brain, which in turn depends on the activity of the gene that codes for the GR. The more GRs there are, the more opportunity cortisol has to bind to them and turn off CRH production.

The Meaney group found that the gene for GR in the hippocampus of high LG mothers has fewer methyl groups on its DNA than the gene for the GR in the brains of low LG mothers. Here it gets a bit complicated, so read the next few sentences slowly and you will catch on. The differences in methylation Meaney found are in the promoter region of the GR gene, a portion of a gene where transcription of mRNA begins. Methyl groups turn down the promoter region, thus turning down the whole gene. Fewer methyl groups bound to the DNA in the promoter region of the gene for GRs means a more active gene and therefore more GR receptors in the high LG mothers' brains than the low LG mothers' brains. The result of this is that when cortisol goes into the brain, it finds more GR receptors to bind to in the high LG mother than in the low LG mother, leading to more robust negative feedback and more vigorous turning down of the release of CRH and the whole HPA axis. When a high LG mother or her offspring are stressed, the cortisol that is released from the adrenal gland more rapidly turns off CRH production in the brain, thus stopping the stress response more quickly. Is it possible that licking and grooming leads to a decrease in GR gene promoter region methylation?

Indeed, that is what Meaney and other scientist believe is the case. When a rat pup born to a low LG mother is taken from the litter and placed with a high LG mother, it grows up to behave just as if it had been born to the high LG mother, with less fear and lower HPA axis activity. And it also has less methylation in the GR gene promoter region. The experience of being licked and groomed a lot does not change the rat pup's genetic code, but it does seem to change how methyl groups regulate the activity of stress-producing hormones in the brain like CRH.

Nessa Carey, in her book *The Epigenetics Revolution*, notes that not all scientists are comfortable with Meaney's methylation hypotheses.[21] She points out that it isn't that the number of methyl groups bound to DNA in the GR promoter regions of

---

[21] Carey N: *The Epigenetics Revolution*. New York, Columbia University Press, 2013.

infant rats goes up because they aren't licked enough by low LG mothers. "It's because DNA methylation has gone *down* in the ones that were licked and groomed the most" (p. 252). But, as we already noted, DNA methylation is very stable, and no one understands how a stimulus like licking and grooming would work to remove methyl groups from DNA binding sites. More recent research has provided some possible answers to this conundrum, and it is widely believed that changes in DNA methylation are indeed responsible for many of the differences observed in the offspring of high and low LG rat mothers.

DNA methylation is one of the three main mechanisms for epigenetic control of gene expression; the other two also appear to affect life-long behaviors. Levels of histone acetylation, for example, play a role in determining whether rodents exhibit depressed-like behaviors when subjected to social defeat stress[22] and maintain chronic fear behaviors.[23] Conversely, environmental enrichment increases histone acetylation in rats—even aging rats—and improves overall brain function and learning ability.[24] Nessa Carey notes that "increased acetylation levels in the brain seem to be consistently associated with improved memory" (p. 258). Eric Nestler and colleagues at the Mount Sinai School of Medicine in New York City, in a series of elegant experiments, have shown that laboratory animals exposed to cocaine have long-lasting increases in histone acetylation of several genes expressed in the brain.[25] He has developed a model of substance abuse that explains how such changes in gene expression can explain the development of craving for abused substances.

RNA interference has similarly been associated with the link between life events and behavior. Stress-related changes in the binding of a long noncoding RNA molecule to a gene in the prefrontal cortex of mice, for example, determines the level of fear behaviors the animals exhibit.[26] Interestingly, the specific gene in this case has been related to risk for schizophrenia in humans.

Much of the animal research on epigenetics involves the early relationships between mothers and their infants, but there is also evidence that noncoding RNA regulation of gene expression that involves fathers also occurs. Tracy Bale and her colleagues at the University of Pennsylvania have shown that stressed male mice have an increase

[22] Golden SA, Christoffel DJ, Heshmati MH, et al.: Epigenetic regulation of RAC1 induces synaptic remodeling in stress disorders and depression. *Nature Medicine* 2013;19:337–344.

[23] Tran L, Schulkin J, Ligon CO, Meerveld BG-V: Epigenetic modulation of chronic anxiety and pain by histone deacetylation. *Mol Psychiatr* 2015;20:1219–1231.

[24] Neidl R, Schneider A, Bousiges O, et al.: Late-life environmental enrichment induces acetylation events and nuclear factor kB-dependent regulations in the hippocampus of aged rats showing improved plasticity and learning. *J Neurosci* 2016;36:4351–4361.

[25] Renthal W, Nestler EJ: Epigenetic mechanisms in drug addiction. *Trends Mol Med* 2008;14:341–350.

[26] Spadaro PA, Flavell CR, Widagdo J, Ratnu VS, et al.: Long noncoding RNA-directed epigenetic regulation of gene expression is associated with anxiety-like behavior in mice. *Biol Psychiatry* 2015;78:848–859.

in noncoding microRNAs on the DNA in their sperm cells.[27] Their offspring demonstrate reduced HPA reactivity to stress. In this case, the life experience of the father alters gene expression in the brain that is passed on to his children.

A fascinating recent development is the discovery that we *Homo sapiens* have traces of Neanderthal DNA in our genes. Until they disappeared for unclear reasons about 50,000 years ago, our species appears not infrequently to have mated with Neanderthals. Since then, we have continued to pass on Neanderthal DNA, and it turns out that the Neanderthal genes produce gene products that regulate our more abundant *Homo sapiens* genes. A recent study showed that the Neanderthal genes are relatively silenced in human brain tissue,[28] but the effects of the Neanderthal genes have been linked to several human traits, such as height, and to the susceptibility to diseases like schizophrenia and systematic lupus erythematosus.

## TRANSLATING EPIGENETICS TO HUMAN BEHAVIOR

Having shown the effect of early life experience on gene expression in the rodent brain, the Meaney research group considered the possibility that the methylation status of glucocorticoid receptor genes might play a role in human emotion and behavior as well. In a remarkable study, they obtained postmortem brain samples from suicide victims, some of whom had a history of childhood abuse and some who did not, and from a control group of people who died of other causes. Just as in the offspring of low LG mothers, they found that the promoter region of GR genes from brains of suicide victims with a history of child abuse had more methyl groups than those of suicide victims without a history of child abuse or from the controls.[29] As expected, there were also fewer glucocorticoid receptors in the hippocampus of the suicide victims with child abuse histories than in the other two groups. Fewer GR receptors in the hippocampus means less opportunity for the HPA axis' negative feedback loop to regulate the release of its anxiety-provoking hormones, CRH and cortisol. The implication is that the experience of being an abused child causes a change in the methylation status of the gene that encodes the GR receptor. This in turn sets loose a system that predisposes an individual to feeling anxious and depressed throughout life and helps explain why being the victim of abuse as a child is the precursor to adult psychopathology like depression and anxiety disorders and to behaviors like suicide. This is a striking piece of evidence that what is found in rodents and monkeys might also apply to humans, that adverse early life experiences—having a mother that doesn't lick and groom much (rat), or having a mother who is distracted by being unable

[27] Rodgers AB, Morgan CP, Leu NA, Bale TL: Transgenerational epigenetic programming via sperm micro-RNA recapitulates effects of paternal stress. *Proc Natl Acad Sci USA* 2015;112:13699–13704.

[28] McCoy RC, Wakefield J, Akey JM: Impacts of Neanderthal-introgressed sequences on the landscape of human gene expression. *Cell* 2017; Epub ahead of print

[29] McGowan PO, Sasaki A, D'Alessio AC, Dymov S, Labonte B, Szyf M, Gustavo Turecki G, Meaney MJ: Epigenetic regulation of the glucocorticoid receptor in human brain associates with childhood abuse. *Nat Neurosci* 2009;12:342–348.

to predict when food will be easily available (monkey), or having been abused by a parent (human)—can permanently change behavior, emotion, and biology and do so by altering the expression level of genes in the brain. The finding gains further support from a study of adolescents who were divided based on psychiatric assessment of their propensity for suicidal behavior into high-risk and low-risk groups. DNA was extracted from blood samples and several differences in methylation status of genes that are active in the CRH pathway were seen between the high- and low-risk for suicide groups.[30]

There are other hints that epigenetic regulation of gene expression may be one way that adverse early life experiences translate into human behavioral patterns and mental disorders. The evidence that exposure to in utero starvation during the Dutch Famine Winter increased the risk for schizophrenia? A Dutch research group found that individuals exposed to the famine prenatally had a decrease in DNA methylation on a specific gene compared to their unexposed siblings 6 decades after the Dutch Famine Winter occurred.[31] A further study of this group of people showed links between in utero exposure to the famine and DNA methylation of several genes.[32]

Another study found that, among 132 adolescents, those who grew up with lower socioeconomic status (SES) had an increase in methylation of a gene that codes for the serotonin transport receptor, the same receptor in the brain that binds the selective serotonin reuptake inhibitor (SSRI)-type antidepressants like fluoxetine (Prozac) and paroxetine (Paxil).[33] During functional brain imaging, these individuals with increased gene methylation also had the highest reactivity of a brain structure involved in fear, the amygdala, when presented with a threatening stimulus. The combination of increased gene methylation and increased amygdala reactivity to threat was in turn linked in these adolescents to a propensity to develop depressive symptoms. Another group has also shown in human men that both early life and recent life stress alters methylation of the serotonin transport receptor gene, changing the gene's expression level and influencing cortisol responses to stress.[34] These are but examples of the increasing evidence that life's experiences, including adversity, change the epigenetic regulation of gene expression in the human brain and thereby influence how we feel and behave.

---

[30] Jokinen J, Bostrom AE, Dadfar A, et al.: Epigenetic changes in the CRH gene are related to severity of suicide attempt and a general psychiatric risk score in adolescents. *EBIO Medicine* 2018;27:123–133.

[31] Heijmans BT, Tobi EW, Stein AD, et al.: Persistent epigenetic differences associated with prenatal exposure to famine in humans. *Proc Natl Acad Sci USA* 2008;105:17046–17049.

[32] Tobi EW, Goeman JJ, Monajemi R, et al: DNA methylation signatures link prenatal famine exposure to growth and metabolism. *Nat Commun* 2014;5:5592.

[33] Swartz JR, Hariri AR, Williamson DE: An epigenetic mechanism links socioeconomic status to changes in depression-related brain function in high-risk adolescents. *Mol Psychiatr* 2017;22:209–214.

[34] Duman EA, Canli T: Influence of life stress, 5-HTTLPR genotype, and SLC6A4 methylation on gene expression and stress response in healthy Caucasian males. *Biol Mood Anxiety Disord.* 2015;14;5:2.

One of the most intriguing links between epigenetic regulation of gene expression and human psychiatric disturbance comes from the work of my good friend and former colleague, Rachel Yehuda of the Mount Sinai School of Medicine. Yehuda is one of the world's experts on the biology of PTSD. Several years ago, she showed that survivors of the Nazi Holocaust, especially those who developed PTSD, have lower levels of cortisol than matched controls. This is a somewhat paradoxical finding since high levels of cortisol are usually found in people who are under stress. Most striking, Yehuda found that the children of Holocaust survivors also had low levels of cortisol, even though they themselves had never been exposed to anything nearly as traumatic as their parents.[35] More recently, Yehuda has also shown an association between methylation of a stress-related gene that codes for a protein called $FKBP_5$ and the risk among the children of Holocaust survivors to develop PTSD.[36] Interestingly, another research group found that the $FKBP_5$ protein is part of a pathway of proteins that controls methylation of other genes and that $FKPB_5$'s activity can be influenced by the SSRI antidepressant paroxetine (Paxil).[37] Paroxetine acts through this pathway to decrease methylation and increase expression of genes that code for proteins that may have important effects in countering depression. Thus, this work on Holocaust survivors with PTSD and their children suggests that biological abnormalities are found in the offspring of survivors who were not themselves exposed to the Holocaust and to the methylation status of a gene linked to depression and the consequent risk that people in these subsequent generations have of developing PTSD. An association between methylation of the $FKBP_5$ gene and childhood adversity among people with major depression has also been reported.[38]

This finding of an increased risk of PTSD in the offspring of Holocaust survivors raises the question of whether experience-induced changes in epigenetic control can be passed on from one generation to the next. If a women undergoes a stressful life event that increases the number of methyl groups bound to a gene that controls its expression in the brain, can she pass on that increase in methylation and change in gene expression to her children, and can they in turn pass these on to a third generation? There is evidence that this can occur in rodents; whether it is the case for the much more complicated human genome is controversial. But we do not need to

[35] Rodriquze T: Descendants of holocaust survivors have altered stress hormones. *Sci Am* March 1, 2015. https://www.scientificamerican.com/article/descendants-of-holocaust-survivors-have-altered-stress-hormones/.

[36] Yehuda R, Daskalakis NP, Bierer LM, Bader HN, Klengel T, Holsboer F, Binder EB: Holocaust exposure induced intergenerational effects on *FKBP5* methylation. *Biol Psychiatry* 2016;80:372–380.

[37] Gassen NC, Fries GR, Zannas AS, et al.: Chaperoning epigenetics: FKBP51 decreases the activity of DNMT1 and mediates the epigenetic effects of the antidepressant paroxetine. *Sci Signal* 2015;8:ra 119.

[38] Tozzi L, Farrell C, Booij L, et al.: Epigenetic changes of FKBP5 as a link connecting genetic and environmental risk factors with structural and functional brain changes in major depression. *Neuropsychopharmacology* 2018;43:1138–1145.

invoke inheritance of acquired epigenetic changes to recognize that, within any in-dividual, experience routinely alters methylation, acetylation, RNA interference, and many other mechanisms that control the level of gene expression in the brain.

Is it possible to change these epigenetic effects of early life stress? It does ap-pear to be in the case of Michael Meaney's rats. His group infused adult rats with HDAC inhibitors that prevent acetyl groups from being removed from histones or with drugs that add methyl groups (in this case the amino acid L-methionine) to the DNA. These maneuvers would be expected to have opposite effects on gene expres-sion, the former increasing and the latter decreasing it. They found that, in fact, the drugs reversed the effects of early licking and grooming when the offspring became adults.[39] It is striking that a pharmacological intervention could reverse the effects of early life experience, but these effects appear to work by reversing the original epige-netic effects of different levels of licking and grooming. Scientists have already begun to consider whether these drugs could be modified for use in humans with psychi-atric illness.

Perhaps more interesting is the possibility that offering a "better" life experience in the form of psychotherapy might also be able to reverse the epigenetic effects of early life trauma. It has already been shown in one study that successful CBT for patients with panic disorder reversed abnormally low methylation levels of a gene coding for a protein called *monoamine oxidase A* (MAOA).[40] In this case, the methylation levels were measured on DNA taken from blood cells and not, of course, from the panic disorder patients' brains. We must be cautious in concluding from one study done on peripheral cells that psychotherapy changed anything in these patients' brains. It is certain that more similar studies will be pursued, and we will get some more definitive answers soon.

## THE USUAL CAUTIONS

I promised in the introduction to this book to refrain from getting carried away by ele-gant experiments and compelling hypotheses, and so some comments on the strength of the findings discussed in this chapter are in order.

There is no question at this point that life experiences are a factor in determining life-long patterns of human emotion, behavior, and the propensity to develop mental illness. We also know that an increase in gene expression in the prefrontal cortex is one of the defining characteristics of the human brain. There is also no question that experiences have physical effects on the brains of laboratory animals at the molec-ular level, including changing the levels of gene expression and protein synthesis. We know that early life adversity can profoundly affect human brain function at a regional

[39] Weaver IC, Meaney MJ, Szyf M: Maternal care effects on the hippocampal transcriptome and anxiety-mediated behaviors in the offspring that are reversible in adulthood. *Proc Natl Acad Sci USA* 2006;103:3480–3485.

[40] Ziegler C, Richter J, Mahr M, et al.: MAOA gene hypomethylation in panic disorder-reversibility of an epigenetic risk pattern by psychotherapy. *Transl Psychiatry* 2016;6:e773.

level.[41] But we cannot as a rule study the molecular biology of brains of living humans, and therefore it is less certain that what is found in animals is also found in humans. Are the epigenetic changes that Meaney found in rat brains applicable to humans, for example?

Certainly, we can point to Meaney and his colleague's findings in suicide victims with a history of child abuse as suggesting they do. We have also noted several other instances in which epigenetic changes are described in humans that are associated with having psychiatric illnesses, enduring traumatic experiences, taking medications, and even undergoing a course of psychotherapy. These findings in humans, however, are made using either blood cells or brain tissue from autopsy samples of people who died under a variety of conditions, not, as in the case of preclinical studies, from brains of either living animals or animals that have been sacrificed under careful laboratory conditions. This limitation means we must be cautious in accepting the idea that life experiences alter the physical structure and function of the brain via epigenetic changes in the regulation of gene expression. Many more studies will be needed to make such conclusions more secure.

For now, the following scenario seems reasonable. Over the course of the 6 million years of evolution since we separated from chimpanzees, we not only added more neurons to the prefrontal cortex of our brains than any other species, we also increased the number of genes in those neurons that are expressed and code for proteins. The sequence of bases on our DNA—our genetic code—makes us human but does not differentiate us very much from each other. Rather, it is the increase in the number of genes expressed that allows each person's individual experiences to establish a unique set of emotions, behaviors, and abilities. This increase in brain gene expression gives us a great deal of flexibility, but it also leaves room for errors that can cause trouble. It makes some of us able to write poetry, others to throw a fastball, and still others to enjoy playing with children. But it also makes some of us prone to worrying about trivial things, getting depressed, or even contemplating ending our lives. The way our experiences determine these things is very likely through the molecular mechanism of epigenetic control over gene expression. As Eric Nestler puts it "There is now robust and growing evidence supporting a role for epigenetic modification as a key mechanism underlying lifelong regulation of gene expression and, consequently of stress vulnerability."[42]

In the next chapter, we will move from the molecular level to the cellular level. When a gene is expressed, something new happens inside a neuron that changes an aspect of how the brain looks and works. We turn now to two of these events: dendritic remodeling and neurogenesis.

[41] Klumpers F, Kroes MCWW, Baas J, Fernandez G: How human amygdala and bed nucleus of the stria terminalis may drive distinct defensive responses. *J Neurosci* 2017; Epub ahead of print

[42] Nestler EJ: Transgenerational epigenetic contributions to stress responses: fact or fiction? *PLoS Biol* 2016 1002426

# 4

## Sadness and Depression
### *Neurons Constantly Change*

People with depression are remarkably intransigent. Our instinct is to cheer them, but they refuse to be cheered. They blame themselves for things for which they could not possibly be responsible, yet cannot be persuaded by facts to abandon their guilt. Depressed people exaggerate their faults and fear that far-fetched catastrophes are about to occur. Logic seems to have no effect on the tenacity of these exaggerated beliefs. Trying to reason with a loved-one with serious depression is frustrating.

In Chapter 3, we saw that adverse life experiences increase the risk for depression and that a possible molecular mechanism for this effect is a change in the epigenetic regulation of gene expression in the brain. The result of changes in activity levels of our DNA molecules is that the proteins for which the genes involved code will not be produced in the normal amounts. What would be the consequences of such a change in gene expression and protein production, and how could it be involved in the inability of depressed people to yield their melancholic view of themselves and the world to logic and reason? In this chapter, we will describe two ways in which aberrant protein production affects the way cells in the brain behave. These processes, *dendritic remodeling* and *neurogenesis*, can explain many aspects of depression and move us from the molecular level of Chapter 3 to the cellular level of brain function. First, we must review a few aspects of how proteins are made and how they influence the way cells function.

Proteins do the work of cells in the body, including neurons in the brain. The messenger RNA (mRNA) that is transcribed from DNA in the neuron's nucleus migrates out of the nucleus and into the cell's cytoplasm. Once there, it joins an assembly comprising two subunits of a structure called the *ribosome* (see Figure 4.1) and another type of RNA called *transfer RNA* (tRNA). This complex takes the building blocks of proteins, called *amino acids*, and strings them together into full-length proteins according to a code embedded in the mRNA. A newly made protein is then often cleaved into several smaller proteins so that the original gene can wind up coding for more than one protein.

The new proteins are now ready to carry out the myriad tasks of our cells. We can think for a moment about these proteins as contents of a house. Just as all houses have roofs, windows, furnaces, and pipes, so all cells have a set of the same proteins that

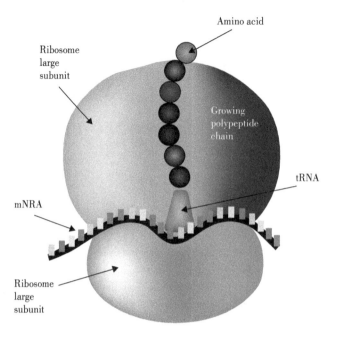

Labels within/around figure:

Amino acid

Ribosome
large
subunit

Growing
polypeptide
chain

tRNA

mNRA

Ribosome
large
subunit

**Figure 4.1** The synthesis of proteins occurs when a messenger RNA (mRNA) molecule travels from the cell's nucleus to the cytoplasm and joins this assembly composed of the two subunits of a ribosome and transfer RNA (tRNA). Amino acids are strung together according to the genetic code on the mRNA into full-length proteins.
Shutterstock.

carry out tasks such as transcribing DNA, making energy, and breaking down waste products. But houses are also specialized to fit their unique environments and the tastes of individual owners. Houses in Seville have red tile roofs, while houses in Paris have grillwork on the windows. My house in New York has a basement, while yours in Florida probably does not. Similarly, cells have proteins necessary for their special functions: in liver cells (hepatocytes), specialized proteins are the enzymes that break down the food and drugs we swallow. In the adrenal gland's endocrine cells, a unique protein is the cortisol that gets released in response to corticotropin from the pituitary gland. Proteins make up the unique smooth muscle cells of the heart (myocardial cells) that make it contract with each heartbeat. Thus, cells have both common and unique proteins, the latter of which allow them to carry out specialized functions like digestion, pumping blood, and remembering facts.

The brain has three main types of cells—glia, endothelial cells, and neurons—each with its own set of specialized proteins. Glial cells include three main subtypes: *astrocytes* that surround and nourish neurons;[1] *glia cells,* including oligodendroglia cells that

---

[1] Astrocytes actually do much more than just facilitate the work of neurons and there is burgeoning research into their many essential functions. They will undoubtedly play a much more important role in a future edition of this book.

make the myelin sheath that surrounds a neuron's axons and microglial cells that serve as the brain's immune system; and *endothelial cells* that line the blood vessels that penetrate the brain and form, along with astrocytes, what is called the blood–brain barrier. The blood–brain barrier is a functional complex that carefully regulates what substances can move from the circulating blood into and out of the brain. It protects the delicate cells of the brain from toxins and infectious particles, and, sometimes unfortunately, blocks many medications that can easily penetrate other organs of the body from entering the brain. This makes designing medications for psychiatric and neurological conditions especially challenging. Of all these cell types, it is the neuron that remembers, senses, and communicates, and it will be the focus our attention in this chapter.

## NEURONS, AXONS, AND DENDRITES

Thanks to Suzana Herculano-Houzel (see Chapter 2), we now know that the human brain has 86 billion neurons, all packed into an organ that weighs about 3 pounds. What does a neuron look like? In some ways, like any other cell. It has a cell body encased in a cell membrane, a nucleus that contains chromosomes made of DNA and proteins called histones, and mitochondria, where the cell's energy is produced. It is the strange projections from the cell body, however, that make the neuron look different from other cells (see Figure 4.2). Most neurons have one axon and many dendrites. Neurons generate electrical signals when they are activated, and it is these signals that carry information from one neuron to another. The neuronal signals leave the neuron's cell body and travel along its axon until they reach a kind of dead end. There is a gap or space between the end of the axon and projections from the next neuron. These projections are the dendrites, prepared to receive electrical signals from another neuron, and the gap between the axon of one neuron and dendrites of another neuron is called the *synapse*. We call the neuron that is sending the signal down the axon the *presynaptic neuron* and the neuron whose dendrites are prepared to receive the signal the *postsynaptic neuron*.

In Figure 4.3, you can see a blown-up version of the synapse, with the signal traveling from left to right. Something must happen for the signal to bridge the synapse: it is the release of chemical messengers called *neurotransmitters* from the presynaptic neuron. The two most abundant neurotransmitters in the brain are the proteins glutamate and gamma aminobutyric acid (GABA). The ones most often talked about in psychiatry are noradrenalin, serotonin, and dopamine. An important one for Alzheimer's disease is acetylcholine. We will have occasion to say much more about these chemicals and many others that bridge the synaptic gap later on. Right now, let's focus on glutamate, an example of what is called an *excitatory neurotransmitter*.

When glutamate is released by a presynaptic neuron, it goes across the synapse until it finds an appropriate receptor on the surface of the postsynaptic receptor. Receptors are specific for individual neurotransmitters, so that there are glutamate receptors, GABA receptors, serotonin receptors, and so forth. Each specific receptor is a unique protein coded for by a gene in the neuron's nucleus. When a molecule of

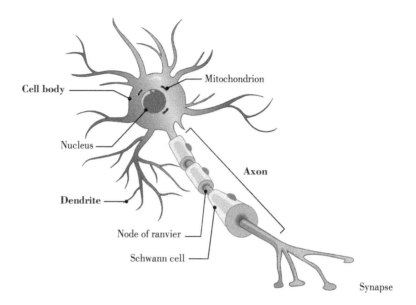

**Figure 4.2** The neuron has a cell body that looks much like that of any other cell, with a nucleus that contains the DNA and mitochondria that produce energy. What makes a neuron unique in appearance are its projections, the axons, which conduct neural signals away from the cell body, and the dendrites, which conduct neural signals toward the cell body. In this image, the Schwann cell and Node of Ranvier refer to parts of the myelin sheath that coats the axon as a kind of insulation that improves nerve conduction.
Shutterstock.

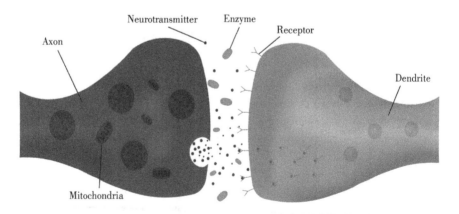

**Figure 4.3** The synapse is the gap between the axon of the presynaptic neuron on the left and one of the dendrites of the postsynaptic neuron on the right. Neurotransmitters, released by the presynaptic neuron, travel across the synapse and bind to receptors on the surface of the postsynaptic dendrite, initiating a chemical process there that allows continued conduction of the neuronal signal.
Shutterstock.

glutamate binds to one of the several types of glutamate receptors, it causes a series of chemical and electrical events that result in the continued propagation of the electrical signal down the postsynaptic neuron's dendrite. In this way, electrical signals in the brain are transmitted from neuron to neuron, carrying all the things we learn, think, see, smell, and hear. They are also transmitted from the brain to every part of our bodies over axons that can be more than 3 feet long. Whenever we want to move an arm, the thought originates in one part of the brain as an electrical signal that is transmitted through axons and dendrites down the spinal cord to the arm muscle in a fraction of a second. Whenever we see something, the image triggers a response in the retina of the eye that becomes an electrical signal propagated along the optic nerve to the occipital region of the brain, where we recognize what it is. Nerves are really axons and dendrites carrying these signals throughout the brain and from the brain to our muscles and our organs, telling them what to do. In turn, sensory neurons in the skin send signals back to the brain with information about things we touch via axons and dendrites. Our ears, noses, and eyes do the same thing for what we hear, smell, and see. In fact, all our organs send signals to the brain so that it can coordinate every aspect of bodily function. The same brain that is responsible for our thoughts, emotions, and behaviors must also ensure that we continue to breathe, that our hearts keep on beating, and that we can digest our food.

With a few exceptions, each neuron has only one axon, but neurons have anywhere from one to several hundred dendrites. Dendrites make up about 90% of neural tissue. Although the exact number is somewhat elusive, it is estimated that each neuron can make anywhere from one to several hundred thousand synaptic connections between axons and dendrites and that there are between 100 and 1,000 trillion total synaptic connections in a single human brain. It is said that if one human brain were to have all its dendrites and axons lined up end to end, it would go from here to the moon and back. While that description is fanciful, it is meant to help us translate the staggering number of brain cell connections into something we can come close to imagining. Given that a typical neuron fires about every 5 to 50 seconds, you can see that the human brain is a mass of highly charged activity, its electrical signals traveling and erupting across a network of axons and dendrites that makes the billions of stars in the Milky Way galaxy seem simple by comparison.

## WHAT CHANGES IN THE BRAIN?

The brain cannot possibly be a static organ because that would make it impossible to learn a new fact or remember a new experience. More than any other organ in the body, the brain must continuously change itself as it translates life's experiences into electrical impulses that stream through billions of neurons and across trillions of synaptic connections.

Dendrites grow from the cell bodies of neurons like tree branches, creating elaborate structures called *dendritic trees* or *dendritic arbors*. If you look closely at a dendrite (Figure 4.4) you will see that there are tiny outcroppings protruding from the surface,

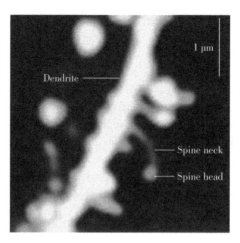

**Figure 4.4** Spines are protrusions along a dendrite, as shown in this picture taken with a laser scanning two-photon microscope. Most spines have a bulbous head and a neck attaching the spine to the body of the dendrite. Axons from presynaptic neurons make synapses with spines on dendrites. Image in public domain, http://en.wikipedia.org/wiki/Image:Spines.jpg

called *spines*. Most dendrites have spines, and most spines have a head that is connected via a neck to the dendrite. There can be as many as five spines per micrometer along a spine (a micrometer is equal to 0.001 millimeters). It is on the dendritic spine that axons from a presynaptic neuron form a synapse. Receptors on the dendritic spine surface receive neurotransmitters released by the incoming axon. This starts the chemical activity that results in an electrical spark, called an *action potential*, that permits the neural signal from the axon to continue propagating down the dendrite. The great number of spines on each dendrite explains how every dendrite can make hundreds to thousands of synaptic connections. It is now understood that dendrites are 10 times more electrically active than the cell body, or soma, of the neuron.[2] Activation of dendrites at the point where they make synapses with axons from other neurons appears to make otherwise subliminal perceptions fully conscious;[3] general anesthesia makes us unconscious by suppressing this dendritic activity.[4] Thus, dendrites play a critical role in our conscious appreciation of the world around us.

Spines were first noticed in the early twentieth century by the great neurobiologist Santiago Ramon y Cajal, but it wasn't until about a decade ago that a new technique called *two-photon laser microscopy* allowed scientists to observe a fascinating aspect of spines: they come and go. In fact, the entire tree of dendrites and their spines are

[2] Moore JJ, Ravassard PM, Ho D, Acharya L, Kees AL, Vuong C, Mehta MR: Dynamics of cortical dendritic membrane potential and spikes in freely behaving rats. *Science* 2017; Epub ahead of print.
[3] Takahashi N, Oertner TG, Hegemann P, Larkum ME: Active cortical dendrites modulate perception. *Science* 2016;354:1587–1590.
[4] Meyer K: The role of dendritic signaling in the anesthetic suppression of consciousness. *Anesthesiology* 2015;122;1415–1431.

capable of constantly expanding and retracting, with spines popping up on the surface of dendrites and then disappearing moment to moment. This means that synaptic connections between neurons can be formed, deleted, and formed again on a continuous basis. The time scale for this is a matter of minutes or less.[5]

The receptors on spines for neurotransmitters can also be resorbed inside the spine, a process called *endocytosis*. Thus, dendrites have multiple ways of connecting, disengaging, and reconnecting to other neurons. Some spines are more stable than others, and therefore some memories are longer lasting than others. Every time we learn something new, see something different, or encounter a new experience, dendrites expand, spines are exposed on the dendritic surface, and new synaptic connections are made. When we sleep, contacts between axons and dendritic spines decrease by about 20%.[6] Normal aging is associated with a gradual decrease in the size of dendritic trees and the number of dendritic spines. The expansion and contraction of dendrites is often referred to as *dendritic remodeling,* and the increases and decreases in synaptic strength caused by what we experience and what we do are called *activity-dependent plasticity*. Strengthening of synaptic connections caused by enlargements of dendrites is called *long-term potentiation* (LTP), and weakening of synaptic connections caused by shrinkage of dendrites is called *long-term depression* (LTD).

Scientists have identified many of the proteins responsible for the brain's remarkable amount of dendritic plasticity.[7] For example, a protein called CPG2 is required for the resorption of receptors on the dendritic surface.[8] Another protein called Integrin α3 is necessary for dendrite and spine stability over time.[9] The list of the proteins involved in dendritic remodeling and synaptic plasticity—and the genes that code for them—keeps getting longer as neuroscientists probe the biology of the dendrite in increasing detail.

One aspect of this story was at first a mystery. Although dendrites are typically shorter than axons, they can nevertheless extend several inches from the neuron's cell body. And, of course, they branch off in many directions. At first, it wasn't clear how proteins synthesized in the cytoplasm of a cell body could travel all the way to the ends of dendrites where synapses occur in time to direct spines to protrude to the surface at the speed necessary to sustain learning and stimulus–response. This mystery was solved when it was shown that mRNA molecules are transported from the cell body and take up permanent residence in distant parts of dendrites, ready to synthesize new

[5] Berning S, Willig KI, Steffens H, Dibaj P, Hell SW: Nanoscopy in a living mouse brain. *Science* 2012;335:551.

[6] Acsady L, Harris KD: Synaptic scaling in sleep. *Science* 2017;355:457.

[7] Martin KC, Zukin SR: RNA trafficking and local protein synthesis in dendrites: an overview. *J Neurosci* 2006;26:7131–7134.

[8] Loebrich S, Benoit MR, Konopka JA, Cottrell JR, Gibson J, Nedivi E: CPG2 recruits endophilin B2 to the cytoskeleton for activity-dependent endocytosis of synaptic glutamate receptors. *Curr Biol* 2016;26:296–308.

[9] Kerrisk ME, Greer CA, Koleske AJ: Integrin α3 is required for late postnatal stability of dendrite arbors, dendritic spines and synapses, and mouse behavior. *J Neurosci* 2013;33:6742–6752.

proteins on a moment's notice.[10,11] As these mRNA molecules move, they become more and more active in translating new proteins.[12]

And it turns out that life events can trigger the genes that code for the mRNA and proteins involved in synapse formation, causing the expansion and retraction of dendrites and their spines.[13] Bruce McEwen of Rockefeller University and others have shown, for example, that rats exposed to chronic stress have retracted spines in two parts of the brain that play key roles in suppressing fear, the prefrontal cortex and the hippocampus,[14] whereas, after conditioned fear training, spines pop out on the surface of rats' dendrites in one of the brain's main fear centers, the amygdala.[15,16] In the frontal cortex, fear conditioning causes elimination of dendritic spines, whereas extinction of conditioned fear increases the number of spines.[17]

Rats that are separated from their mothers during infancy are more anxious and have permanently enlarged dendritic trees with more spines in the amygdala, but a single episode of exposure to an enriched environment as adults reverses both the behavioral and dendritic changes.[18] Stress thus disrupts synaptic connections in parts of the brain that can control fear, like the prefrontal cortex, while increasing synaptic connections in a part of the brain that is needed to learn to fear, the amygdala. On the other hand, a positive experience—like becoming a father—increases the number of dendritic spines in the prefrontal cortex of marmoset monkeys compared to fatherless males.[19] And an experimental antidepressant reversed

[10] Schuman EM, Dynes JL, Steward O: Synaptic regulation of translation of dendritic mRNAs. *J Neurosci* 2006;26:7143–7146.

[11] Martin KC, Zukin SR: RNA trafficking and local protein synthesis in dendrites: an overview. *J Neurosci* 2006;26:7131–7134.

[12] Iwasaki S, Ingolia NT: Seeing translation. *Science* 2016;352:1391–1392.

[13] Gorman JM, Docherty JP: A hypothesized role for dendritic remodeling in the etiology of mood and anxiety disorders. *J Neuropsychiatry Clin Neurosci* 2010;22:256–264.

[14] Radley JJ, Sisti HM, Hao J, Rocher AB, McCall T, Hof PR, McEwen BS, Morrison JH: Chronic behavioral stress induces apical dendritic reorganization in pyramidal neurons of the medial prefrontal cortex. *Neuroscience* 2004;125:1–6.

[15] Magarinos AM, McEwen BS, Flugge G, et al.: Chronic psychosocial stress causes apical dendritic atrophy of hippocampal CA3 pyramidal neurons in subordinate tree shrews. *J Neurosci* 1996;16:3534–3540.

[16] Radley JJ, Johnson LR, Janssen WG, Martino J, Lamprecht R, Hof PR, LeDoux JE, Morrison JH: Associative Pavlovian conditioning leads to an increase in spinophilin-immunoreactive dendritic spines in the lateral amygdala. *Eur J Neurosci* 2006;24:876–884.

[17] Lai CS, Franke TF, Gan WB: Opposite effects of fear conditioning and extinction on dendritic spine remodeling. *Nature* 2012;483:87–91.

[18] Koe AS, Ashokan A, Mitra R: Short environmental enrichment in adulthood reverses anxiety and basolateral amygdala hypertrophy induced by maternal separation. *Transl Psychiatry* 2016;6:e729.

[19] Kozorovitskiy Y, Hughes M, Lee K, Gould E: Fatherhood affects dendritic spines and vasopressin via receptors in the primate prefrontal cortex. *Nat Neurosci* 2006;9:182–189.

structural remodeling in the amygdala of mice exposed to chronic stress, making them more resilient.[20]

Psychiatrist Norman Doidge nicely summarizes the effects of enriched environments and learning on brain growth:

> Animals raised in enriched environments—surrounded by other animals, objects to explore, toys to roll, ladders to climb, and running wheels—learn better than genetically identical animals that have been reared in impoverished environments. . . . Mental training or life in enriched environments increases brain weight by 5 percent in the cerebral cortex of animals and up to 9 percent in areas that the training directly stimulates. . . . For people, postmortem examinations have shown that education increases the number of branches among neurons. (p. 43)[21]

We can now lay out a scenario for how life events affect dendritic structure, cause dendritic remodeling, and modify synaptic connections. As explained in Chapter 3, various forms of stress and fear-learning cause methyl groups to bind to DNA and acetyl groups to bind to histone proteins that surround DNA. This changes the activity level of genes in key regions of the brain like the prefrontal cortex, hippocampus, and amygdala. When the result of these epigenetic effects is to turn down the activity of genes that code for proteins involved in dendritic activity, less mRNA is transcribed, resulting in reduced synthesis of proteins necessary to maintain the health of dendrites and their spines. Spines disappear from the surface of the dendrites and the dendritic tree atrophies,[22] leaving axons from presynaptic neurons with fewer places to make synaptic connections. The brain becomes relatively disconnected.

Some of the connections that stress disrupts are between structures that are far apart in the brain. For example, as we will explain in more detail in a later chapter, there are extensive connections between the prefrontal cortex and the amygdala. The prefrontal cortex can suppress fear memories stored in the amygdala when these connections are intact.[23] But stress can disrupt these connections, leaving the amygdala isolated and without sufficient brakes on its capacity for creating new fear memories. An uncontrolled amygdala is believed to be the source of the excessive fears that plague people with depression and anxiety disorders and make them beyond the reach of reason and logic. Now let us consider a typical case of major depression and see how this might work.

[20] Lau T, Bigio B, Zelli D, McEwen BS, Nasca C: Stress-induced structural plasticity of medial amygdala stellate neurons and rapid prevention by a candidate antidepressant. *Mol Psychiatr* 2017;22:227–234.

[21] Doidge N: *The Brain that Changes Itself.* New York, Penguin, 2007.

[22] Francis TC, Chandra R, Gaynor A, et al.: Molecular basis of dendritic atrophy and activity in stress susceptibility. *Mol Psychiatr* 2017;22:1512–1519.

[23] Quirk GJ, Likhtik E, Pelletier JG, et al.: Stimulation of medial prefrontal cortex decreases the responsiveness of central amygdala output neurons. *J Neurosci* 2003;23:8800–8807.

# DEPRESSION DISCONNECTS THE BRAIN

Marjorie is having a tough time. She got married right out of college and now, 8 years later, is having trouble remembering why. Her husband, Rich, is no longer the "fun" guy he was back then but instead seems intent on doing as little of anything as possible. He has never had a steady job but constantly concocts get-rich schemes that never pan out. Meanwhile, Marjorie works long hours as an account executive to support herself, her husband, and their 3-year-old son. Her husband is home all day, supposedly watching the boy, but Marjorie worries that Rich pays little attention to him. She can't afford day care for her son on her salary, so she does her best to play with him after work, along with having to clean the house and cook dinner every night. Marjorie periodically yells at Rich to do more of the household chores since he has nothing else to do, but he always insists he is too busy with his various "projects." Marjorie thinks constantly of leaving her husband, but she simply doesn't have the energy to find a new place to live.

The straw that breaks the camel's back is the sudden death of Marjorie's mother, the one person she felt close to and who tried to help. Her mother was only in her early 60s but had diabetes and one day just dropped dead of a stroke. Marjorie feels devastated but maintains her composure through the funeral. In the succeeding weeks, she does her best to comfort her father, with whom she has always had a strained relationship, while continuing to work and care for her child and home. But about 6 months after her mother died, she begins to feel the strain to be unbearable. She is always exhausted, her son seems constantly cranky, and her husband either watches television or surfs the Internet all day and all night. The one person she had in her life to talk to when she couldn't stand things any longer was now gone.

At first, Marjorie thinks maybe she is getting some kind of flu. Her head hurts all the time and she feels drugged, like she just needs to go to sleep. But at night she just tosses and turns, worrying about the bills, her marriage, and her son's development. She only gets a few hours of sleep, waking up hours before she must each morning. Her appetite slowly disappears. At work, her co-workers and boss notice that she seems distracted and less energetic than usual. She makes several mistakes filling out paperwork for her clients.

One year after her mother's death, Marjorie feels like a thoroughly useless person. Nothing she does is right, she thinks, and nothing matters. There is nothing for her to look forward to. She begins to feel like a bad mother and wonders if her son would be better off if she were gone and her husband found a better wife. Maybe someone sexier would appeal to her husband, she thinks, and decides the marital problems are all her fault. Then, 18 months after her mother's death, Marjorie takes an overdose of the sleeping pills her internist prescribed for her. Fortunately, such overdoses are rarely fatal, and she is merely in a deep sleep when her husband finds her in the bedroom and calls 911. After waking up, Marjorie is transferred from the emergency department to the inpatient psychiatry unit.

When asked by a hospital staff member why she took the overdose, Marjorie mumbles "it would be better for everyone if I were dead." When asked why that is so, she answers, "because I screw up everything, I'm useless. Everything I do is wrong." She cries and asks to be left alone. She requests discharge from the hospital but cannot promise she won't try to kill herself again.

Marjorie remains in the hospital for 6 weeks, during which time she is given antidepressant medication and daily psychotherapy. For the first 2 or 3 weeks, she continues to feel hopeless. She talks as little as possible and does not interact voluntarily with any of the other patients or the staff. She barely eats or sleeps at night and spends her days sitting in a chair near her hospital room.

It is only after 3 weeks that her mood starts to lighten, and then, little by little, she begins to eat and sleep, to talk with more animation, and finally to be able to express all her fears and worries. Now, for the first time, the psychotherapist working with her feels it is possible to make some progress and to get a commitment from Marjorie not to attempt suicide again. Marjorie recognizes that no other mother would be better for her son and is discharged with a careful plan to continue medication under the supervision of a psychiatrist and to begin regular outpatient psychotherapy.

Marjorie is fortunate, once discharged, to be referred to an experienced and skilled psychotherapist who is trained in both cognitive behavioral and psychodynamic psychotherapy techniques. Dr. Martin helps Marjorie understand the nature of the stresses in her life, going back to her childhood, when she lived with a dismissive and absent father. Marjorie comes to recognize that she is not at fault for her marital problems and decides to seek a divorce. She also realizes that she must replace her mother with other people in her life and begins to make friends at work and church. Over time, Marjorie figures out how to be kinder to herself and to seek out better relationships.

There are many aspects of interest with Marjorie's case. Her diagnosis of major depressive disorder is clear, as are the multiple stresses in her life—a difficult father, bad marriage, young child, financial strains, and death of a cherished mother. Her hospital treatment was successful, and she fortunately responded to antidepressant medication.

But I want to focus on the intransigence of her worldview before she began to respond to treatment. As you read about Marjorie, I am sure you recognized immediately that she is quite a strong person, able to work long hours to support a family, raise a child with an uninvolved husband, and continue a warm relationship with her mother. Yet, once depression set in, Marjorie could not be consoled or persuaded that her guilt was misplaced. She was mired in a hopeless, negative state in which her basic vegetative functions—sleep, appetite, libido, energy—were shut down. No amount of reason touched her.

We can speculate that the series of stressful life events Marjorie experienced from early life through the death of her mother affected the way her brain functions. These events increased her levels of the stress hormone corticotropin releasing hormone (CRH; see Chapter 3 for more about CRH), activated the primitive and emotional parts of her brain like the amygdala, and downregulated genes in the reasoning and reward centers of her brain. With the imbalance between brain regions, the fear centers of Marjorie's brain were left unchecked and hyperactive, mediated in part by the excitatory neurotransmitter we mentioned earlier, glutamate.

During times of high levels of stress, glutamate may become overactive in the brain. Too much glutamate is toxic to neurons, and so, to protect themselves, John Docherty and I speculated in 2010[24] that neurons adaptively retract dendrites and dendritic spines, thus decreasing the number of available glutamate receptors. But this shrinking of the dendritic arbor also causes a loss of synaptic connections, and so primitive parts of Marjorie's brain and more evolved reasoning parts became disconnected. The prefrontal cortex is now less able to suppress the amygdala, and so Marjorie is mired in fear and catastrophic thinking. Interestingly, a drug that blocks the ability of glutamate to bind to its postsynaptic receptor, ketamine, is showing great promise as a novel antidepressant in clinical trials now being conducted.

Psychotherapy is a kind of positive experience in which patients learn to recognize their fears and reassert the brain's control over them. Docherty and I further speculated that the psychotherapeutic process results in a reversal of the depression-induced dendritic atrophy, with a corresponding revitalization of synaptic connections. Antidepressants may also stimulate dendritic branching and spine formation. As already mentioned, animal studies consistently show that both enriched environments and antidepressant medications contribute to the health of dendrites and synaptic connections.[25]

When we deal with molecular changes in the brain, like epigenetic regulation of gene expression, and cellular changes, like dendritic remodeling, we are well below the ability of modern brain imaging techniques to visualize these processes in a living, human brain. Everything we have said so far is based on solid evidence from the basic neuroscience laboratory. We know that stress causes dendritic and spine retraction and that positive experiences reverse those changes from studies on rodents and non-human primates. But we cannot see dendrites sprouting or retracting in a human brain with even the most powerful brain imaging technology currently available.

One validation for the dendritic remodeling hypothesis comes from the laboratory of Kalanit Grill-Spector of Stanford University. She and colleagues used a brain imaging technique called *quantitative magnetic resonance imaging* (qMRI) to compare two brain regions between a group of children, aged 5 to 12 years, and a group of adults, aged 22 to 28 years. One region studied, the fusiform gyrus, is involved in our ability to recognize faces, and the other, the collateral sulcus, is involved in the recognition of places and locations. The researchers found that the fusiform gyrus was about 12% larger in adults than in children, but no differences were found in the collateral

---

[24] Gorman JM, Docherty JP: A hypothesized role for dendritic remodeling in the etiology of mood and anxiety disorders. *J Neuropsychiatry Clin Neurosci* 2010;22:256–264.

[25] Hajszan T, MacLusky NJ, Leranth C: Short-term treatment with the antidepressant fluoxetine triggers pyramidal dendritic spine synapse formation in rat hippocampus. *Eur J Neurosci* 2005;21:1299–1303.; Galimberti I, Gogolla N, Alberi S, et al.: Long-term rearrangements of hippocampal mossy fiber terminal connectivity in the adult regulated by experience. *Neuron* 2006;50749–763.; Bessa JM, Ferriera D, Melo I: The mood-improving actions of antidepressants do not depend on neurogenesis but are associated with neuronal remodeling. *Mol Psychiatr* 2009;14:764–773.

sulcus.[26] This may explain why we get better at recognizing faces as we get older. The research group did a series of calculations and also looked at postmortem data from humans and anatomical data from monkeys and concluded that the growth in fusiform gyrus volume from childhood to adulthood is most likely caused by an increase in the size of dendritic arbors. Thus, this study implies that our continuous exposure to new people and need to remember and recognize new faces causes the dendrites in the fusiform gyrus to grow new synaptic connections.

Brain imaging studies have also demonstrated a decrease in connectivity among various brain regions in people who experience chronic stress or depression, and these are consistent with the notion of dendritic remodeling as a factor in depression. Researcher's including Rockefeller's Bruce McEwen and B. J. Casey, the latter then at Cornell Weill Medical School, used a brain imaging technique that allows visualization of the strength of connections between brain regions in humans. They showed that chronic psychosocial stress causes a reversible disruption in connections between the frontal and parietal cortices, a network known to be important for attention. The authors concluded that their findings "can be easily understood within the framework of rodent studies showing alterations in dendritic arborization . . . [which may disrupt] long-range corticocortical connections between the [prefrontal cortex] and more distant areas" (p. 916).[27] After a month without stress, they found that the connections were reinstated, again suggesting underlying dendritic plasticity and remodeling in response to stress in humans that mirrors what is found in laboratory animals.

Postmortem studies are also consistent with the idea that stress and depression negatively affect dendritic health. Steven Arnold, a psychiatrist and neuropathologist, and colleagues at the University of Pennsylvania collaborated with scientists who are conducting the Rush University Religious Orders Study. For more than two decades, over 1,000 members of religious orders agreed to annual medical and psychological examinations and to donating their brains to the project after death. Arnold's team examined 72 of these brains and found that high levels of anxiety and depression during life were associated with decreased dendritic and spine density in the hippocampus at postmortem brain examination.[28]

An even more enduring disruption in spine formation may be involved in severe psychiatric illnesses like schizophrenia. A human gene curiously named "disrupted in schizophrenia 1" (DISC1) has been found to be altered—or mutated—in patients with schizophrenia. Researchers from Cardiff University in Wales and the US National

---

[26] Gomez J, Barnett MA, Natu V, et al.: Microstructural proliferation in human cortex is coupled with development of face processing. *Science* 2017;355:68–71.

[27] Liston C, McEwen BS, Casey BJ: Psychosocial stress reversibly disrupts prefrontal processing and attentional control. *Proc Natl Acad Sci USA* 2009;106:912–917.

[28] Soetanto A, Wilson RS, Talbot K, Un A, Schneider JA, Sobiesk M, Kelly J, Leurgans S, Bennett DA, Arnold SE: Association of anxiety and depression with microtubule-associated protein2-and synaptopodin-immunolabeled dendrite and spine densities in hippocampal CA3 of older humans. *Arch Gen Psychiatry* 2010;67:448–457.

Institutes of Health showed that disrupting *DISC1* in neonatal mice caused a decrease in spine formation and in the activity of a receptor for the neurotransmitter glutamate.[29] Deficiencies in glutamate transmission have been linked to schizophrenia and decreased spine density has been found in postmortem samples of the prefrontal cortex from people with schizophrenia and bipolar disorder.[30] While *DISC1* is only one of many genes implicated in schizophrenia, this work raises the possibility that dendritic pathology could be an important component of the illness. One study even showed that an antipsychotic medication, olanzapine, reversed dendritic spine loss in an animal model of schizophrenia.[31]

## MAKING NEW NEURONS

There is another way in which neurons in the brain may respond to experience, and this one came as quite a surprise. Classic biology textbooks tell us that, at birth, humans have all the neurons in the brain and spinal cord they will ever have. During fetal life, stem cells called *radial glial cells* rapidly divide in the developing embryo and create the central nervous system. Stem cells continue to be active in every part of the body after birth except, it was thought, the brain and spinal cord. In humans, most neuronal cell division is completed during the second trimester of pregnancy, months 4 through 6.

Unlike cells in other parts of the body—and indeed the two other types of cells in the brain—neurons in adult mammals were thought incapable of mitosis, the process by which a cell divides to form two new cells. Neurons in the brain are therefore called *postmitotic*. If you cut your skin or break a bone, skin and bone cells will divide and repair the injury. Even nerves outside of the central nervous system, like those that convey pain signals from the skin when you touch something hot, can divide and repair an injury throughout life. But sadly, if you transect your spinal cord, it cannot repair itself because the neurons on either side of the cut cannot divide and bridge the gap. The same seemed true of neurons in the brain.

Adult lizards and birds can regenerate neurons in their brains and spinal cords. In the 1980s, Fernando Nottebohm showed that songbirds grow new neurons every year in order to learn and sing new songs. Next time you call someone a "birdbrain," remember that birds, unlike humans, have this amazing capacity to regenerate their brains that humans seem to lack.

The idea that adult mammals never grow new brain cells was challenged, however, when Nazi Holocaust survivor Joseph Altman reported a startling

---

[29] Greenhill SD, Juczewski K, de Haan AM, Seaton G, Fox K, Haringham NR: Adult cortical plasticity depends on an early postnatal critical period. *Science* 2015;349:424–427.

[30] Konopaske GT, Lange N, Coyle JT, Benes FM: Prefrontal cortical dendritic spine pathology in schizophrenia and bipolar disorder. *JAMA Psychiatry* 2014;71:1323–1331.

[31] Wang HD, Deutch AY: Dopamine depletion of the prefrontal cortex induces dendritic spine loss: reversal by atypical antipsychotic drug treatment. *Neuropsychopharmacology* 2008;33:1276–1286.

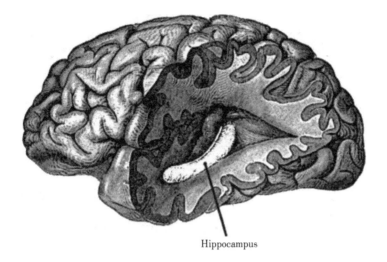

Hippocampus

**Figure 4.5** The hippocampus is shaped like a seahorse and is found buried deep inside the temporal lobe of the brain. This drawing is from Henry Gray's classic textbook *The Anatomy of the Human Body* (Philadelphia, Lea and Febiger, 1918).

Image in public domain, https://commons.wikimedia.org/wiki/File:Gray739-emphasizing-hippocampus.png

discovery: new neurons are created in a few parts of the brains of adult rats.[32] The finding immediately sparked controversy, with many prominent neuroscientists hanging on to the neuronal postmitotic idea. It took 30 years before scientists finally proved to everyone's satisfaction that new neurons are indeed born in adult brains and called the process *neurogenesis*. Then, a flurry of work made neurogenesis one of the hottest areas in neuroscience, and the details of the process became clearer. Neurogenesis in the adult brains of mammals appears mainly restricted to three regions (although there are continuous reports that it has been detected in other areas as well): the hippocampus, which is critical for learning and memory; the subventricular zone, which lines the fluid-filled spaces of the brain, called the ventricles; and the olfactory bulb, which is important for the sense of smell that is so vital for rodent survival but somewhat less important for humans (unless you work in the perfume industry).

Because of its critical role in learning and memory, the most interesting neurogenesis research has focused on a part of the hippocampus (Figure 4.5) called the *dentate gyrus*. The hippocampus is central to the consolidation of memory, including committing what we learn to long-term memory. It is also necessary for contextual memory—remembering the physical places where things we experienced happened. The hippocampus is part of a group of brain regions sometimes called the *limbic system*

[32] Altman J: Are new neurons formed in the brains of adult mammals? *Science* 2002;135: 1127–1128 (1962).; Altman J, Das GD: Autoradiographic and histological evidence of postnatal hippocampal neurogenesis in rats. *J Comp Neurol* 1965;124: 319–335.

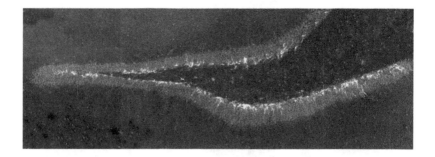

**Figure 4.6** In this section of dentate gyrus from a rat hippocampus, BrdU injected into the animal's brain before the animal is euthanized is made to fluoresce. Under a confocal microscope some of the BrdU is seen within neurons. These neurons must have been dividing in order to have been incorporated into the neuronal DNA, proving that neurogenesis has occurred.
Shutterstock.

that is very similar from rodents through primates, including humans and also plays an important role in the experience and regulation of emotion. The dentate gyrus is one portion of the hippocampus, and it is here that neurogenesis occurs throughout life in mammals including humans.

The method used to identify newly born neurons is intriguing. A type of nucleotide base, bromodeoxyuridine (BrdU), that is known to incorporate into the DNA of dividing cells, is injected into a rodent hippocampus and then made to fluoresce in brain slices. These brain slices are examined under a confocal microscope. Doing this reveals BrdU incorporated into the DNA of neurons in the hippocampus, something that can only happen if the neurons were dividing while the animal was still alive. Further studies showed that these new neurons develop into mature neurons, growing axons and dendrites and hooking up with other neurons (Figure 4.6).[33] These new neurons become part of new synaptic connections in the brain, which also entails some disrupting of existing connections. Thus, neurogenesis is also associated with forgetting[34] and has been linked to the phenomenon of *infantile amnesia*, whereby we do not have memories of our first 2 or 3 years of life.

Perhaps most striking are findings that stress and injury to the brain decrease hippocampal neurogenesis. Elizabeth Gould of Princeton University, one of the pioneers of neurogenesis research, and her group showed that disrupting previously stable social hierarchies in rat colonies led to a decrease in hippocampal neurogenesis.[35] On the other hand, exercise and enriching the environment increases the rate

[33] Van Praag H, Schinder AF, Christie BR, Toni N, Palmer TD, Gage FH: Functional neurogenesis in the adult hippocampus. *Nature* 2002;415:1030–1040.
[34] Akers KG, Martinez-Canabal AL, Restivo L, et al.: Hippocampal neurogenesis regulates forgetting during adulthood and infancy. *Science* 2014;344:598–602.
[35] Opendak M, Offit L, Monari P, et al.: Lasting adaptations in social behavior produced by disruption and inhibition of adult neurogenesis. *J Neurosci* 2016;36:7027–7038.

of neurogenesis in rodent brains.[36] And enriched environments also promote dendritic growth in newly formed neurons.[37] Because stress is such an important factor in the risk for depression and anxiety disorders, it immediately occurred to scientists that perhaps neurogenesis is suppressed in the hippocampus of patients with those conditions.

How can we tell if neurogenesis occurs in human brains? We cannot inject BrdU into a person's head and then retrieve his brain for study. At the same time, brain imaging techniques cannot see down to the level of individual cells, let alone identify those that are only recently born. An ingenious way was found, however, to prove that neurogenesis does occur in adult human brains. In 1998, Fred Gage, an eminent neuroscientist at the Salk Institute in La Jolla, California, teamed up with a group of doctors at the Sahlgrenska Hospital in Sweden to study patients with terminal brain tumors. The patients consented to have an infusion of BrdU, and, when they died, their families consented to having Gage and the Swedes remove the brains. The research team found BrdU incorporated into DNA in the dentate gyrus of the recently deceased patients, proving that neurogenesis does indeed occur in the human brain.[38] Enthusiasm was somewhat tempered in 2013, when a group of scientists used carbon dating on autopsy samples of human hippocampus to estimate the exact extent of neurogenesis. It turns out that about 700 new neurons are born in the human hippocampus every day, so that about 1.75% of neurons turn over annually.[39]

Is that seemingly small number of new neurons sufficiently robust to be a factor in stress-related psychiatric illnesses? There are two compelling reasons to believe that neurogenesis plays a role in human psychiatric illness. First, as we have already noted, stress blocks neurogenesis, and, second, antidepressant medications enhance neurogenesis.[40] Rene Hen and members of his laboratory at Columbia University showed that antidepressants like fluoxetine (Prozac) increase BrdU incorporation into the rat dentate gyrus. This group and others have also shown that antidepressants reverse depression-like behaviors in mice and other rodents. When Hen and his colleagues disabled the neurogenesis system by selectively irradiating the mouse hippocampus, however, they found that antidepressants lost that ability on depression-like behaviors.[41] These and studies like them led to the conclusion that antidepressants

[36] Nokia MS, Lensu S, Ahtiainen JP, et al.: Physical exercise increases adult hippocampal neurogenesis in male rats provided it is aerobic and sustained. *J Physiol* 2016;594:1855–1873.

[37] Alvarez DD, Giacomini D, Yang SM, et al.: A disynpatic feedback network activated by experience promotes integration of new granule cells. *Science* 2016;354:459–465.

[38] Eriksson PS, Perfilieva E, Bjork-Eriksson T, Alborn A-M, Nordborg C, Peterson DA, Gage FH: Neurogenesis in the adult human hippocampus. *Nature Med* 1998;4:1313–1317.

[39] Spalding IL, Bergmann O, Alkass K, et al.: Dynamics of hippocampal neurogenesis in adult humans. *Cell* 2013;153:1219–1227.

[40] Hanson ND, Owens MJ, Nemeroff CB: Depression, antidepressants, and neurogenesis: a critical reappraisal. *Neuropsychopharmacology* 2011;36:2589–2602.

[41] Santarelli L, Saxe M, Gross C, et al.: Requirement of hippocampal neurogenesis for the behavioral effects of antidepressants. *Science* 2003;301:805–809.

like the widely used selective serotonin reuptake inhibitors (SSRIs, including fluoxetine [Prozac], sertraline [Zoloft], and escitalopram [Lexapro]) require neurogenesis to work.[42] Coupled with findings that stress and depression are associated with decrease in the size of the hippocampus in humans,[43] and that electroconvulsive therapy for patients with depression increases hippocampal volume in synchrony with clinical improvement,[44] a great deal of excitement arose around the hypothesis that enhancing neurogenesis might be a way to treat depression in humans.

There are, however, several reasons to question the neurogenesis hypothesis. First, there is no evidence that neurogenesis occurs in the prefrontal cortex. Although learning, memory, and emotional control are obviously of great relevance to depression, patients with depression suffer from the kind of cognitive disturbances we saw earlier in Marjorie that can only be ascribed to the prefrontal cortex. It is hard to believe that a process located only in the hippocampus and involving only a very small percentage of hippocampal neurons could explain everything we see in a person with serious depression.

Second, not all studies replicate the findings of the Hen group on the relationship between antidepressants and neurogenesis. For example, one group of investigators inactivated hippocampal neurogenesis with the chemical methylazoxymethanol acetate (MAM), but this did not prevent antidepressants from blocking the behavioral effects of chronic stress.[45] Even Hen's group showed that neurogenesis is not required for environmental enrichment to reduce learning or anxiety-like behavior in rodents.[46] It may be that neurogenesis is necessary for antidepressants to work, but it is not at the root of what causes depression or necessary for relieving depression by nonpharmacological means.

Third, neurogenesis is also associated with adverse events in the brain. For example, neurogenesis occurs in the hippocampus after someone has had a stroke. Atypical-appearing neurons are born in this case, and they seem to play a role in the loss of memory after stroke.[47] Thus, we cannot assume that neurogenesis is always a positive occurrence.

[42] Samuels BA, Anacker C, Hu A, et al.: 5-HT1A receptors on mature dentate gyrus granule cells are critical for the antidepressant response. Nat Neurosci. 2015;18:1606–1616.

[43] Sheline YI, Wang PW, Gado MH, Csernansky JG, Vannier MW: Hippocampal atrophy in recurrent major depression. Proc Natl Acad Sci USA 1996;93:3908–3913.

[44] Joshi SH, Espinoza RT, Pirnia T, et al.: Structural plasticity of the hippocampus and amygdala induced by electroconvulsive therapy in major depression. Biol Psychiatry 2016;79:282–292.

[45] Bessa JM, Ferriera D, Melo I: The mood-improving actions of antidepressants do not depend on neurogenesis but are associated with neuronal remodeling. Mol Psychiatr 2009;14:764–773.

[46] Meshi D, Drew MR, Saxe M, Ansorge MS, David D, Santarelli L, Malpani C, Moore H, Hen R: Hippocampal neurogenesis is not required for behavioral effects of environmental enrichment. Nat Neurosci 2006;9:729–731.

[47] Woitke F, Ceanga M, Rudolph M, et al.: Adult hippocampal neurogenesis poststroke: More new granule cells but aberrant morphology and impaired spatial memory. PLoS One September 14, 2017; 0183463.

Finally, there is reason to question whether neurogenesis, even if it occurs to a significant degree in humans, persists into adulthood. One hint of this came from a mouse study that showed that the creation of new neurons actually depletes the supply of stem cells in the brain.[48] There might be enough stem cells to keep neurogenesis going through the short lifespan of mice, but the authors wondered if they could last through the much longer human lifespan. Indeed, in a study of 59 samples of post-mortem human hippocampus, scientists found lots of neurogenesis during prenatal life, but declining amounts through childhood. By adulthood, they could not detect any evidence of neurogenesis.[49] The human study has proven controversial and some scientists question its conclusions.

Thus, there has recently been some lowering of enthusiasm for the neurogenesis story, although it remains an active area of study, particularly in schizophrenia research.[50] By contrast, the hypothesis that dendritic remodeling, which occurs in every part of the human brain and has an important role in translating stressful life experiences into mood and anxiety disorders, remains fully in play. Picture the brain of a depressed or highly anxious person as dendritic trees shrink, dendrites pull away from synaptic connections, and dendritic spines disappear from the dendritic surface. Then think of someone like Marjorie undergoing a successful psychotherapy in which she is fully engaged with the therapist, figuring out how early life experiences influenced her emotional development, and recognizing the way her catastrophic thinking forces her to live with gloomy pessimism. Her dendrites begin to sprout again, spines reappear on dendritic surfaces in key brain areas like the prefrontal cortex and hippocampus, new synaptic connections are made. Now when her therapist points things out to Marjorie, she is fully able to make use of the new insights because her brain is "connected up" again.

Is this a simplistic, reductionistic way of looking at things? I propose instead that it is a way of understanding how a complicated process like psychotherapy induces complex changes in the brain, leading to structural changes at the cellular level that promote insight and recovery. There are many genes and hundreds of proteins potentially involved in this process. Essentially, if the dendritic remodeling hypothesis is correct, we can say that therapeutic communications induce enhanced communication throughout the brain by promoting the growth of new and strengthened synaptic connections. This seems anything but simple.

[48] Obernier K, Cebrian-Silla A, Thomson M, et al.: Adult neurogenesis is sustained by symmetric self-renewal and differentiation. *Cell Stem Cell* 2018;22:221–234.
[49] Sorrells SF, Paredes MR, Cebrian-Silla A, et al.: Human hippocampal neurogenesis drops sharply in children to undetectable levels in adults. *Nature* 2018;fff:377–381.
[50] Kempermann G, Krebs J, Fabel K: the contribution of failing adult hippocampal neurogenesis to psychiatric disorders. *Curr Opin Psychiatry* 2008;21:290–295.

# 5

## Brain Imaging
### *What We Can and Cannot See*

Doctors love new gadgets, but the excitement over this brand-new brain imaging machine exceeded the usual enthusiasm. I still remember the day on morning rounds in 1977, when I was a pediatric intern at what is now the Columbia University Medical Center. After we presented a case to our senior resident, she told us "I am going to see if we can get an M-E scan for this child." What is an "M-E scan?" we wondered.

It turns out she was referring to the brand-new computed axial tomography (CAT) machine that was then manufactured by the EMI company, the same company that made the Beatles' records in those days. The "M-E" (our way of pronouncing "EMI") scan quickly became known as the CAT scan, a revolution in radiology 40 years ago, but now a routine procedure in virtually all hospitals and many outpatient settings in the United States. Why was this such a big development?

The human brain is an extraordinarily difficult thing to study. Ordinary X-rays of the head show us almost nothing about the brain. Whenever a patient had head trauma or some neurological symptoms like a headache or weakness in a leg, we would order ordinary X-rays of the skull, which would show us if there was a skull fracture or if the brain was shifted from its proper position by some kind of mass. But ordinary skull X-rays were useless in telling us much about the many substructures of the brain and spinal cord. A CAT scan of the head, on the other hand, takes X-rays in multiple, thin slices called *tomograms*. Then, a computer puts the slices together to show the brain in three dimensions. It allows us to see things that formerly would only be apparent at surgery, like tiny brain tumors, strokes, and abnormalities in blood vessels that surround and penetrate the brain. To us in the late 1970s, the pictures of the brain taken with the CAT scanner were exquisite in their details of brain anatomy.

CAT scans are now obtained for all parts of the body, making the detection of many diseases far easier than could be made with ordinary X-rays. I've had several CAT scans of my abdomen following surgery for a gastrointestinal tract obstruction. The procedure is quick and painless and enabled my doctors to see exactly where the obstruction was in order to plan surgery at precisely the right spot.

But CAT scans are of little help to us in psychiatry. Unlike the situation with neurology, in which many diseases involve relatively large structural abnormalities like brain tumors and areas of dead or infarcted tissue that occur in a stroke, we were always pretty sure that nothing that big was the cause of depression or schizophrenia. At the level of gross anatomy—what can be seen if we look at a dissected brain with the unaided eye—the brains of people with mental illness look pretty much the same as anyone's brains. CAT scans do not reveal anything more remarkable.

## OUR PROTECTED, SEQUESTERED BRAINS

If even a new brain imaging technique like CAT scanning that yielded such exquisite pictures of brain anatomy couldn't help us understand what the brain was doing in psychiatric illness, perhaps, we hoped, we might find out something about mental illness if we looked instead at bodily fluids like blood, urine, and cerebrospinal fluid (CSF), the fluid that bathes the brain. Doctors routinely order blood and urine tests looking for abnormalities in most organs of the body. A simple blood test can reveal anemia, abnormal kidney or liver function, or even a heart attack. Urine tests are used to tell us if a patient has a bladder infection or a serious complication of diabetes. When meningitis, an infection of the lining of the brain and spinal cord, is suspected, physicians perform a lumbar puncture or "spinal tap" to obtain a CSF sample and can quickly learn if that suspicion is correct. These tests work because the organs of our body are in direct communication with the circulating blood, taking in oxygen and nutrients in exchange for carbon dioxide and waste products. Almost everything in the blood winds up getting filtered by the kidneys into the urine. Bacteria and viruses that infect the brain get swept up into the CSF along with inflammatory cells trying to eradicate them.

Almost nothing in the blood, urine, or CSF, however, turns out to be useful in telling us anything about psychiatric disorders. Psychiatrists order blood tests only when they are concerned that what seems to be a psychiatric symptom is really caused by a different medical condition. Some types of confusion, for example, can be the result of liver or kidney abnormalities, and psychotic symptoms might stem from a brain tumor. Depression is the result of abnormal levels of thyroid hormone in a case here or there. These disorders can be detected by blood, urine, and CSF samples and by X-rays and CAT scans. But, in the clear majority of cases, these diagnostics are completely normal even in people with the most severe psychiatric disturbances.

The reason for this frustrating state of affairs is called the blood–brain barrier (BBB). No organ is more important to life than the brain, and it is therefore protected behind a veritable physiological wall that carefully moderates what gets in and out. Many toxic and infectious substances that easily pass into other organs of the body simply can't enter the brain because they are too big or have the wrong electrical charge or chemical structure. Without the BBB, our brains would be vulnerable to all kinds of environmental dangers. The protection is well worth its downsides.

But those downsides are substantial. Perhaps the most problematic is that many drugs that are effective in treating diseases of organs like the lungs, heart, and liver cannot pass through the BBB and get into the brain. This includes some chemotherapy drugs used to treat cancer and some of the medications used to treat HIV infection. Primary and malignant tumors in the brain are especially resistant to drug treatment because of the BBB. The virus that causes AIDS—HIV—readily penetrates the brain, but the antiretroviral drugs that have been so successful in treating HIV-positive people often cannot follow the virus into the brain. Many strategies have been tried to loosen the BBB to medications without opening it to dangerous substances, but these attempts have so far been largely unsuccessful. An interesting development, however, may make gene therapy for brain diseases more easily accomplished. The benign viruses, called viral vectors, that are used in gene therapy to insert reparative genes into diseased cells do not readily cross the human BBB and therefore have to be given in high doses with attendant greater risks for adverse effects. Scientists have now discovered a small set of amino acids—the building blocks of proteins—that can be grafted onto the coating of these viral vectors that make it easier for them to cross the BBB and deliver a potentially curative gene.[1]

For psychiatric research, the BBB also causes problems. It is likely that what is wrong with people with illnesses like schizophrenia, panic disorder, depression, and bipolar disorder involves events that occur inside the neuron and between neurons at the synapses. In the previous two chapters, we have detailed some of those molecular and cellular events that are believed to translate stressful life events into vulnerability to mental illness. We have already noted that these molecular and cellular events are too small to be detected by CAT scans or even seen with light microscopes.

Because of the BBB, the chemicals involved in these processes—hormones, neurotransmitters, and enzymes—do not leave the brain and enter its surrounding circulating blood either. Although we can detect substances in blood, urine, and CSF like the neurotransmitters dopamine and serotonin, neurohormones like CRH and oxytocin, and some of the proteins that make neurons function, their levels in these "peripheral" bodily fluids do not exactly reflect their levels in the brain. For example, given that many antidepressants increase the amount of serotonin in brain synapses, it would be logical to speculate that perhaps depression involves abnormally low levels of serotonin. Serotonin is present in peripheral nerves throughout the body and in platelets in the bloodstream and is not terribly difficult to measure in blood, urine, or CSF. Many scientists have tried doing this, but it turns out that no one has ever found any meaningful differences in serotonin levels between depressed and nondepressed people in any bodily fluid. The amount of serotonin in blood seems to have very little to do with how much is in brain synapses: the BBB makes sure that serotonin synthesized by neurons in the brain stays in the brain.

Of course, the BBB is not a cement wall, but rather a dynamic relationship among several types of cells and proteins. As shown in Figure 5.1, capillaries throughout the body are lined by endothelial cells that permit substances to pass from the blood into various organs, but, in the brain, these endothelial cells are stitched together to form

---

[1] Blake HA, Storey CM, Murlidharan G, et al.: Mapping the structural determinants required for AAVrh.10 transport across the blood-brain barrier. *Molecular Therapy* 2017;28:510–523.

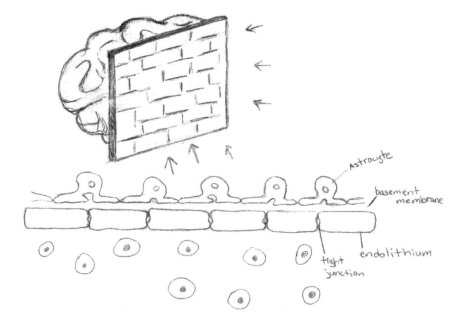

**Figure 5.1** The top of this illustration shows a brain securely protected by the wall known as the blood–brain barrier. The bottom shows what actually makes up the blood–brain barrier. A capillary in the brain (shown here at the very bottom with red blood cells flowing through) is lined by endothelial cells (endothelium) that are tied together to form tight junctions. A basement membrane further strengthens the separation between the blood and the brain. The basement membrane and endothelial cells on the blood side, together with brain cells called astrocytes that interface with them, make up the blood–brain barrier that protects the brain from exposure to toxic and infectious substances.
Illustration by Catherine DiDesidero.

what are called *tight junctions*. The arms of another brain cell type, astrocytes, surround the tight junctions, providing them with nutrients. In order to freely pass from capillary blood through the tight junctions into brain cells, substances must be very small and *lipophilic*, meaning they dissolve in fat but not in water. Alcohol is a perfect example of a small and very lipophilic molecule that easily and rapidly crosses through the BBB, explaining why we get drunk so easily. Psychiatric drugs like antidepressants are specially designed to be sufficiently lipophilic to cross the BBB, but most drugs do not have this ability.

The brain needs nutrients that circulate in the blood to function, of course. In order to get them across the endothelial cells, the BBB has a set of proteins called *transporters* that can grab selected substances that the brain needs out of the capillary blood and pull them through the tight junctions. This is how the brain gets its main source of energy, glucose, and necessary hormones like insulin. Most of the amino acids, the building blocks of proteins, must be actively transported from the blood into the brain in this manner. But there are also transport proteins that have the reverse effect and actively prevent substances from getting into the brain. These transport proteins literally pump out whatever the brain doesn't want as they try to cross the BBB. One of these "reverse" active transporters, called *P-glycoprotein*, prevents some cancer drugs from crossing the BBB.

The inability to harness blood and urine tests to help make diagnoses has been a major impediment to progress in psychiatry. Another limitation is the obvious fact that we cannot routinely obtain biopsy samples of brain tissue. When a dermatologist is unable to identify the cause of a rash, she may cut out a small sample of it and have it analyzed in the laboratory. Kidney and liver specialists can insert needles to grab samples of tissue as well. Cardiologists insert tubes into blood vessels and thread them all the way into the heart to get pictures and measure pressures in the various chambers of the heart. Only in the direst circumstances, however, do neurosurgeons attempt to biopsy the brain. Hence, we rarely have brain tissue to study from people with psychiatric illness. Postmortem samples can be used for research, but the brain quickly deteriorates after death, making obtaining them a very complicated and expensive undertaking.

Before brain imaging, psychiatric researchers resorted to several strategies to try to figure out what the brain does. In one of my own research studies, we tried to figure out what was going on in the brain by one very indirect method. In this case, we knew that when people have panic attacks—the abrupt onset of extreme fear, trembling, and heart racing that occur in patients with panic disorder, depression, and many other psychiatric disorders—they often hyperventilate. We also knew that the speed and depth at which we breathe is controlled by neurons in the lowest part of the brain, called the *brain stem*. Ordinary air that we breath has almost no carbon dioxide in it, but mixing a small amount of carbon dioxide into room air will make any individual breath very fast and very deeply. This does not bother most people, but we and others discovered that it makes panic disorder patients very anxious and often causes a panic attack. We asked patients with panic disorder to agree to breathe carbon dioxide, knowing they might have a panic attack, to enable us to study what goes on physiologically during the attacks. Then we treated them with either medication or psychotherapy and repeated the carbon dioxide breathing experiment, finding that the second time around carbon dioxide still made the patients breathe fast but no longer was capable of making them panic.[2]

By studying the response of patients and normal control volunteers to carbon dioxide breathing and making some calculations, we could speculate about what might be going on in the brain during a panic attack. This led my mentor, Donald Klein, to write a famous paper in which he proposed that patients with panic disorder have an abnormal "suffocation alarm" in the brain that can be reset by successful treatment.[3] In a classic case of a mentee trying to outmaneuver a mentor, I developed a competing

[2] Gorman JM, Martinez J, Coplan JD, Kent J, Kleber M: The effect of successful treatment on the emotional and physiological response to carbon dioxide inhalation in patients with panic disorder. *Biol Psychiatry* 2004;56:862–867.

[3] Klein DF: False suffocation alarms, spontaneous panics, and related conditions. An integrative hypothesis. *Arch Gen Psychiatry* 1993;50:306–317.

hypothesis that nevertheless also attempted to use the carbon dioxide experiments to extrapolate to how the brain was responding during panic attacks.[4] Unsurprisingly, neither of these ideas is entirely correct because they are based on a great deal of theorizing about how the brain was working when in fact we had no direct look at the brain itself.

## A NEW WINDOW TO BRAIN FUNCTION

Fortunately, brain imaging technology advanced very quickly through the last decades of the twentieth century, and our frustrations with studying living human brains seemed about to yield to two exciting new brain imaging technologies: positron emission tomography (PET) and the many varieties of magnetic resonance imaging (MRI). A great deal of the work we will be discussing in the next few chapters involves MRI scanning, but PET has provided some important insights, and we will touch on it briefly first.

When the universe was created in the Big Bang 13.7 billion years ago, two kinds of matter emerged, called *matter* and *anti-matter*. The three main components of the atom—protons, neutrons, and electrons—therefore all have corresponding anti-matter particles. Whenever a subatomic particle collides with its corresponding anti-matter particle, the two annihilate and a gamma ray is created that shoots out in both directions perpendicular to the collision path of the particles. Fortunately for us, and for entirely unclear reasons, the Big Bang created more matter than anti-matter and therefore the universe survives.

The anti-matter particle of an electron is called a *positron,* and it is the basis for PET scanning. Some radioactive compounds emit positrons. An example is a form of glucose called fluorine-18 fluorodeoxyglucose (FDG). When FDG is injected into the vein of someone having a PET scan, it travels to the brain where it is taken up by brain cells and releases positrons in proportion to the metabolic activity of the neuron. These positrons collide with electrons to form gamma rays, which are detected by sensors distributed in a circle around the individual's head. A computer then constructs a three-dimensional image of the brain that reveals which regions are the most active. FDG-PET scanning can be used to detect malignant tumors in the brain and elsewhere because they are generally more metabolically active than normal tissue.

The application of PET scanning of most interest in psychiatry involves radio-actively labeling compounds that bind to specific neurotransmitter receptors in the brain. For example, in a series of experiments, with some of which I was a collaborator, Mark Laruelle and Anissa Abi-Dargham, then both at Columbia University, used a radioactive compound, or ligand, that binds to a receptor for the neurotransmitter dopamine (the $D_2$ receptor). It has long been suspected that some of the acute symptoms

---

[4] Gorman JM, Kent JM, Sullivan GM, Coplan JD: Neuroanatomical hypothesis of panic disorder, revised. *Am J Psychiatry* 2000;157:493–505.

experienced by psychotic patients, like hallucinations and delusions, are the result of excessive release of dopamine in a brain circuit called the *mesolimbic pathway*. These investigators used PET scanning to show that, in fact, actively psychotic patients had increased release of dopamine in this pathway compared to nonpsychotic people and that the higher the level of dopamine released, the greater the chance the patient would respond to antipsychotic medications.[5] On the other hand, patients with schizophrenia who are not acutely psychotic do not show this increase in dopamine release. This work helped to secure the "dopamine hypothesis" of psychosis. More recently, a PET scan study showed that increased dopamine is present in acutely psychotic patients whether they have schizophrenia or bipolar disorder.[6] This is an important finding because it challenges our current psychiatric diagnostic system, indicating that symptoms like psychosis have a biology that cuts across our current *Diagnostic and Statistical Manual* (DSM-5) diagnostic schemes.

As another example, it was known from laboratory experiments that the commonly prescribed antidepressants called selective serotonin reuptake inhibitors (SSRIs) bind to a specific receptor that sits on the presynaptic membrane of neurons in the brain. The result of the binding of the medication to this receptor—called the *serotonin reuptake transport receptor*—is to increase the amount of serotonin in the synapse. Using PET scanning and the SSRI antidepressant paroxetine (Paxil), we visualized this phenomenon in the brains of living humans with anxiety disorders and measured the degree of binding of the antidepressant to its receptor.[7] Many other neurotransmitter receptors can be imaged in this way, including those for opioids, leading to important observations about the mechanism of action of various medications.

PET scanning is a wonderful tool, but the radioactive tracers are expensive to purchase, the equipment is costly to maintain, and the patient is exposed to radiation, which limits the number of times any individual can have a PET scan for research purposes. MRI, on the other hand, while not cheap, does not involve radiation and has become a very important technology for neuroscience research. It has also become the target of derision from some sources, as we will see.

[5] Abi-Dargham A, Rodenhiser J, Printz D, Zea-Ponce Y, Gil R, Kegeles LS, Weiss R, Cooper TB, Mann JJ, Van Heertum RL, Gorman JM, Laruelle M: Increased baseline occupancy of D2 receptors by dopamine in schizophrenia. *Proc Natl Acad Sci USA* 2000;97:8104–8109; Laurelle M, Abi-Dargham A, Gil R, Kegeles L, Innis R: Increased dopamine transmission in schizophrenia: Relationship to illness phases. *Biol Psychiatry* 1999;46:56–72.
[6] Jauhar S, Nour MM, Veronese M, et al.: A test of the transdiagnostic dopamine hypothesis of psychosis using positron emission tomographic imaging in bipolar affective disorder and schizophrenia. *JAMA Psychiatry* 2017;74:1206–1213. doi:10.1001
[7] Kent JM, Coplan JD, Lombardo I, Hwang DR, Huang Y, Mawlawi O, Van Heertum RL, Slifstein M, Abi-Dargham A, Gorman JM, Laruelle M: Occupancy of brain serotonin transporters during treatment with paroxetine in patients with social phobia: a positron emission tomography with 11C McN 5652. *Psychopharmacology (Berl)* 2002;164:341–348.

# THE MANY FACES OF MRI

Magnetic resonance imaging—the MRI scan—was developed in the early 1970s and won the Nobel Prize for its inventors. We thought the pictures of the brain taken by CAT scans were amazing, but the detail offered by an MRI scan of the brain is even better. Structural MRI scans, also called anatomical MRI scans, also allow us to see the brain in three dimensions, with excellent differentiation between tissue and fluid. Brain tumors, strokes, abscesses, and many other physical abnormalities are seen with great resolution. Neurologists rely heavily on MRI scans to confirm what they think may be going on in a patient's brain. Some old-time neurologists even complain that the new generation eschew the elegant neurological exam that was once the only way to tell where in the brain an abnormality might be; the MRI scan gives a more definitive answer to the localization question.

The brain, like the rest of the body, is mostly water, and a water molecule is made of two hydrogen atoms and one oxygen atom. When a person's head is placed in the MRI scanner tube, the scanner's powerful magnet applies a strong magnetic field that causes the nuclei of the hydrogen atoms—which are composed of one proton each—to line up and spin in neat row-like conformations. Next, the scanner sends a radio frequency wave through the protons, which causes them to flip and spin in different directions. When the field is turned off, the protons gradually return to the previously aligned spin. Protons in different types of tissue return to that spin, or relax, at different speeds, a process called *precession*. Precession sends out radio signals at different frequencies that detectors in the scanner can measure and turn into 3D images, like the one shown in Figure 5.2. The magnets in an MRI machine come in different strengths and are measured in units called the *Tesla* (T). Most of the work I did involved 1.5 T MRI magnets, but today 3.0 T magnets are in general use in research, and some centers have 7 T magnets. Even a 1.5 T magnet is thousands of times stronger than the earth's magnetic field. (Don't go near an MRI machine with credit cards in your pocket: they will be erased.) In general, the stronger the magnet, the greater the resolution of the images created by the MRI scanner. To my eye, modern MRI scans of the brain using high-strength magnets are worthy of museum exhibits. They are just beautiful.

Another very attractive feature of MRI scanning is that, unlike CAT scans, MRI does not involve radiation. This means that it is safe to obtain MRI scans as many times as needed, either for clinical or research purposes. There are a few limitations to MRI scans, however. They are generally more expensive than CAT scans, take a longer period of time than a CAT scan requires, and make more noise. Some people are claustrophobic of being in the narrow MRI tube, listening to the banging noise for prolonged periods of time. In clinical medicine, there is no question that MRI scanning is overused: every person complaining of a headache or back ache seems to get one, even though in these situations they rarely show anything that affects how a patient is actually treated. Cutting down on the rampant overuse of MRI scans is one of the most important strategies to bring the cost of US healthcare down from its ridiculous heights.

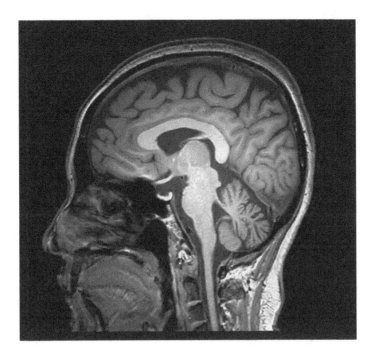

**Figure 5.2** A magnetic resonance imaging (MRI) scan showing structural details of the human brain.
Shutterstock.

Structural MRI scans have proved to be of some, albeit limited, value in psychiatric research. Few mental health conditions affect the gross size, volume, or shape of brain structures, but there have been a few important findings. Patients with schizophrenia have enlarged fluid-filled spaces of the brain, called *ventricles*, although the differences between them and people without schizophrenia are subtle and not useful for diagnostic purposes. Still, the finding of enlarged ventricles in schizophrenia was one of the first pieces of evidence linking the illness to physical abnormalities in the brain and suggesting that the problem is most likely linked to abnormal brain development rather than loss of brain tissue, called *atrophy*, later in life. Atrophy of the brain is seen in the various types of dementia, like Alzheimer's disease, but, by the time this can be seen on a structural MRI scan, it is usually already obvious that the patient is suffering from dementia.

Studies consistently show that men have larger brain volumes than women, but this structural MRI finding turns out to be of limited value. The largest structural brain imaging study ever done, involving 2,750 women and 2,466 men, showed that although the male brain was a bit bigger than the female brain, there is a great deal of overlap between men and women, and, when other factors were controlled for, the differences became unimpressive.[8] While the study has some intriguing findings, the bottom line

[8] Ritchie SJ, Cox SR, Shen X, et al.: Sex differences in the adult human brain: evidence from 5,216 UK Biobank participants. *bioRxiv beta* https://doi.org/10.1101/123729

is that if you look at a structural MRI of a person's brain, there is no way to tell if it's male or female.

In the next chapter, we will discuss functional abnormalities in the brains of people who are excessively fearful, but it is worth noting that a recent study showed that people with high levels of anxiety have smaller volumes of a part of the brain called the *inferior frontal cortex*, located right behind the temples.[9] Smaller inferior frontal cortex volume was associated in this study with a bias to view things with a negative tinge. While there are many possible ways to interpret a finding like this, one speculation is that people born with smaller inferior frontal cortex volumes are less able to suppress the more primitive parts of the brain that evolved to alert us to dangerous situations. Such individuals are therefore prone to see everything as a potential threat.

Another series of structural MRI studies I find interesting was discussed by Kimberly G. Noble, a neuroscientist at Columbia University's Teachers College, in her article in *Scientific American*. Studies show that children raised under adverse conditions have smaller brain volumes than children raised under better conditions. "We found," Noble explains, "that both parental educational attainment and family income were associated with differences in the surface area of the cerebral cortex" (p. 47).[10] She describes work from other laboratories showing that "less supportive and more hostile parenting appears to lead to worse outcomes—in this case, a smaller hippocampus" (pp. 48–49). While brain scans cannot be used to discern retrospectively who was affected by such adverse parenting during childhood, this kind of work makes clear that environmental influences affect physical brain growth. As a diagnostic tool for psychiatry, structural MRI is not useful. But as a tool to demonstrate the importance of early childhood environments, it is invaluable.

## IMAGING THE LIVING, FUNCTIONING HUMAN BRAIN

Despite a few promising insights from structural MRI studies, psychiatric researchers reasoned that it is more likely mental illnesses involve abnormalities in how the brain functions than in its absolute size, shape, or volume. An analogy might be to think of type 1 or juvenile-onset diabetes, in which the pancreas fails to make insulin. A structural MRI scan of the pancreas of someone with type 1 diabetes looks normal. The abnormality occurs at the level of cells that function abnormally. In diabetes, we can measure levels of glucose and insulin by simple blood tests and infer that the pancreas is not functioning normally. As we have already said, blood tests are not helpful in understanding psychiatric disease, so is there a way to test the function of different parts of the human brain?

[9] Hu Y, Dolcos S: Trait anxiety mediates the link between inferior frontal cortex volume and negative affective bias in healthy adults. *Soc Cogn Affect Neurosci* 2017;12:775–782.
[10] Noble KG: Brain trust. *Sci Am* March, 2017, 45–49.

The answer to this question comes from a variation on structural MRI scanning that has revolutionized psychiatry, psychology, and neuroscience—functional magnetic resonance imaging (fMRI). When a structure or region of the brain is activated, its metabolic demand increases abruptly, and the circulatory system responds by increasing blood flow selectively to that part of the brain. Hemoglobin is the molecule in the blood that carries oxygen; tissues extract oxygen from hemoglobin to meet their metabolic needs, and this turns hemoglobin from its oxygenated state, called *oxyhemoglobin*, to its deoxygenated state, called *deoxyhemoglobin*. It turns out that deoxyhemoglobin has greater magnetic resonance than oxyhemoglobin, so that as oxygenated hemoglobin rushes to an activated brain area and displaces deoxygenated hemoglobin, the strength of the magnetic resonance signal changes. An MRI scan can pick up on the relative change in magnetic resonance as oxygenated blood rushes to an active brain region and is turned into deoxyhemoglobin and thus show us what parts of the brain are activated on a moment-to-moment basis.

The computer programs that analyze fMRI data divide the brain into three-dimensional boxes called *voxels* that are a few millimeters in each direction. There are around a million neurons in each voxel.[11] Changes in activity can be localized with great resolution to specific subregions of the human brain. Scientists have become increasingly sophisticated at administering special tasks to people while in the scanner to understand how different emotions, thoughts, and sensory processes affect activity levels of different parts of the brain. For example, if we show people pictures of frightening scenes like houses burning or people with injuries, we can see the amygdala lighting up on the fMRI scan. If we show people disgusting pictures, another part of the brain lights up, the anterior insula. Doing complicated math activates parts of the prefrontal cortex. Functional MRI scans can show how a task activates a circuit in the brain or how, in response to a task, one brain region suppresses the activity of another. Functional maps of brain activity have been made for a wide range of emotions, cognitive processes, and tasks, and we even have a functional map of the parts of the brain that are active when we are given a specific task but just day dreaming, the so-called *default network*. Figure 5.3 shows an example of fMRI in which a color-coded map indicates exactly which structures in the brain have been activated during a specific task.

A good example of the kind of insights into brain function that fMRI can give us for use in psychiatry is a recent study in which investigators attempted to elucidate subtypes of depression based on brain activation patterns. We know that depression is not just one illness; one patient we diagnose with depression may be anxious, have trouble sleeping, and lose weight because of no appetite. Another with the same depression diagnosis may be sleeping all the time, overeating, and too slowed down to worry about anything. Treating these patients is largely trial and error: we know

[11] https://blogs.scientificamerican.com/observations/whats-a-voxel-and-what-can-it-tell-us-a-primer-on-fmri/

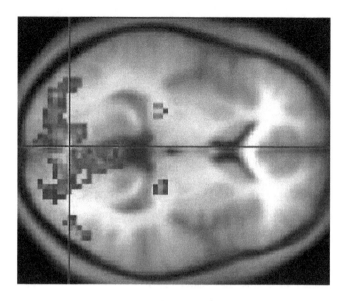

**Figure 5.3** A functional magnetic resonance imaging (fMRI) scan. The areas of the brain shown in color have been activated compared to other parts of the brain. In this case, the colored regions are in the back (posterior) part of the brain, corresponding to the occipital lobe. This part of the brain is activated whenever we see something. In this manner, functional maps of brain activity can be made for a wide range of emotions, cognitions, and sensory processes.

From *Textbook OpenStax Anatomy and Physiology*, Published May 18, 2016, https://cnx.org/contents/FPtK1zmh@8.25:fEI3C8Ot@10/Preface

that antidepressant medications and some psychotherapies like cognitive behavioral therapy (CBT) work equally well, so which should we pick first? And if we decide to start with antidepressant medication, which one of the many drugs is the patient most likely to respond to? If we had some objective way of distinguishing among different types of depression, we might make headway in knowing beforehand where to start treatment.

In fact, scientists from a consortium of medical centers obtained fMRI scans from 1,885 patients with depression—a remarkable feat given the difficulty in recruiting patients to studies like this and of synchronizing analyses of scans obtained from so many different MRI machines—and found they could identify four distinct subtypes based on the pattern of connections among brain regions.[12] The subtypes also predicted response to at least one type of treatment for depression, called *transcranial magnetic stimulation* (TMS). The investigators point out that these depression subtypes could not have been figured out just on the basis of different symptom patterns. We also must say that any study, no matter how exciting, needs to be replicated before we take it too seriously. But this one clearly has the potential

---

[12] Drysdale AT, Grosenick L, Downar J, et al.: Resting-state connectivity biomarkers define neurophysiological subtypes of depression. *Nature Med* 2017;23:28–38.

to advance our ability to diagnose and treat patients with depression. And, as we will see in the next chapter, the findings fit in well with theories about abnormal brain connections as a cause of depression.

## CAN MRI SCANS READ OUR MINDS—YET?

Chapter 6 will include some very fascinating fMRI findings, but fMRI is not without controversy. Some of these concerns involve the technical details of image acquisition and data analysis.[13] The field was in a flutter not long ago when a Swedish research team concluded that three software packages commonly used to analyze fMRI are highly prone to false positives.[14] Not all scientists agree with that conclusion, but it is always smart to be cautious when reading a paper involving fMRI imaging for several reasons.

First, there are some questions about exactly how closely coupled brain activity is to blood flow. There is a lag time between activation of a brain region and increase in blood flow to that area, and even though that lag may be less than 1 second, it can still cause problems for experiments in which different pictures are shown to the experimental subject in a rapid sequence. Remember also that we can change our thoughts in much less than a second. Furthermore, there are a few instances in which the increase in blood flow to a region is not accompanied by a proportional increase in neural activity and vice versa.[15]

Second, motion by the subject, including breathing, causes *artifact*, which can be dealt with using mathematical corrections but can still distort the fMRI picture. Also, different tasks or emotions often activate overlapping brain regions. Sometimes, for instance, a paper might report that a particular task activates "areas of the brain known to be involved in decision-making under conditions of uncertainty." This sounds great, except that only the day before we read a paper in which a completely different task activated the very same brain structures, only that time the regions involved were described as "areas of the brain known to be involved in discriminating important from unimportant stimuli." In other words, fMRI conclusions sometimes sound like that adage of the man who throws darts against a blank wall and then draws bull's-eyes around the places where each dart falls.

Third, fMRI studies are challenging to perform. It takes a big grant to do them because the scans are expensive. Some people find the confinement in the MRI tube and all the noise the machine makes too uncomfortable and either refuse to participate or demand the study be stopped before all the data are collected. For these reasons, fMRI studies tend to involve small numbers of subjects who are not necessarily

[13] Miller G: Brain scans are prone to false positives, study says. *Science* 2016;353:208–209.
[14] Eklund A, Nichols TE, Knutsson H: Cluster failure: why fMRI inferences for spatial extent have inflated false-positive rates. *Proc Natl Acad Sci USA* 2016;113:7900–7905.
[15] O'Herron P, Chhatbar PY, Levy M, Shen Z, Schramm AE, Lu Z, Kara P: Neural correlates of single-vessel haemodynamic responses in vivo. *Nature* 2016;534:378–382.

representative of the general population.[16] These problems make the results some-what unstable and have led to an inability to replicate some published fMRI studies.

Even the most distinguished neuroscientists have their concerns about overinterpreting MRI scans in psychiatric research. In a penetrating article on the limitation of brain imaging, Daniel Weinberger—one of the great psychiatric researchers of our time—and Eugenia Radulescu, his colleague at Johns Hopkins University School of Medicine, pointed to a host of potential confounders that bedevil the interpretation of brain scan data. "The overarching purpose of this cautionary note," they wrote, "is to encourage a discussion about a widely and tacitly recognized, though mostly ignored, 'inconvenient' truth: that conventional MRI does not allow us to make firm inferences about the primary biology of mental disorders and that we need to acknowledge this as a starting point in realizing the full value of MRI studies in psychiatry" (p. 28).[17]

Weinberger and Radulescu are particularly concerned about "resting-state" fMRI studies in which no task is given to the imaging subject. Instead, the subject is told to try to think about nothing. We all know that telling someone to think about "nothing" is an invitation to obsess about everything. If I say or write, "don't think about your breathing," the audience or readers are then obligated to think about every breath they take for the next few moments.

Let's take another kind of concern that I worried about when involved in imaging research. Imagine that two people are asked to have a resting-state fMRI for a research project, one with a diagnosed anxiety disorder and the other a control subject with no history of psychiatric illness. The two are told to think of nothing during the scan, and they do their best. We find a big difference in brain activation patterns between the two—the anxious patient has an increase in amygdala activity let us say—and we ascribe that to the anxiety disorder itself. But what we don't know is that the anxious patient had terrible headaches as a child and a pediatric neurologist, fearing her patient might have a brain tumor, ordered an MRI scan. The child found the whole procedure of having an MRI scan traumatic. Now, years later, being placed in the same tube activates unconscious memories of the headaches, the fear of serious illness, and the frightening MRI scan she had as a child. The difference between the two subjects in the research study may reflect a traumatic memory in one and not the biology of an anxiety disorder after all. In other words, we cannot control for the myriad of different memories and emotional states that people bring into the scanner, all of which can add uncontrolled artifacts to the data.

There are also policy and philosophical worries about brain imaging, including concerns that fMRI will be used to make critical decisions about people's lives, even though the science is not yet strong enough to justify doing so. A fascinating recent

---

[16] LeWinn KZ, Sheridan MA, Keyes KM, Hamilton A, McLaughlin KA: Sample composition alters associations between age and brain structure. *Nat Commun* 2017 8:874.

[17] Weinberger DR Radulescu E: Finding the elusive psychiatric "lesion" with 21st-century neuroanatomy: a note of caution. *Am J Psychiatry* 2016;173:27–33.

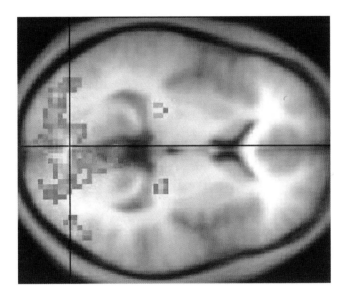

**Figure 5.3** A functional magnetic resonance imaging (fMRI) scan. The areas of the brain shown in color have been activated compared to other parts of the brain. In this case, the colored regions are in the back (posterior) part of the brain, corresponding to the occipital lobe. This part of the brain is activated whenever we see something. In this manner, functional maps of brain activity can be made for a wide range of emotions, cognitions, and sensory processes.

From *Textbook OpenStax Anatomy and Physiology*, Published May 18, 2016, https://cnx.org/contents/ FPtK1zmh@8.25:fEI3C8Ot@10/Preface

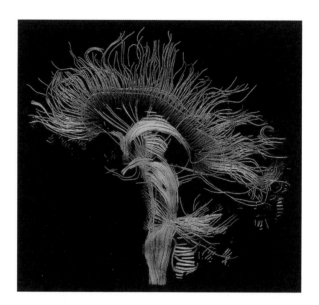

**Figure 5.5** Visualization of a diffusion tensor imaging (DTI) measurement of a human brain. Depicted are reconstructed fiber tracts that run through the mid-sagittal plane. Especially prominent are the U-shaped fibers that connect the two hemispheres through the corpus callosum (the fibers come out of the image plane and consequently bend toward the top) and the fiber tracts that descend toward the spine (blue, within the image plane).

Image from Thomas Schultz. Courtesy of Gordon Kindlmann at the Scientific Computing and Imaging Institute, University of Utah, and Andrew Alexander, W. M. Keck Laboratory for Functional Brain Imaging and Behavior, University of Wisconsin-Madison.

paper, for example, showed that it may be possible to tell whether people commit illegal acts on purpose or impulsively without making a conscious choice to do so. A team of researchers from Vanderbilt, Virginia Tech, and Yale Universities asked 40 volunteer subjects to decide whether they would carry a suitcase across a checkpoint, varying the probability in the simulation that one of the suitcases contained illegal drugs and that there would be a guard present to search the suitcases. The subjects therefore had more certainty in some of the scenarios than others whether a suitcase did or didn't have contraband in it. They obtained fMRI scans from the subjects as they made their choices and showed distinct differences in the pattern of brain region activation between choices made "knowingly"—that is, when the subjects could be certain whether they were choosing to carry suitcases with illegal drugs in the— versus "recklessly."[18] While the study is quite impressive, it is worrisome that it could be interpreted as providing an actual tool for courtroom use. Deciding whether a criminal acted out of cold, calculating deliberateness or reckless impulsivity is crucial for determining penalties but is an extremely difficult task for juries. Having an objective tool to guide making such decisions would be great, but this study involved 40 carefully picked, presumably noncriminal volunteers given a simulated situation and imaged at exactly the moment they made their choices. This is nowhere near ready for use in deciding any convicted criminals' fate, but one wonders how long it will take for lawyers to clamor for their clients' brain scans to be entered into evidence. As federal judge Jed S. Rakoff puts it "the point is that neuroscience is at a stage where it may be able to provide helpful insights to the general development of the law, but not much, if anything, in the way of evidence about individuals in particular cases" (pp. 31–32).[19]

Julia Gottwald and Barbara Sahakian mull this kind of problem over in their book *Sex, Lies, and Brain Scans: How fMRI Reveals What Really Goes on in our Minds.*[20] They point out that fMRI scans can reveal that a person is lying with greater accuracy than traditional lie detectors. But, they note, the fMRI scanner cannot tell that a delusional person who thoroughly believes he committed a crime actually did no such thing or that a criminal who truly believes he is innocent is in fact guilty. Clearly, fMRI is not ready for routine courtroom use.

Even more contentious are claims that fMRI can reveal the neural basis for human characteristics like empathy and altruism. An important study showed that the strength of connections between three brain regions, the anterior cingulate cortex (ACC), anterior insula (AI), and ventral striatum (VS), can distinguished whether altruistic acts are made because subjects expected something in return (reciprocity) or

---

[18] Vilares I, Wesley MJ, Ahn W-Y, et al.: Predicting the knowledge-recklessness distinction in the human brain. *Proc Natl Acad Sci USA* 2017;114:3222–3227.

[19] Rakoff JS: Neuroscience and the law: don't rush in. *New York Review of Books*, May 12, 2016, p. 30–32.

[20] Gottwald J, Sahakian B: *Sex, Lies, and Brain Scans: How fMRI Reveals What Really Goes on in our Minds.* Oxford, Oxford University Press, 2017.

because they identified with the suffering of another person (empathy). The authors of the study stated:

> Motives are purely mental constructs that are not directly observable. Here we show, however, that distinct motives have a distinct neurophysiological representation in the brain. Although the empathy and the reciprocity motive increase the frequency of altruistic acts by the same amount relative to the baseline condition, they are associated with different patterns of brain connectivity that enabled us to predict the different motives with relatively high accuracy. (p. 1078)[21]

What a remarkable statement! It is not hard to discern altruistic acts. Every time we see someone drop coins in a homeless person's cup or help a stranger with a disability cross the street, we witness them. But how do we know the motives behind such acts? We may not even know our own motives when we act with altruism. Did I put that coin in the cup because I really feel for the plight of homeless people or because it makes me feel like a good person? Was I unconsciously hoping that someone would see me help the disabled person and think "what a nice guy he is to do that?" Now we are told that we can stick a person's head in the MRI scanner and readily distinguish among these different motives. To some, that represents substantial scientific progress, but to others it seems to make the very essence of "humanness" subject to technology and computers. The motives behind our actions are fundamental aspects of each individual's human character, not something into which we necessarily want a machine to delve.

Similarly, we like to think that many things go into making one person "smarter" than the next, including genetics, social environment, and education. What does it mean, then, when an MRI study shows that IQ is related to how densely connected are the major "hubs" in the brain between different regions?[22] Can we interpret this finding as meaning that "mere" structural aspects of how our brains are connected determine how intelligent we are?

Brain imaging is quickly moving to areas beyond understanding how the brain functions in health and disease. The technology has been used in studies that purport to show differences in brain regional activity between people who have a "high level of moral reasoning" and those at a lower level[23] and even to predict how people will respond to crowdfunding appeals, a use of brain imaging referred to as "neuroforecasting."[24] One commentator in *Scientific American*, a PhD candidate, went

---

[21] Hein G, Morishima Y, Leiberg S, Sul S, Fehr E: The brain's functional network architecture reveals human motives. *Science* 2016;351:1074–1078.

[22] Seidlitz J, Vasa F, Shinn M, et al.: Morphometric similarity networks detect microscale cortical organization and predict inter-individual cognitive variation. *Neuron* 2018;97:231–247.

[23] Fang Z, Jung WH, Korczykowski M, et al.: Post-conventional moral reasoning is associated with increased ventral striatal activity at rest and during task. *Sci Rep* 2017;7:7105.

[24] Genevsky A, Yoon C, Knutson B: When brain beats behavior: neuroforecasting crowdfunding outcomes. *J Neurosci* 2017;37:8625–8634.

so far as to sound the alarm that the use of technologies like brain imaging may lead to "brainjacking."[25] Marcello Lenca calls for steps to "protect all of us from harmful manipulations of our neural activity through the misuse of technology."

Some of these reservations seem to reflect more fear of a new technology than a true understanding of what brain imaging can do and how it works. In his book *Against Empathy*, Yale psychologist Paul Bloom issues a familiar complaint: "Nowadays, many people only seriously consider claims about our mental lives if you can show them pretty pictures from a brain scanner. . . . There is a particular obsession with localization, as if knowing where something is in the brain is the key to explaining it" (pp. 59–60).[26] Bloom does not give any data to support this statement: How many people is he complaining about, and to what extent do these people "only consider" brain imaging data to be the sole important reflections of human mental life? While it is true that the images generated by brain scans are often elegant, to dismiss them as "pretty pictures" seems a bit cavalier. They are, as I have explained, the result of some quite remarkable advances in physics and engineering, enabling us to visualize the details of brain structure and function with previously unimaginable resolution. Nor is it accurate to say that any serious neuroscientist thinks that simply identifying the location in brain where something happens is sufficient to explain how the brain works. This book is, in part, all about explaining the many levels at which neuroscientists look to understand brain function, from molecules to cells to structures. Bloom is falling victim to the "reductionist" fear that somehow brain imaging is part of a neuroscientific conspiracy to take all the mystery out of the human mind.

Still, he is identifying a concern that all of us must be vigilant about: overselling what brain imaging can do. It is clearly premature to say that brain imaging can tell who is really selflessly altruistic or telling the real (as opposed to subjective) truth or even who is a man or woman. We must go very slowly in inferring brain function from brain scans.

Despite these reservations, it is very clear that fMRI has enabled us to trace important patterns of brain activity and make inferences about the way the brain develops in children and adolescents, how the brain works when we are frightened or feeling pleased, and some of the abnormalities in brain function in disorders like depression and obsessive compulsive disorder. Ever-evolving advances in the sophistication of MRI machines, in the statistical techniques used for analyzing brain imaging data, and in study design have progressively lessened the negative impact of confounds like movement artifact and emotional state that hamper fMRI interpretation. In Chapters 3 and 4, we observed some of the ways in which life's experiences affect the brain on the molecular and cellular level, respectively. In Chapter 6, we will have the opportunity to see how brain imaging research, mostly involving fMRI, allows us to see life's experiences affecting the way brain regions function and connect with each

[25] Lenca M: The right to cognitive liberty. *Sci Am* August 2017, 10.
[26] Bloom P: *Against Empathy: The Case for Rational Compassion*. New York, HarperCollins, 2016.

other. In discussing this research, I will concentrate on findings that have been persistently replicated and seem robust against the many technical challenges to fMRI integrity enumerated earlier. And I will stay clear of research purporting to tell us anything about our deepest motivations and belief systems. We New Yorker Yankee fans assume that Boston Red Sox fans have much smaller brains than ours, but we will leave that kind of speculation for another day.

Before delving into the way the brain is connected, I want to mention two other MRI variants that are important in psychiatric research, *diffusion tensor imaging* (DTI) and *magnetic resonance spectroscopy* (MRS).

## ALMOST LIKE A BIOPSY

In Chapter 4, we paid considerable attention to the dendrite, the tree-like appendages on neurons that receive input signals from the axons of presynaptic neurons. We barely mentioned the axons themselves, however, even though they are responsible for conducting neuronal signals over long stretches of territory. Neurons have many dendrites, but each neuron generally has only one axon, which may travel many feet to its targets. These targets are either the dendrites of the next neuron across a synapse, muscle fibers, or glands. Axons are what we refer to as nerves or nerve fibers. An important feature of about 80% of axons is a fatty coating around them called *myelin*. The myelin sheath, produced by a type of glial cell called the *oligodendrocyte*, insulates the axon and thereby increases the speed of electrical conduction through it (see Figure 5.4). Multiple sclerosis (MS) is the most common form of demyelinating disease in which the myelin sheath is stripped off the axons, resulting in markedly slowed neural conduction and a variety of neurological consequences.

The human brain is incompletely myelinated at birth, which explains in part why newborn babies cannot walk or talk. During the first 2 years of life, there is a massive increase in myelination of brain tracts, thus increasing the speed of neural conduction and connecting brain regions to each other and to muscles and organs throughout the body. As you watch a baby learn to grasp objects, sit-up, crawl, and finally walk you can picture myelin being laid down along axons in her brain, hooking up the brain regions that coordinate movement to the muscles in hands and legs. After age 2, the speed of myelination slows but is not complete until late adolescence or even early adulthood. It may be that the speed of adolescent brain fiber myelination partly determines how quickly a teenager develops mature judgment and values. A good reason not to try teenage offenders as adults is that their brains have not yet sufficiently myelinated to give them an adult's ability to make sound judgments.

Myelin has a whitish appearance and therefore the parts of the brain composed of myelinated nerve tracks are called *white matter*. The parts of the brain that contain neurons, their dendrites, and other cells have a pinkish-gray appearance and are therefore called *gray matter*. White matter tracts connect the gray matter regions of the brain. The fibers in white matter lie in parallel to each other, like cables in long-distance electrical power wires. DTI uses a combination of magnetic signals and complicated mathematical calculations to measure the integrity of the white matter fibers.

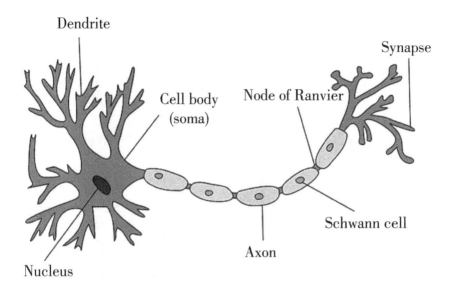

Dendrite

Synapse

Cell body (soma)

Node of Ranvier

Nucleus

Axon

Schwann cell

**Figure 5.4** A cell body, or soma, on the left of this image, has a long axon that looks something like a chain of sausages. The axon is surrounded by a myelin sheath that has indentations or gaps called Nodes of Ranvier. On the right side of this image, the axon terminates in several branches, which then form synapses with dendrites on another neuron, with a muscle fiber or with cells in a gland. In multiple sclerosis (MS), the myelin sheath is attacked by immune cells, causing demyelination and slowing of the speed and efficiency of the neuron's electrical conduction system.
From Quasar Jarosz at English Wikipedia.

DTI images like the one shown in Figure 5.5 provide beautiful pictures of white matter tracts in the brain. Jeremy Coplan and I, working with colleagues at Mount Sinai School of Medicine and the State University of New York, Downstate Medical School, used DTI to show that connections between brain regions are disrupted in monkeys who were exposed to very early life stress.[27] DTI can show the massive disruption of axons in patients with severe MS. It can also show the relative strength of axonal connections between gray matter regions as brains develop. Finally, there are some psychiatric conditions in which disruptions of brain connectivity may play a central role. Abnormalities in white matter integrity may play an important role in schizophrenia, for example, and DTI is being used to define the extent of these disruptions.

A final variant of MRI for us to consider is MRS. Some chemical metabolites in brain tissue have distinctive magnetic frequency signals that can be detected with MRS. Instead of giving a picture of the brain, MRS yields a spectral graph that shows the relative concentrations of these chemicals in different regions of the brain. It is

[27] Coplan JD, Abdallah CG, Tang CY, Mathew SJ, Martinez J, Hof PR, Smith EL, Dwork AJ, Perera TD, Patnol G, Carpenter D, Rosenblum LA, Shungu DC, Gelernter J, Kaffman A, Kackowski A, Kaufman J, Gorman JM: The role of early life stress in development of the anterior limb of the internal capsule in nonhuman primates. *Neurosci Lett* 2010;480:93–96.

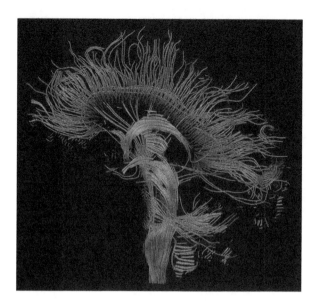

**Figure 5.5** Visualization of a diffusion tensor imaging (DTI) measurement of a human brain. Depicted are reconstructed fiber tracts that run through the mid-sagittal plane. Especially prominent are the U-shaped fibers that connect the two hemispheres through the corpus callosum (the fibers come out of the image plane and consequently bend toward the top) and the fiber tracts that descend toward the spine (blue, within the image plane).

Image from Thomas Schultz. Courtesy of Gordon Kindlmann at the Scientific Computing and Imaging Institute, University of Utah, and Andrew Alexander, W. M. Keck Laboratory for Functional Brain Imaging and Behavior, University of Wisconsin-Madison.

something like what would happen if scientists could get a little piece of brain tissue from many different sites in a living human brain and put the pieces into a chemical analyzer. It is almost as if we could biopsy the brain.

But not quite: only a few chemicals give robust enough signals for the MRS technique to identify and measure, and these are not necessarily the ones in which we are most interested. One of them is called *N-acetyl aspartate* (NAA), which is believed to represent the integrity of neurons. Reductions in NAA concentration may mean that a specific part of the brain is undergoing a loss of function. MRS is sometimes used to help evaluate certain brain tumors and infections.[28] My research group reported some interesting findings with MRS in both our monkeys who had been exposed to early life stress[29] and humans with generalized anxiety disorder.[30]

---

[28] Gujar SK, Maheshwari S, Bjorkman-Burtscher I, Sundgren PC: Magnetic resonance spectroscopy. *J Neuroophthalmol* 2005;25:217–226.

[29] Coplan JD, Mathew SJ, Abdallah CG, et al.: Early-life stress and neurometabolites of the hippocampus. *Brain Res* 2010;1358:191–199.

[30] Mathew SJ, Mao X, Coplan JD, et al.: Dorsolateral prefrontal cortical pathology in generalized anxiety disorder: a proton magnetic resonance spectroscopic imaging study. *Am J Psychiatry* 2004;161;1119–1121.

MRS has not yielded the kind of information that fMRI or even DTI have for psychiatric researchers, but I mention it because it is likely that, in time, it will become more sophisticated and able to measure concentrations of chemicals in the brain in which we are more interested, like neurotransmitters and neurohormones. The important thing to remember about brain imaging is that it is developing at a very rapid pace. The magnets used for MRI keep getting bigger and stronger and the resolution of the images sharper.

The kind of brain imaging that scientists use to probe emotions, cognitive tasks, and sensory perception is a relatively new technology and will surely get better and better. It is true that what it can do is frequently exaggerated. We cannot read minds with fMRI or see neural signals travel down a nerve fiber bundle with DTI. All these techniques require that we make assumptions about how the signal is being generated and that we use complicated computer algorithms to turn the signals into pictures. Hence, those who complain that we have gone too far in interpreting brain function based on PET and fMRI scans are not entirely wrong.

It is going too far, however, to liken brain scanning to phrenology, as some have done. Sahakian and Gottwald nicely put that canard to rest when they write "when scientists use language carefully and keep the vast complexity of the brain in mind, fMRI is far from phrenology. It can reveal new and intriguing information about the human brain."[31] If we apply some caution and skepticism, then, it is clear that PET and MRI have given us some incredible new insights into brain function. In the next chapter, we will discuss how these insights lift us from the level of molecules and cells to that of whole-brain structures as they respond to the environment and communicate with each other. I will try my best not to exaggerate the meaning of these findings, but I hope you will also agree that there is a great deal about which to be enthused.

[31] Gottwald J, Sahakian B: *Sex, Lies, and Brain Scans: How fMRI Reveals What Really Goes on in Our Minds*. Oxford, Oxford University Press, 2017, p. 122.

# 6

## Making Connections
### *Where Does Fear Come From?*

The Brain—is wider than the Sky
For, put them side by side,
The one the other will include
With ease, and you beside—
—Emily Dickinson

Close your eyes and wave your arms around and around. No matter how fast you do that, you know exactly where your arms are at every moment. Signals that tell our brains the positions of our muscles in space are among the fastest neural impulses transmitted by the nervous system, with speeds exceeding 250 miles per hour. Other signals are slower. If you touch a hot stove, you will withdraw your hand instantaneously, but there is a delay before you actually feel and record the pain. Even slower are our thoughts: those neural signals travel at a relatively sluggish 50 miles an hour. None of this comes close to the speed of electricity, and it is not surprising that computers can do calculations faster than we can, but the image we have of neural signals buzzing around our brains is definitely accurate.

Our brains are always active, even when we sleep. Without the constant barrage of external stimuli, sleep allows us to consolidate memories from the day. You have surely found that you are more likely to remember things you experienced during the day if you get a good night's sleep. While awake but not engaged in a specific task, a group of brain regions called the *default network* is nevertheless active, allowing us to daydream and reflect on our own thoughts. Neural signals are always traveling from one neuron to the next and from one part of the brain to another, traveling over roads comprised of axons and dendrites, carrying messages that may be conscious or unconscious, some trivial and some novel.

In Chapter 4, we saw how neurons in the brain extend and retract dendrites to make and disrupt connections with other neurons. In Chapter 5, we further explained that each neuron has a single axon that conducts neural impulses, often over great distances, to dendrites extending from another dendrite. Between the tips of an axon from one neuron and the protrusions called spines on dendrites from another neuron, there is an empty space called the synapse that the neural impulse traverses by means of chemical messengers called neurotransmitters.

You can think of a neural impulse carrying a piece of information as a traveler moving along an axon who suddenly comes upon a gap in the road. The traveler requests the assistance of a neurotransmitter to transport him across the gap, or synapse, and together they dock on a receptor sitting on the membrane of a dendritic spine on the next neuron. The traveler can then continue his journey along the dendrite to the new neuron's cell body and then down another axon. These neural impulses can be tracked and measured in the laboratory by placing electrodes right into the axons, cell bodies, and dendrites of neurons in living animals or preparations of neurons extracted from an animal's brain. Neurologists do this with their patients when they perform tests called *electromyograms* (EMGs) and *nerve conduction studies* detect abnormalities in the way peripheral nerves and muscles handle neural signals. Another technique, the *electroencephalogram* (EEG), involves placing electrodes on the scalp that detect electrical signals emitted from the brain. Abnormalities in these signals can help diagnose neurological conditions like epilepsy.

## A LITTLE—VERY LITTLE—BRAIN ANATOMY

At first glance, the organ that houses all this remarkable activity may not seem up to the task. The human brain looks fairly unimpressive at first when it is examined in the medical school neuroanatomy lab. The average adult brain weighs only about 3 pounds and is around 6 inches long. It is gray in color, with grooves called sulci and bumps called gyri, giving it a wrinkled appearance. Of course, that little 3-pound organ packs in more than 80 billion neurons, and those grooves and bumps increase the surface area of the brain (see Figure 6.1), giving us more space to make connections among all those neurons, more than a trillion of them.

The nervous system is built for communication, both internally and with the outside world. The pathways that permit the latter are mostly well-understood. When we see something, for instance, the light that bounces from the object to our eyes causes a chemical reaction in neurons that sit in the back of the eye, the section called the *retina*. The retina turns the light image into electrical signals that are transmitted via the optic nerve all the way to the back of the brain, a section called the *occipital lobe*. There, the signals are processed to tell us what it is we are looking at, its shape and color, and its relationship to objects around it. That signal is then sent to other parts of the brain that tell us whether we have seen the object before, what significance it has, and whether an action is required. Finally, the image is consolidated into a memory. Similar pathways turn what we hear, touch, and smell into electrical signals that travel to other parts of the brain for interpretation and storage. The regions of the brain that process external stimuli are highly specialized to perform these functions, and damage to one of them disrupts only its specific sensory pathway. Thus, damage to the occipital lobe impairs vision but does not affect hearing or smell, whereas damage to a part of the temporal lobe of the brain affects hearing but not vision.

Other regions of the brain are similarly specialized to perform specific functions. The largest part of the human brain, the cerebral cortex, is the outermost layer and

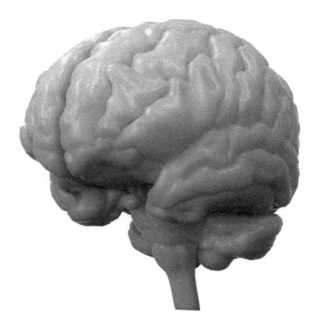

**Figure 6.1** The human brain weighs only about 3 pounds and is about 6 inches long. The large section with the grooves and bumps is the cerebral cortex. Each brain has two nearly identical cerebral cortices, the right and left hemispheres. In most people, including most left-handed people, the left hemisphere is "dominant." In this model, the basal ganglia are shown underneath the front of the cortex, but it is really located deep in the middle of the brain. The cerebellum protrudes from the back of the brain, underneath the cortex. The brain stem connects the brain to the spinal cord. Shutterstock.

is divided into four lobes (see Figure 6.2). An area in the frontal lobe, traditionally called *Broca's area*, is required for speech production, whereas an area in the temporal lobe, traditionally called *Wernicke's area*, enables us to understand the speech of others. Although these terms are considered outdated, students are still taught that damage to Broca's are renders a person unable to speak but still able to understand what others say, whereas damage to Wernicke's area has the opposite effect. Unlike most other specialized areas, which are represented on both sides of the brain, Broca's and Wernicke's areas are found on only one side of the brain, usually the left.

We know about these specialized brain areas mostly because damage to them knocks out a specific function. Before brain imaging became as sophisticated as it is today, neurologists determined where in the brain a problem existed, like a stroke or tumor, by figuring out which of a patient's functions were disturbed. If the patient could not move the right hand, this meant that the lesion must be somewhere in the pathway that starts in a region on the left side of the brain that controls right-hand movement (many pathways that start on one side of the brain cross to the other side of the body before reaching their targets) and then progresses down the spinal cord to the right arm and hand. If the patient could not see, the pathway from the eye to the optic nerve to the occipital lobe's visual center must be involved. Medical students

# HUMAN BRAIN ANATOMY

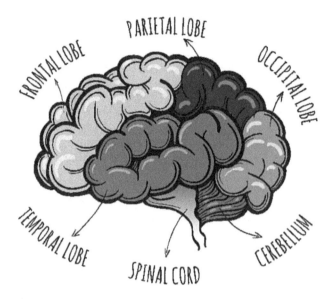

**Figure 6.2** The cerebral cortex of the brain is divided into four lobes: frontal, parietal, occipital, and temporal. The cerebellum, located under the cerebral cortex, is critical for coordination of movement and several cognitive functions. The brain stem is the bulging structure underneath the temporal love in this drawing, connecting the brain to the spinal cord. The brain stem is further subdivided into the midbrain, the pons, and the medulla oblongata.

Shutterstock.

thus learned brain anatomy by memorizing which functions of the body derive from which brain regions. Neurologists often know exactly where in the brain a tumor is located before getting the results of an MRI scan by examining the patient and determining what functions have been lost.

We now know, however, that mapping functions to specific areas of the brain tells us only one part of the brain communication story. Many of the things we do depend on complicated interactions among multiple brain regions. Our ability to pay attention to something, to experience emotions like love and fear, and to make decisions based on new and old information cannot be mapped onto a single brain region but rather require intact connections between parts of a region and among several regions. These regions are found in subdivisions of the lobes of the cerebral cortex and of other parts of the brain such as the basal ganglia, cerebellum, and brain stem. The brain imaging techniques we described in the previous chapter, especially functional magnetic resonance imaging (fMRI), enable us to visualize connections in living human brains and show us which networks are active when we are not thinking of anything special, when we are angry or performing an altruistic act, or when we are listening to a recording of a newborn baby crying. Because these things involve thought and emotion, it is no surprise that multiple brain regions are involved and that disruptions of connections among them can cause abnormalities in the way we think and feel. Every human being has his or her own, unique set of connections among brain regions, called the *functional connectome*. We inherit the basic blueprint of the connectome from our parents, and therefore some of what makes us individuals is implanted in how our brains are hooked up at birth.[1] Upon this basic blueprint, however, our subsequent life experiences shape and alter brain connections so that they ultimately reflect both what we are born with and what we experience. Imaging studies are now able to elucidate how the connectome works in both normal brains and in the brains of people with a wide array of mental illnesses. A compelling example is work that shows the way connections between brain regions grow during early childhood to permit the acquisition of important developmental cognitive milestones.

## CONNECTIONS FORM AS BABIES DEVELOP

Just as infants learn to sit up and walk, they also must master certain critical forms of perception and awareness. One of these is called *theory of mind* (ToM), our ability to understand that other people have their own thoughts that are independent from ours. Between 3 and 4 years of age, children develop ToM and first realize that other people's thoughts and minds can be different from theirs. ToM is necessary for our ability to function in social groups; without it, we would be effectively socially isolated. It turns out that it is the maturation of a connection between two parts of the brain between ages 3 and 4 that allows ToM to develop. The arcuate fasciculus is one of the white matter fiber bundles, composed of myelinated axons, that runs through the brain. It connects a region in the back of the temporal lobe called the *precuneus* and a region in the frontal lobe, the prefrontal cortex. An fMRI study showed that the maturation of this connection accompanies the development of ToM capability in young children.[2]

Here we have both a powerful example of the way connections between brain regions are required for complex cognitive abilities and of the use of a brain imaging technique, in this case fMRI, to delineate them. Scientists are now slowly piecing together how many different aspects of infant and early childhood development follow directly on the maturation of connections between regions in the brain. As dendrites sprout and myelin is laid down around axons, connections in the baby's brain develop and the speed of neural transmission increases. Because this happens at different rates among individual babies, the acquisition of new talents varies; some walk at 10 months and others at 14 months. Boasting about a baby's early development or worrying about later development is usually pointless; sooner or later, the requisite brain connections are made, and, except for rare exceptions, all of us learn to walk.

---

[1] Miranda-Dominguez O, Feczko E, Grayson DS, Walum H, Nigg JT, Fair DA: Heritability of the human connectome: a connectotyping study. *Netw Neurosci* November 2, 2017.
[2] Wiesmann CG, Schreiber J, Singer T, Steyinbeis N, Friederici AD: White matter maturation is associated with the emergence of Theory of Mind in early childhood. *Nat Commun* 2017;8:14692.

In Chapter 5, we also discussed some of the limitations of brain imaging. One way to give us more confidence in what we see on an fMRI scan is to detect the same pathways at work in the brains of laboratory animals. We can monitor the activity in networks during specific activities in mice and rats in several ways that we cannot with humans. Electrodes can be placed at specific spots in the rodents' brains and recordings made of which neurons fire during specific activities. We can disrupt pathways in the animals' brains with surgery or drugs and then see what happens. Or we can use some marvelous techniques in mice that involve knocking out or activating genes in specific pathways to see which ones are required for which functions. Most recently, scientists use a new technique called *optogenetics*. Developed by Karl Deisseroth and colleagues at Stanford University, optogenetics involves using genetics to insert proteins into neurons in specific pathways in a living animal's brain that are activated or deactivated by shining light at specific wavelengths on them. Investigators can therefore precisely control a selected neuronal group in a specific part of the brain by shining light on the animal's head and then seeing whether activating or deactivating different pathways results in changes in the animal's behavior. When the results of these laboratory experiments in animals fall in line with results from human brain imaging studies, we believe we can say that a specific set of pathways in the human brain is specifically activated during a specific task.

The limitation here, of course, is that mice and rats cannot perform many of the tasks that humans do, nor do we know a lot about rodents' emotional life. If we are interested in understanding how the brain works when we read something—of great interest to scientists who study reading problems in children—we can easily stick humans into the MRI machine, ask them to read from texts on projected images, scan their brains while they read, and study the resulting fMRI pictures. Obviously, none of the basic neuroscientist's most sophisticated tools will ever enable us to know what brain regions a rat activates when he or she reads a book.

Similarly, we may want to study why some people respond more strongly to an infant's cries than do others. We can play recordings of babies crying while imaging the brains of new mothers and fathers and determine with sophisticated psychological instruments how much they were disturbed by the crying. Exactly how much emotion a mouse attaches to its pups crying is much harder to determine.

We therefore will focus for now on examples of human behavior and emotion that can be modeled with some degree of accuracy in rodents so that we can reasonably correlate what happens in their brains to what happens in ours. It turns out that one emotion has been very instructive in this endeavor: fear.

## FEAR AND THE LABORATORY RAT

It is hard to know what prelinguistic human infants or animals other than humans think about or feel, but certain things seem intuitive. We know that babies and pets feel pain when they get an injection. A dog withdraws its paw from a hot object in the same way that we pull our hand away, and we can reasonably assume the dog feels the pain of the hot object in the same way that we do. In fact, such an inference is still an assumption: we don't know for sure whether the dog feels the pain sensation exactly as we do. The dog cannot describe its sensations to us, but from it actions, vocalizations, and facial expressions it is a very good assumption that physical pain is the same sensation for dog, cats, babies, and adult humans.

Fear comes in many varieties for us. We experience very primitive fears, like the startle sensation we exhibit when we hear a sudden, unexpected loud noise or the reaction we have when we first see a rattlesnake in a cage at the zoo. Fear of snakes and spiders is present in 6-month-old infants and seems to be of evolutionary origin.[3]

We also have more complicated fears, like whether we are studying hard enough for a test or saving enough money for retirement. The primitive ones tend to involve responses to immediately present stimuli whereas the complicated ones often involve things that will happen in the future. When there is a real threat, we say the fear is "rational" or "adaptive." Jumping when we hear a sudden bang or getting scared at first when we see a snake are evolutionarily determined and reflexive responses shared by all animals (except snakes themselves, I suppose). It is also perfectly reasonable to have fears about our future condition. Without the fear of failing or being destitute, who would study for a test or save money for retirement? Fear, of course, is a motivating factor that ensures that we avoid things that are dangerous and make sensible plans for future contingencies.

We say that fears are "irrational" or "maladaptive" when they exceed the severity of the threat, when no real threat is present, or when they interfere with our lives. Once you know the snake is in the cage in the zoo and can't get to you, it becomes less reasonable to fear it. We stop jumping when we realize the loud noise is just the clanging of the pipes as the heat comes up. People who get scared even of pictures of snakes have a snake phobia. People who jump at every little noise are, well, jumpy. A student who studies hard and gets good grades but lives in constant fear that she is going to flunk out of school clearly has excessive worries. A 25-year-old who contributes to her company's pension plan but nevertheless can't sleep at night worrying that she will be broke when she is 70 similarly has a problem.

Fear is a component of most psychiatric illnesses, including, but not limited to, those we call anxiety disorders. Patients who worry constantly to the point that they are miserably unhappy all the time have generalized anxiety disorder. People who have repetitive, sudden outbursts of intense fear, heart pounding, inability to breathe, and sweating have panic disorder. Phobias are fears and avoidance of things that aren't really dangerous. When a person has panic attacks every time she is with other people or must speak up at a meeting for work, we might diagnose social anxiety disorder.

Patients with depression fear they have done something terrible, even when they haven't; patients with schizophrenia may have paranoid delusions and fear that others are trying to harm them; patients with anorexia nervosa fear they are fat when they are in fact emaciated; and patients with posttraumatic stress disorder (PTSD) avoid

---

[3] Hoehl S, Hellmer K, Johansson M, Gredeback G: Itsy bitsy spider . . . infants react with increased arousal to spiders and snakes. *Front Psychol* October 18, 2017.

otherwise innocuous places that remind them of the scene in which the original traumatic event occurred. Fear is a ubiquitous symptom for mental disorders, and therefore researchers would like to know what is going on in the brains of people who seem needlessly and excessively afraid.

We have learned a lot, as we will see, from fMRI and positron emission tomography (PET) scan studies about connections among brain regions that are activated when humans are fearful, but we would feel much more secure about these findings if we had an animal model with corresponding brain activation patterns. We know that rats aren't concerned about SAT scores or retirement funds, but can we develop an animal model that is useful for understanding the anatomy and biology of an emotion like fear? And does the biology of fear in the animal match in any way the biology of human fear?

The very idea of studying the biology of any human emotion in a rodent might seem far-fetched, so it took a genius to figure out how to do it. Joseph LeDoux (Figure 6.3), a neuroscientist at New York University, pioneered research that has immeasurably advanced our understanding of how fear works. In doing so, he stimulated the work of countless other scientists, including many who study humans. Perhaps no other area in neuroscience demonstrates so clearly the power of using an animal model to help focus human research. LeDoux should win the Nobel Prize for his seminal research.

In the laboratory, rats are smart and cooperative. If you put one in a special cage and play some loud tones, the rat will look toward the source of the noise and continue doing whatever it had been doing. But if you give the rat a small electric shock right

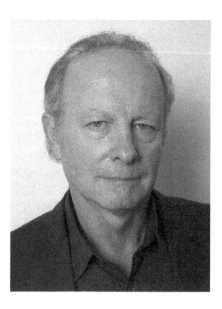

**Figure 6.3** Neuroscientist Joseph LeDoux, Center for Neural Science, New York University. LeDoux has revolutionized the study of emotion with his seminal studies of the biology of conditioned fear.

Image obtained from Dr. LeDoux.

after one of those loud noises, it will suddenly freeze in place. Its heart rate, respiratory rate, and blood pressure zoom up, and its adrenal glands pour out the rat version of the human hormone cortisol, called *corticosterone*.[4] After a few seconds, the rat begins to move around again. But now, if you play the loud tone again—without the shock— the animal immediately freezes and all the physiological changes again occur. For the rest of its life, the tone alone will cause this reaction, even if the rat never receives another electric shock. We call this phenomenon *classical* or *Pavlovian conditioning*. The shock is the unconditioned stimulus (UCS) because the rat freezes without ever having experienced it before. The tone is the conditioned stimulus (CS) because the rat only freezes when the tone is associated with a shock. Freezing and the physiological changes are the conditioned responses (CR).

LeDoux wondered if he could determine the brain pathways that are necessary for conditioned fear to occur in a rat. Using electrophysiology (placing recording electrodes directly into the animal's brain), lesion studies in which a selected area or fiber tract is destroyed, and other techniques, LeDoux and his laboratory co-workers traced the flow of information that begins with the rat hearing the loud tones after it has undergone *fear conditioning*. The message is relayed from the rat's ears to a structure called the *auditory thalamus*, which is a kind of processing center for what we hear and many other sensations, and then to an almond-shaped structure buried in the temporal lobe called the amygdala (Figure 6.4).[5] The amygdala is part of what some anatomists called the limbic system of the brain, a broad grouping of structures involved in emotional responses and memory. Although the designation "limbic system" may no longer be precise enough for anatomical purposes, it is still used to describe a network in the brain that is fairly consistent in size, shape, and function from lower mammals all the up through monkeys, apes and humans.

The amygdala is itself comprised of several subsections. Information from the auditory thalamus first enters the amygdala through its lateral nucleus (LA) and is then transferred to the central nucleus (CA). Like humans, mice and rats differ in their baseline or trait levels of anxiety. Highly anxious mice have stronger propagation of neural signals from the LA to the CA than do less anxious mice.[6] From the CA, fear information is transferred to regions of the brain directly responsible for the various parts of the conditioned fear response. An area of the brain stem called the *periaqueductal gray area* (PAG) turns the amygdala signal into freezing; when the hypothalamus and other

[4] In humans, cortisol is the predominant hormone released by the adrenal gland during a fear response. The rat adrenal also synthesizes cortisol, but the related hormone corticosterone is more abundant. They are both members of a class of chemicals called glucocorticoids. We refer to cortisol throughout to refer to any glucocorticoid released by the adrenal gland in response to fear, threat, or stress.

[5] LeDoux J: *The Emotional Brain: The Mysterious Underpinnings of Emotional Life*. London, Weidenfeld & Nicolson, 1997; LeDoux J: Emotional circuits in the brain. *Ann Rev Neurosci* 2000;20:155–184.

[6] Avarbos C, Sotnikov SV, Dine J, Markt PO, Holsboer F, Landgraf R, Eder M: Real-time imaging of amygdalar network dynamics in vitro reveals a neurophysiological link to behavior in a mouse model of extremes in trait anxiety. *J Neurosci* 2013;33:16262–16267.

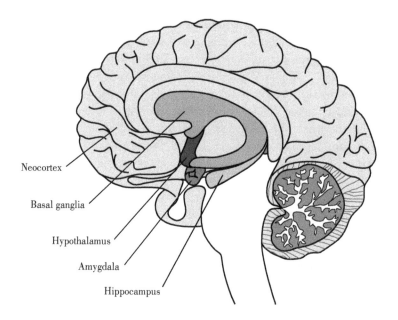

**Figure 6.4** The amygdala is shown in its place deep in the brain, adjacent to the hippocampus on one side and the basal ganglia on the other. It has connections to all the other brain regions shown here. The portion of "neocortex" shown here is the same as the prefrontal cortex.
Shutterstock.

parts of the brain stem get the information, it provokes the increase in vital signs like heart rate, breathing, and blood pressure; transfer from the CA to the hippocampus and hypothalamus causes the release of the brain hormone corticotrophin releasing hormone (CRH), which results in the adrenal glands increasing release of cortisol into the peripheral blood.

CRH is synthesized and released by the hippocampus when an animal is exposed to stressful situations. In Chapter 3, we reviewed work by Jeremy Coplan, Leonard Rosenblum, and me in which we showed that when female monkeys with young infants are exposed to uncertainty about their source of food, their infant offspring grow up to be anxious and to have elevated levels of CRH. Ned Kalin, a psychiatrist and neuroscientist at the University of Wisconsin, Madison, and his team injected the gene that encodes CRH directly into the amygdala's of five young rhesus monkeys and showed that these animals developed an anxious temperament compared to monkeys that did not undergo the gene insertion procedure.[7] Thus, our work and Kalin's paint an interesting picture of early life stress leading to overstimulation of the CRH system, hyperactivity of the amygdala, and chronic anxiety.

---

[7] Kalin NH, Fox AS, Kovner, et al.: Overexpressing corticotropin-releasing factor in the primate amygdala increases anxious temperament and alters its neural circuit. *Biol Psychiatry* 2016;80:345–355.

This, then, is one brain circuit relevant to fear: auditory thalamus to amygdala to hypothalamus, hippocampus, and brain stem. If the amygdala is damaged in the laboratory rat, it will still freeze when it gets an electric shock but never learn to associate a tone (or anything else) with the shock and therefore cannot be fear-conditioned. If the connection between the CA and the PAG is lesioned, the rat can be successfully fear-conditioned, and its heart rate and blood pressure will go up when it hears the tone, but it will not freeze when the tone is sounded. LeDoux has called this pathway the "low road" because it is automatic, fast, and unconscious.

We can imagine this low road of fear transmission occurring in any of us during a sudden threat like an impending car crash. If you have ever been driving a car and suddenly realized that another car is about to smash into you, this situation will seem all too familiar. You suddenly feel a wave of fear come over you when you recognize a crash is inevitable, and events happen in a whiz until you feel and hear the impact. You are at least emotionally dazed for a few moments, so that everything seems unreal. Then you begin to return to reality. You can still feel your heart pounding and realize you are gasping for air. You feel terrified and wonder why you didn't brake harder or swerve more forcefully to avert the crash. But, in fact, you were frozen in place, unable to take any meaningful action in the split seconds before impact. In this situation, you are no different from the laboratory rat who is hearing the tone that reminds it of the shock. There is laboratory evidence to support the existence of the "low road" pathway in the human brain that rapidly, but crudely, sends threat signals to the amygdala.[8] A study of two patients with a rare genetic condition called *Urbach-Wiethe syndrome,* in which calcium deposits develop in the amygdala on both sides of the brain and disrupt its function, showed that they had reduced anxiety-like behavior, as if they had been given an antianxiety drug like chlordiazepoxide (Librium).[9]

The "high road," by contrast, involves transmission of the signal from the auditory thalamus to the prefrontal cortex and then to the amygdala. This adds a conscious element to the fear experience, and, the more developed the prefrontal cortex, the more opportunity there is for the conscious brain to modify how we respond to a frightening experience. The next time you approach the intersection where that car running through the stop sign hit you, you have more than just a wave of fear. This time, you recall the crash and say to yourself, "I know I have the right of way here and the other guy has the stop sign, but I am going to slow down anyway just in case there is another idiot in a hurry." Fear, in this case, is processed by your prefrontal cortex, and, instead of freezing, you take a sensible, protective action. Synchronized electrical oscillations between the prefrontal cortex and the amygdala are necessary for many aspects of fear

[8] Mendez-Bertolo C, Morati S, Toldeano R, et al.: A fast pathway for fear in human amygdala. *Nature Neurosci* 2016;19:1041–1049.

[9] Korn CW, Vunder J, Miro J, Fuentemilla L, Hurlemann R, Bach DR: Amygdala lesions reduce anxiety-like behavior in a human benzodiazepine-sensitive approach-avoidance conflict test. *Biol Psychiatry* 2017;82:522–531.

processing and expression. Scientists can stimulate this pathway using the technique of optogenetics and induce fear in laboratory animals.[10]

The human prefrontal cortex receives and sends messages to the amygdala. It records what the amygdala finds fearful for future use. Under some circumstances, the prefrontal cortex can suppress amygdala activity and reduce fear and anxiety. This happens, for example, when we use our reasoning capacities and decide that something that frightened us is not really a threat. Stimulating a portion of the prefrontal cortex in humans with a technique called transcranial magnetic stimulation (TMS) reduced response to fearful stimuli in one study.[11] There is evidence that genetic variations between people are associated with different levels of activation of the inner or medial portion of the PFC (mPFC) when fear cues are presented. Those who have inherited one genetic variant have stronger mPFC responses, less amygdala response, and less fear than those who have inherited a different genetic variant.[12] Also, individuals with a thicker mPFC seem to inhibit fear more readily after extinction training.[13] It seems that the powerful human prefrontal cortex can override the automatic fear response generated by the amygdala and that some people are naturally more adept at this than others. What animal correlates do we have for this phenomenon?

We have no way of knowing what rats think when they hear the tone that has become a CS and makes them freeze, but we can see their prefrontal cortex in action in another part of the fear-conditioning process. Fear of a conditioned stimulus like a loud tone can be extinguished if the CS is presented repeatedly without any UCS, in the present case without any shock. Eventually, the rat learns that the tone and shock are not paired and stops freezing to the tone. A direct connection from the rat's mPFC to its amygdala (see Figure 6.5) is required for conditioned fear extinction to occur.[14] If we disrupt the pathway of nerve fibers from the mPFC to the amygdala, even repeated presentations of the tone without the shock fails to extinguish conditioned fear: the rat will still freeze when it hears the tone no matter how many times it is played without an accompanying shock. A fascinating aspect of conditioned fear extinction is that it does not erase the original conditioned fear memory. Instead, extinction creates a new memory—tone and shock are not paired—that exists in the amygdala alongside the original memory—tone and shock are paired—essentially forever.[15] For a time after

[10] Karalis N, Dejean C, Cahudun F, et al.: 4-Hz oscillations synchronize prefrontal-amygdala circuits during fear. *Nat Neurosci* 2016;19:605–612.

[11] Notzon S, Steinberg C, Zwanzger P, Junghofer M: Modulating emotion perception: opposing effects of inhibitory and excitatory prefrontal cortex stimulation. *Biological Psychiatry Cognitive Neuroscience and Neuroimaging.* 2018;3:329–336.

[12] Tupak SV, Reif A, Pauli P, et al.: Neuropeptide S receptor gene: Fear-specific modulations of prefrontal activation. *Neuroimage* 2013;66:353–360.

[13] Hartley CA, Fischl B, Phelps EA: Brain structure correlates of individual differences in the acquisition and inhibition of conditioned fear. *Cereb Cortex* 2011;21:1954–1962.

[14] Quirk GJ, Garcia R, Gonzalez-Lima F: Prefrontal mechanisms in extinction of conditioned fear. *Biol Psychiatry* 2006;337–343.

[15] Quirk GJ, Pare D, Richardson R, Herry C, Monfils MH, Schiller D, Vicentric A: Erasing fear memories with extinction training. *J Neurosci* 2010;30:14993–14997.

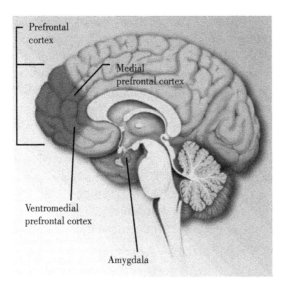

**Figure 6.5** This image shows the brain as we see it when it is cut in half and we look at the inside surface. We see the ventromedial prefrontal cortex (vmPFC), the part of the prefrontal cortex located in front (ventral) and in the middle (medial) of the brain. Also shown is the amygdala. These two brain structures can inhibit activity of each other.

From the National Institute of Mental Health.

the extinction protocol is accomplished, the new memory dominates the old and the animal no longer freezes when it hears the tone. But, over time, this can change. The original fear memory can spontaneously recover its dominant position. And if the animal is exposed to acute stress, including receiving an electric shock, freezing to the tone is reinstated. This is believed to be what happens when a patient with a phobia, like fear of heights, is successfully deconditioned by guided exposure to higher and higher places until the phobic fear is extinguished. At some point after the successful behavioral therapy, the patient may relapse, perhaps because of some new stressful life experience, and the original fear of heights once again dominates the more recently acquired extinction of fear. We have more to say about this in Chapter 8.

The amygdala has become famous in popular culture as the "seat of fear" in the brain, but, as usual when we are delving into neuroscience, things are more complicated. The amygdala is also activated by pleasurable stimuli.[16] We needn't worry here about how the amygdala accomplishes this feat of responding to both positive and negative events. Our point in this chapter is to show how the amygdala fits into a network of connected brain regions that mediate the emotion of fear in animals and humans. Activity in the prefrontal cortex inhibits the amygdala[17] and

[16] Douglas A, Kucukdereli H, Ponserre M, et al.: Central amygdala circuits modulate food consumption through a positive-valence mechanism. *Nat Neurosci* 2017;20:1384–1394.
[17] Rosenkranz JA, Moore H, Grace AA: The prefrontal cortex regulates lateral amygdala neuronal plasticity and responses to previously conditioned stimuli. *J Neurosci* 2003;23:11054–11064.

vice versa.[18] When fear signals are especially strong, the amygdala dominates and the mPFC is relatively silent, but, over time, the mPFC can regain its status and inhibit the amygdala's automatic fear-inducing properties. The balance between these two structures is delicate and varies from situation to situation and among individuals. One study, for example, showed that people with suicidal thoughts have a prefrontal cortex that is relatively disconnected from other parts of the brain, perhaps representing an inability to assert reason over emotion.[19] On the other hand, in one study stimulating the PFC with TMS reduced anxiety and avoidance among patients with height phobia (acrophobia) during behavioral therapy.[20] Thus, the more scientists can learn about how the mPFC interacts with other brain regions, the more we can understand how normal fears develop and what goes wrong in the brains of people with fear-based psychiatric illnesses.

The mPFC and the amygdala are not the only connected brain regions involved in conditioned fear, however.

## LOCATION, LOCATION, LOCATION

Let's go back a moment to the original fear-conditioning protocol. Fear conditioning is accomplished by placing the mouse or rat into a specialized, box-like chamber. Once the animal is conditioned to freeze to the CS, in this case a loud tone, you can put it back into the original chamber a day or more later and then, even without playing the tone, the animal freezes. In this case, the animal has a memory for the place or context in which fear conditioning occurred. This is called *contextual conditioning*, and it turns out to be dependent on activity in a part of the brain adjacent to the amygdala called the hippocampus (see Figure 6.4).[21]

We discussed the hippocampus in Chapter 4 because it is one of the few sites in the adult mammalian brain where neurogenesis—the birth of new neurons—can occur. The hippocampus is critical for many aspects of memory and is one of the first parts of the brain to degenerate in patients with Alzheimer's disease. If the connection between the amygdala and the hippocampus is severed, a rat can acquire conditioned fear but not contextual fear. That is, it will learn to freeze to a tone that has been paired with a shock but not when placed back into the conditioning chamber. A specific group of neurons in the hippocampus fire whenever an animal is placed in a naturally fear-provoking environment, like an open field for a mouse or rat (or the

[18] Garcia R, Vouimba R-M, Baudry M, Thompson RF: The amygdala modulates prefrontal cortex activity relative to conditioned fear. *Nature* 1999;402:294–296.

[19] Just MA, Pan L, Cherkassy VL, et al.: Machine learning of neural representations of suicide and emotion concepts identifies suicidal youth. *Nat Hum Behav* October 30, 2017.

[20] Hermann MJ, Katzorke A, Busch Y, et al.: Medial prefrontal cortex stimulation accelerates therapy response of exposure therapy in acrophobia. *Brain Stimul* 2017;10:291–297.

[21] Foster JA, Burman MA: Evidence for hippocampus-dependent contextual learning at postnatal day 17 in the rat. *Learn Mem* 2010;17:259–266.

Boston Red Sox' field, Fenway Park, for me most likely).[22] Furthermore, neurons in the hippocampus involved in contextual fear have the unusual property of "double projection."[23] A neuron generally has only one axon that carries its electrical signals away from the cell body toward the next neuron with which it forms a synapse. The axons of hippocampal contextual fear neurons, however, bifurcate, with one branch going to the amygdala and the other to the mPFC. Thus, whenever a contextual fear trigger is presented to the fear-conditioned animal, neurons that have encoded the memory of the association between context and shock (UCS) fire and simultaneously stimulate both the amygdala and the mPFC, causing a coordinated behavioral response.

The fear-conditioning network now has three brain structures in it: amygdala (acquisition), mPFC (extinction), and hippocampus (context), but there are more. If the rat in the conditioning chamber is given some control over its fate, say, having access to an escape hatch so it can run out of the chamber when the tone is sounded, the neural signal is rerouted. It still travels from the ear to the auditory thalamus and then to the lateral nucleus of the amygdala, but now, instead of being transferred to the central nucleus and then to the brain stem, hypothalamus, and hippocampus, it is rerouted from the lateral nucleus to another part of the amygdala, the basal nucleus, which doesn't project to the brain stem. Instead, the neural signal is sent to a completely different part of the brain, the striatum. The result is that when the tone is subsequently sounded, the animal freezes less because it has learned it can escape without a shock, even if the escape option is no longer made available.[24] In laboratory animals, optogenetic stimulation of the circuit from the amygdala to the striatum during fear extinction reduces the return of fear that often occurs at some point after extinction has been accomplished.[25]

We will have occasion to talk a great deal more about the striatum in Chapter 7 because it is part of what is sometimes referred to as the "reward pathway" of the brain. But it also plays a key role in movement. It is contained within the structures collectively called the *basal ganglia* (see Figure 6.4), part of which is the site of the degeneration that causes Parkinson's disease.

This ability to reroute the fear signal when an active escape option is provided figures into our ideas about how some forms of psychotherapy work. In 2001, shortly after the World Trade Center terrorist attacks on September 11, Joe LeDoux

[22] Jimenez JC, Su K, Goldberg AR, et al.: Anxiety cells in a hippocampal-hypothalamic circuit. *Neuron* 2018;97:670–683.

[23] Kim WB, Cho J-C: Synaptic targeting of double-projecting ventral CA1 hippocampal neurons to the medial prefrontal cortex and basal amygdala. *J Neurosci* 2017;37:4868–4882.

[24] Cain CK, LeDoux JE: Escape from fear: a detailed behavioral analysis of two atypical responses reinforced by CS termination. *J Exp Psychol Anim Behav Process* 2007;33:451–463.; Boeke EA, Moscarello JM, LeDoux JE, Phelps EA, Hartley CA: Active avoidance: neural mechanisms and attenuation of Pavlovian conditioned responding. *J Neurosci* 2017;37:4808–4818.

[25] Correia SS, McGrath AG, Lee A, Graybiel AM, Goosens KA: Amygdala-ventral striatum circuit activation decreases long-term fear. *Elife* 2016;pii: e12669.

and I published an editorial in the *American Journal of Psychiatry* titled "A Call to Action: Overcoming Anxiety Through Active Coping."[26] In the article, we wondered whether what we know about the neurobiology of active coping could be applied to interventions to help people with psychological wounds from the 9/11 trauma. "In practice," we wrote, "the approach suggested from the laboratory studies requires that patients develop strategies that enable them to 'do something' whenever they are entertaining dysphoric thoughts or are avoiding necessary or meaningful activities" (p. 1955). Writing this piece with LeDoux figured importantly in the development of my ideas about the neurobiology of experience and psychotherapy, and I will come back to these points in Chapter 8. It was the beginning of my reflecting on how psychologists who use behavioral therapy techniques like exposure might be rerouting their patients' neural circuits, strengthening useful ones like those from the mPFC to the amygdala and from the amygdala to the striatum and weakening harmful ones like the one from the amygdala to the brain stem.

We still have one more brain structure to add to the fear network, and this arises from a laboratory that has also done seminal work in the basic science of fear. Michael Davis, now at Emory University, measures "fear potentiated startle" instead of freezing in his laboratory to quantify the strength of the response to a conditioned fear stimulus. Exposure to a sudden, unexpected tone will elicit a startle response in rat and human alike. If that tone has been paired with a truly aversive stimulus like an electric shock, then subsequent tones will enhance the startle response. Rats will jerk their legs when they hear a sudden tone, and this jerking is "potentiated" if the tone has been previously paired with a shock. Similarly, humans will blink when an unexpected loud tone sounds, and the eye blink is even more forceful if that tone has been previously paired with a shock. Davis and his colleagues showed that fear potentiated startle involves activation of the same pathways, including the amygdala, as does conditioned freezing studied in LeDoux's lab.

But Davis found that while the lateral amygdala to central amygdala to brainstem pathway mediates response to immediate fearful stimuli, a projection from the amygdala to a different brain structure is responsible for more slowly developing responses to sustained stress. This structure has the somewhat awkward sounding name of *bed nucleus of the stria terminalis* or BNST; it is often referred to as a part of the "extended amygdala."[27] Davis and other have argued that activation of the BNST may be more closely linked to psychiatric disorders like social anxiety disorder and PTSD than is the amygdala. These conditions do not evolve suddenly but rather develop

---

[26] Ledoux JE, Gorman JM: A call to action: overcoming anxiety through active coping. *Am J Psychiatry* 2001;158:1953–1955.

[27] Walker DL, Toufexis DJ, Davis M: Role of the bed nucleus of the stria terminalis versus the amygdala in fear, stress, and anxiety. *Eur J Pharmacol* 2003;463:199–216.; Walker DL, Davis M: Role of the extended amygdala in short-duration versus sustained fear: a tribute to Dr. Lennart Heimer. *Brain Struct Funct* 2008 213:29–42.; Lebow MA, Chen A: Overshadowed by the amygdala: the bed nucleus of the stria terminalis emerges as a key to psychiatric disorders. *Mol Psychiatr* 2016;21;450–463.

over time and then can be sustained for a lifetime if left untreated. The BNST has not entered the popular imagination as has the amygdala, perhaps because of its less inviting name, and not all scientists in the field agree with the proposal that immediate and sustained fear responses involve the amygdala and BNST respectively and exclusively. A brain imaging study did show that the BNST responded to anticipation of receiving an electric shock, whereas the amygdala responded more when the shock was actually delivered.[28] The study also showed that the amygdala and BNST are functionally connected to each other and to a number of other brain regions, so that it is likely that as much activity within these connections as within the amygdala and BNST themselves mediates differences in their roles in fear. It was also shown that disrupting a specific pathway from the amygdala to the BNST by optogenetic stimulation disrupted the expression of long-lasting, sustained fear in rodents.[29] Brain imaging technology is developing rapidly, and, as we can resolve smaller and smaller structures, we should know for certain whether the distinction between amygdala and BNST in mediating immediate and chronic fear is valid.

We can now draw a somewhat complete brain circuit that serves an emotion common to all animals, fear. The circuit involves connections among the amygdala, hippocampus, medial prefrontal cortex, striatum, and BNST. We can locate our ability to see an object to an area in a single part of the occipital lobe of the brain, but a complex emotion like fear appears to involve a network of interacting brain regions that sometimes stimulate and sometimes inhibit each other. When a stroke damages the back of a person's brain and she loses vision in an eye, neurologists are called in to find the precise area of damage, recommend treatment, and predict what will happen over time. The neurologist's examination, especially when assisted by a specialist called a neuro-ophthalmologist, will make clear what has happened to the patient, and a CAT scan or structural MRI scan will show precisely where the damage has occurred.

But when a patient comes to the emergency room during an acute panic attack, physical examination will not be especially helpful and brain scans show nothing abnormal. This is because the problem does not involve destruction of brain tissue but instead an imbalance in the way different parts of the fear circuit are communicating with each other. We can use fMRI and PET scanning to help elucidate those imbalances. But before we reconstruct how fear evolves in the brain on the larger scale of connections among structures and regions, let's first make full use of what basic scientists have told us about this circuit and delve down into the molecular and cellular levels that were the topics of Chapters 3 and 4.

[28] Klumpers F, Kroes MCW, Baas JMP, Fernandez G: How human amygdala and bed nucleus of the stria terminalis may drive distinct defensive responses. *J Neurosci* 2017:37:9645–9656.
[29] Asok A, Draper A, Hofman AF, Schulkin J, Lupica CR, Rosen JB: Optogenetic silencing of a corticotropin-releasing factor pathway from the central amygdala to the bed nucleus of the stria terminalis disrupts sustained fear. *Molecular Psychiatry* 2018;23:914–922.

# FEAR ACTIVATES GENES, PROTEINS, AND DENDRITES

The beauty of having an animal model that is at least a close approximation of a human behavior or emotion is that it enables neuroscientists to examine the molecules and cells involved. Once scientists like Joe LeDoux, Mike Davis, Greg Quirk, and others understood the pathways involved in conditioned fear, they could use their basic neuroscience laboratories to trace out all the steps that hearing that tone takes. Consequently, we now know the details about genes and their products that are involved in the acquisition, consolidation into memory, and extinction of conditioned fear.

Just as acquisition of conditioned fear can be prevented by physically lesioning the amygdala, injecting chemicals that inhibit activation of genes and synthesis of new proteins directly into the amygdala renders an animal unable to learn to associate any conditioned stimulus with any unconditioned stimulus.[30] Such animals will freeze every time an electric shock is applied but will not freeze to tones no matter how many times they are paired with shocks.

Crucial to this process are genes in the amygdala that code for proteins involved in the activity of the neurotransmitter glutamate. Although psychiatric drugs traditionally focus on neurotransmitters called dopamine, serotonin, and noradrenaline, glutamate is the brain's most abundant neurotransmitter. At synapses throughout the brain, glutamate is released from the presynaptic neuron, crosses the synapse, and binds to one of several types of postsynaptic receptors, exciting the postsynaptic neuron and causing the further propagation of neural signals. Loss of glutamate function causes a variety of abnormalities depending on what part of the brain is involved. Low levels of glutamate have been linked to the cognitive abnormalities in schizophrenia. Higher than normal levels, on the other hand, are toxic to neurons and a factor in the damage that occurs during strokes and traumatic brain injury. Abnormally high glutamate has also been linked to depression, and a drug currently used for anesthesia that blocks glutamate from binding to one of its receptors, ketamine, is now being tested as a possible treatment for patients with depression.

In Chapter 3, we explained that the activation of genes in response to any experience we undergo can be caused by one of several epigenetic mechanisms that turn a previously silent gene on and initiate the processes of messenger RNA transcription that ultimately leads to protein synthesis. Studies show that this is exactly what happens during fear conditioning and fear extinction. When the rat hears the tone and then gets the shock, changes in the binding of methyl groups to DNA in neurons in the amygdala activate genes that code for several proteins, including glutamate receptors. These changes in epigenetic status are permanent unless other, more powerful experiences or drugs are administered that override them and silence the gene again.[31]

---

[30] Schafe GE, LeDoux JE: Memory consolidation of auditory Pavlovian fear conditioning requires protein synthesis and protein kinase A in the amygdala. *J Neurosci* 2000;20:RC96.

[31] Zoykic IB, Sweatt JD: Epigenetic mechanisms in learned fear: implications for PTSD. *Neuropsychopharmacology* 2013;38:77–93.

Injecting drugs into the amygdala that block the formation of glutamate receptors or the ability of glutamate to bind to its receptors inhibits both the acquisition and the extinction of conditioned fear.[32] One interesting aspect involves one of the many varieties of glutamate receptor, called the *N-methyl-D-aspartate* (NMDA) receptor. The NMDA receptor is in turn comprised of several subunits, one of which is called the NR2B subunit, and it turns out that activation of NR2B-containing NMDA receptors in the lateral amygdala is required for fear conditioning acquisition and for fear-conditioning extinction.[33] During the time I worked with LeDoux and his group, I had the opportunity to ask them to conduct experiments to address clinical observations we could not study directly in humans at the molecular level. One of these is the curious fact that antidepressants have immediate effects on neurotransmitters in the brain but take weeks before they work on clinical symptoms. The selective serotonin reuptake inhibitor (SSRI) antidepressants, for example, block the activity of the serotonin receptor at which they are directed after just a few doses, but depressed and anxiety disorder patients generally take 2 weeks or longer to get better. Sometimes the patients even feel a bit worse after the first few doses.

In the laboratory, we gave an SSRI—citalopram—to rats undergoing fear conditioning. We found that after the first 9 days of receiving citalopram, the rats given active citalopram froze longer to auditory tones after fear conditioning than those given a placebo drug. But after several weeks of citalopram—a very long period in the lives of rats—the reverse occurred, and the rats given real citalopram froze for shorter periods of time, indicating that they had become less fearful. We were struck by the further finding that only after the longer period of administration was there a reduction in NR2B-subunits in the rats who received citalopram, but there was no change in the rats who received placebo. Thus, the rats' response to citalopram followed exactly the time course that we see in human patients treated with SSRI antidepressants—worse at first and then responsive—and the time needed for NR2B subunit downregulation mirrored this effect as well.[34]

There are changes on the cellular level, as described in Chapter 4, that accompany these molecular effects. Adverse experiences like fear and stress causes a retraction of dendrites and dendritic spines in most parts of the brain, like the prefrontal cortex. But in the amygdala, fear conditioning causes dendrites to sprout,

[32] Bermudo-Soriano C, Perez-Rodriguez MM, Vaquero Lorenzo C, Baca-Garcia E: New perspectives in glutamate and anxiety. *Pharmacol Biochem Behav* 2012;100:752–754.

[33] Rodrigues SM, Schafe GE, LeDoux JE: Intra-amygdala blockade of the NR2B subunit of the NMDA receptor disrupts the acquisition but not the expression of fear conditioning. *J Neurosci* 2001;21:6889–6896.; Sotres-Bayon F, Bush DE, LeDoux JE: Acquisition of fear extinction requires activation of NR2B-containing NMDA receptors in the lateral amygdala. *Neuropsychopharmacology* 2007;32:1929–1940.

[34] Burghardt NS, Sigurdsson T, Gorman JM, McEwen BS, LeDoux JE: Chronic antidepressant treatment impairs the acquisition of fear extinction. *Biol Psychiatry* 2013;73:1078–1086.

making new connections among neurons in the various subnuclei of the amygdala.[35] When an animal becomes fearful then, it makes stronger connections in the fear-enhancing parts of the brain like the amygdala, while connections in fear-inhibiting areas like the medial prefrontal cortex weaken. Functionally, this means that fear acquisition and expression become easier and fear extinction becomes harder. Naturally more anxious mice, for example, have stronger connections between the lateral amygdala and the central amygdala than do less anxious mice.[36] On the other hand, enriching the environments in which the animals live for 2 weeks—a kind of intensive rodent psychotherapy—not only decreased anxiety levels in rats exposed to the stress of being repeatedly immobilized but also reduced the enlargement of the dendritic arbor in the amygdala usually seen after this kind of stress.[37] Such work suggests to us that psychotherapy may induce similar structural changes in people suffering with psychiatric illnesses as well. We will come back to this possibility in Chapter 8.

## FROM GENES TO CONNECTIONS: FEAR'S WHOLE PICTURE

With this explanation of molecular and cellular events involved in fear conditioning, we can now build a picture from the bottom up of how the experience of a fearful event changes the structure and function of the brain in a laboratory animal. The rat is placed in a conditioning chamber and listens to some loud tones, which startle it and send signals from its ears to its thalamus and then to the temporal lobe areas necessary for hearing. Then, however, one of the tones is terminated with a mild electric shock, and that signal goes from the thalamus to both the amygdala and the medial prefrontal cortex. Genes in neurons of the amygdala that had been quiet are now activated by changes in the binding of epigenetic regulators to DNA and other structural elements. New proteins are synthesized, including those that are used in the excitatory glutamate neurotransmitter system, like the NMDA receptor and its NR2B subunit. Dendrites in the amygdala extend their branches and sprout new spines, increasing the strength of neural connections within the amygdala itself. The neural signal in the lateral amygdala moves swiftly to the central amygdala, where a permanent memory trace of the association of shock with tone is consolidated through a process involving multiple genes and proteins. From there, the neural signal travels to the hypothalamus and the

---

[35] Yasmin F, Saxena K, McEwen BS, Chattarji S: The delayed strengthening of synaptic connectivity in the amygdala depends on NMDA receptor activation during acute stress. *Physiol Rep* 2016;4:ouuLe13002.

[36] Avrabos C, Sotnikov SV, Dine J, Markt PO, Holsboer F, Landgraf R, Eder M: Real-time imaging of amygdalar network dynamics in vitro reveals a neurophysiological link to behavior in a mouse model of extremes in trait anxiety. *J Neurosci* 2013;33:1626–16267.

[37] Ashokan A, Hegde A, Mitra R: Short-term environmental enrichment is sufficient to counter stress-induced anxiety and associated structural and molecular plasticity in basolateral amygdala. *Psychoneuroendocrinology* 2016;69:189–196.

brain stem, causing freezing; increases in heart rate, blood pressure, and breathing; and release of stress hormones. The signal is transmitted to the hippocampus, where a memory trace of the place or context in which the fear conditioning occurred, including its exact smell, color, and geometry, is recorded. The hippocampus is also stimulated to release the stress hormone CRH.

The signal also goes from the thalamus to the mPFC via the "high road," which tries to suppress the amygdala, but the amygdala also sends inhibitory signals to the mPFC and thus overrides mPFC control.[38] Now, every time the rat hears the tone, the memory of the shock is activated in the amygdala and the signal to freeze and the enhancement of the potentiation of the startle response occur. If the animal is simply placed back in an identical looking and smelling conditioning chamber, the contextual memory of where the shock was first felt is triggered in the hippocampus and the rat also freezes. If the animal is exposed to a continuous series of stressful events, the BNST is activated and long-term avoidant and fearful responses evolve.

If the rat is presented with tones repeatedly without shocks, eventually the mPFC regains its control and stimulates a memory in the amygdala of tone without shock that exists side by side with the fear memory and, at least for a while, inhibits the amygdala so that tones no longer cause freezing or enhancement of potentiated startle. Extinction of conditioned fear requires many of the same genes to be activated and proteins to be synthesized as acquisition of conditioned fear and can therefore be blocked by the same manipulations. Even after successful extinction, fear memory can be reinstated at any time. If, on the other hand, the animal is taught that it can terminate the tone without a shock by taking an action, the neural impulse is rerouted from the amygdala to the striatum, and freezing to the tone is decreased and even in some cases eliminated, at least for a while. At every step of the way along these pathways, genes are being activated and silenced and new proteins synthesized. Dendrites expand and retract, forming and breaking off connections among neurons within and between brain regions. In the case of a part of the hippocampus, new neurons are born to store some of the new fear memory traces by the process called neurogenesis (see Chapter 4).

We will mention here briefly one other aspect of fear conditioning that will become more important in Chapter 8, when we consider the biology of psychotherapy. After extinction of conditioned fear, it is possible to revive the whole system of freezing to tones and reinstate or reactivate the consolidated fear memory. Now, however, a curious thing happens to the previously consolidated fear memory—it becomes labile. If, within a brief window of time, drugs are administered that prevent memory reconsolidation, the fear memory can be permanently erased. This phenomenon of reviving a fear memory and then erasing it has some interesting implications for psychoanalytic psychotherapy, which we will review in Chapter 8.

[38] Garcia R, Vouimba R-M, Baudry M, Thompson RF: The amygdala modulates prefrontal cortex activity relative to conditioned fear. *Nature* 1999;402:294–296.

# BUT IS IT TRUE FOR US TOO?

As these molecular, cellular, and systems insights about fear in the laboratory rodent were being established, it became irresistible for us to speculate about how they might translate into human behavior. I will use a personal experience as an example of our thinking. Two days after Hurricane Gloria hit Eastern Long Island in 1985, my intrepid late father-in-law decided to go for a swim in the Atlantic Ocean. Not wanting to seem less courageous than a man many decades my senior, I plunged in with him. But the waves were still enormous and unsynchronized, and we quickly ran into trouble. We swam too far out and were exhausted; the swim back was frightening, and I was thrown back by the undertow and dragged along the bottom of the ocean over and over again. I finally reached shore, only to hear my father-in-law yelling for help. Fortunately, some strong teenage boys were sitting on the beach, and they managed to pull him to safety. We both were close to drowning.

After that experience, which lasted only minutes, and even though I have been swimming in the ocean since I was 5 years old, I became phobic of the ocean. Merely wading in to my waist, even on a day when the water was calm and virtually without waves, made me apprehensive, and I could no longer plunge in and swim. I realized these fears were irrational; after all, I wasn't trying to swim in the ocean right after a hurricane again. Nevertheless, I begged my wife to go in with me, which might strike most wives as a bit ridiculous, but she is a psychiatrist and understands these things better than most. Over several months, we engaged in a kind of behavioral desensitization therapy in which we would start walking into the ocean together, and I would gradually go farther and farther without her by my side. Eventually, my phobia extinguished and I am again able to swim out into the ocean. But I have noticed that I pay more attention to the waves than I used to and am certain that the slightest difficulty will reactivate my phobia.

This seems to me almost exactly like the rat in the fear-conditioning chamber. A single adverse experience in which near drowning was paired with a previously innocuous stimulus—swimming in the ocean—made me avoidant. After Hurricane Gloria, every time I tried to get off my feet and swim in the ocean I froze in place and felt my chest heaving and my heart pounding. Only by repeatedly exposing myself to the waves and learning that, absent a recent hurricane, there is no danger was I able to resume swimming in the ocean, but the experience is no longer as carefree as it once was even though my rational brain tells me that my fears are totally neurotic.

Could it be that I now have a memory trace of conditioned fear to the ocean permanently resident in my central amygdala? I am not afraid to swim in pools or lakes, so is there a contextual fear memory of the ocean lodged in my hippocampus? Is my prefrontal cortex trying to suppress my fears but always vulnerable to an abrupt reemergence of amygdala- and hippocampal-driven phobic avoidance?

When my colleagues and I thought through situations like this, it made us wonder if the amygdala and other parts of the "fear circuitry" might be acting abnormally in psychiatric illnesses that include large components of irrational fear, like panic disorder, PTSD, social anxiety disorder, and depression. Too much amygdala activity seemed somehow involved in anxiety and depression, whereas evidence emerged that too little amygdala activity might be associated with a pathological absence of fear. Juvenile offenders who are callous and unemotional have been shown to have a smaller amygdala than children without these traits.[39]

We also realized that animal studies were delineating networks that might be relevant to other forms of human psychopathology. For example, a pathway from a part of the prefrontal cortex called the *orbitofrontal cortex* (OFC) to the front or ventral part of the striatum has been shown to be involved in both patients and animals with abnormal repetitive behaviors. In this case, the link began with studies of humans with obsessive compulsive disorder (OCD) who persistently showed hyperactivity in the OFC–ventral striatum pathway.[40] It turns out that it isn't OCD per se in which this circuit is overactive, but disorders characterized by any form of abnormal repetitive behavior, including tics, Tourette's syndrome, eating disorders, and substance abuse.

Next, basic scientists showed that they could induce repetitive behaviors in laboratory animals by stimulating this pathway. Optogenetics allows scientists to insert light-sensitive genes into specific brain pathways. When light of a specific color is then directed at the animals' head, these genes are turned on and the specific pathway activated. Optogenetic stimulation of the mouse OFC–striatal pathway produces repetitive grooming behavior.[41] Multiple studies in both humans and animals have now nailed down the relevance of this pathway to repetitive behaviors.[42] In Chapter 7, we will discuss pathways that in both humans and animals are involved in reward and social attachment. Increasingly, then, pathways in humans and animals seem to align in the formation of complex behaviors and emotions.

On the human side, except for the few instances in which we have postmortem brain samples that can be studied and the even fewer times we can stimulate brain regions during brain surgery required to treat diseases, our ability to understand how brain function is tied to behavior and emotion relies on what we can see with the brain imaging techniques described in Chapter 5. In fear research our attention turned to assessing whether the amygdala brain circuits involved in conditioned fear in rats applied to both normal and abnormal fear in humans. How well, then, do fMRI and PET scan studies correlate in fearful humans with what we know happens in the brains of fear-conditioned rodents?

[39] Aghajani M, Klapwijk ET, van der Wee NJ, et al.: Disorganized amygdala networks in conduct-disordered juvenile offenders with callous-unemotional traits. *Biol Psychiatry* 2017;82:283–293.

[40] Rauch SL, Carlezon WA Jr: Illuminating the neural circuitry of compulsive behavior. *Science* 2013;340:1174–1176.

[41] Ahmari SE, Spelman T, Douglass NI, Kheirbek MA, Simpson HB Deisseroth K, Hen R: Repeated cortico-striatal stimulation generates persistent OCD-like behavior. *Science* 2013;340:1234–1239.

[42] Gorman JM, Nathan PE: Challenges to implementing evidence-based treatments. In Peter E. Nathan and Jack M. Gorman, eds. *A Guide To Treatments That Work.* 4th ed. New York, Oxford University Press, 2015, p. 6.

# THE AMYGDALA AND THE FEARFUL HUMAN

In the previous chapter, I promised to be careful in how much credence I attach to fMRI and PET studies. They are fraught with technical problems and difficulty in replicating findings. The link between the fear network we have described so far in animals and fear and anxiety in humans, however, is based on solid neuroimaging research. It is not that every study shows that the amygdala is responsible for every anxiety disorder or that the area is entirely free of conflicting findings. But the number of studies showing that connections among the mPFC, amygdala, and hippocampus are central to our experience of fear is now overwhelming.[43]

Elizabeth Phelps is an extraordinarily clever cognitive psychologist who works with Joe LeDoux at New York University. Phelps has designed studies that use fMRI to establish whether the brain networks known to underlie conditioned fear in rodents also operate in humans. In one such study, she and her colleagues first asked volunteers to set the level of an electric shock they found uncomfortable but not painful.[44] Next, they were shown a series of blue and yellow squares on a computer screen, one color of which was at first paired with a shock and the other was not, called the CS+ and CS−, respectively. Then the researchers measured the volunteers' response to seeing the squares without any shocks. A physiological measure called skin conductance was used to measure the subjects' level of fear. Skin conductance is based on the same principle as the lie detector test. Emotional arousal, like fear, causes imperceptible perspiration that is detected by electrodes placed on the skin. Although the ability of this method to accurately differentiate lies from truthful statements is debatable, it reliably tells us if an individual is emotionally aroused. As expected, if the blue square had been paired with the shock (CS+) but not the yellow square (CS−), then blue squares even without shock subsequently evoked greater skin conductance response than yellow squares. The human subjects had acquired conditioned fear exactly like the rats in the conditioning chamber. Remarkably, then, the brain imaging data showed that conditioned fear acquisition was accompanied by increased activity in the amygdala, again, just like in the rats.

A day later, Phelps conducted an extinction trial on the same subjects in which they were repeatedly shown blue and yellow squares, both without shocks. The blue squares lost their ability to evoke increased skin conductance responses, and fMRI scans showed activation of the ventral portion of the mPFC. Once again, the findings almost exactly mirrored what LeDoux, Davis, Quirk, and other basic neuroscientists had shown with fear conditioning in their laboratories.

Phelps and her group have also validated in humans the preclinical finding that giving a subject a sense of control reroutes the conditioned fear signal to the ventral

[43] Fullana MA, Harrison BJ, Soriano-Mas C, Vervliet B, Cardoner N, Avila-Parcet A, Radua J: Neural signatures of human fear conditioning: an updated and extended meta-analysis of fMRI studies. *Mol Psychiatr* 2016;21:500–508.

[44] Phelps EA, Delgado MR, Nearing KI, LeDoux JE: Extinction learning in humans: Role of the amygdala and vmPFC. *Neuron* 2004;43:897–905.

striatum.[45] The group used methods like those just described, except that this time the research subjects in one group could use an arrow on the keyboard to avoid shocks by moving the CS+ signals (the blue or yellow squares) through a tunnel on the screen. Not only did the group given control over the shocks demonstrate lower skin conductance responses on subsequent CS+ presentations, but fMRI showed activation of the striatum. They also noted that active control attenuated fear more than did passive extinction, a point with implications for our consideration of the biology of psychotherapy in Chapter 8.

This kind of work has been replicated multiple times, and studies consistently show that, in normal humans, the amygdala is activated during the acquisition and expression of conditioned fear, the hippocampus is needed for the expression and acquisition of contextual fear, and the mPFC kicks in during extinction. An intriguing study took advantage of the fact that patients with epilepsy sometimes undergo a study in which electrodes are placed into their brains to map out the electrical focus that is causing their seizures. Investigators at the University of California, Irvine showed nine such epilepsy patients pictures of fearful and peaceful faces while recording signals directly from their brains with these electrodes.[46] While looking at frightening faces there was flow between electrodes in one direction, from amygdala to hippocampus. No such unidirectional flow occurred while looking at peaceful faces. During fear processing, then, the amygdala seems to take over the rest of the brain. Nevertheless, the prefrontal cortex tries to assert its control and put reason into the mix; accordingly, fMRI studies have shown the mPFC inhibiting the amygdala during fear-evoking tasks in human subjects.[47] I have already mentioned in this chapter genetic and volume differences that accompany the strength with which the human mPFC can control the amygdala.

The ability to activate the PFC and control the amygdala is an important component in our ability to rein in our emotions.[48] As one group of scientists from Columbia University concluded "when confronted with distressing stimuli, greater responses in brain regions associated with emotional reactivity and cognitive control can be used to identify people who are likely to regulate their emotional responses. . . and predict whether regulation is chosen for a given stimulus" (p. 2587).[49] It seems that individual differences in which structure, the prefrontal cortex or the amygdala, is more able to inhibit the other help to determine who will be more resilient in the face of a threat and who will develop an anxiety disorder or depression.

[45] Boeke EA, Moscarello JM, LeDoux JE, Phelps EA, Hartley CA: Active avoidance: neural mechanisms and attenuation of Pavlovian conditioned responding. *J Neurosci* 2017;37:4808–4818.
[46] Zheng J, Anderson KL, Leal SL, et al.: Amygdala-hippocampal dynamics during salient information processing. *Nat Commun* 2017;8:1443.
[47] Cha J, DeDora D, Nedic S, et al.: Clinically anxious individuals show disrupted feedback between inferior frontal gyrus and prefrontal-limbic control circuit. *J Neurosci* 2016;36:4708–4718.
[48] Dore BP, Weber J, Ochsner KN: Neural predictors of decisions to cognitively control emotion. *J Neurosci* 2017;37:2580–2588.
[49] Ibid.

This is confirmed by studies by Justin Kim and Paul Whalen of Dartmouth University who used diffusion tensor imaging (DTI), the technique mentioned in Chapter 5 that measures the strength of brain fiber connections between brain regions, and showed that stronger mPFC to amygdala connections predicted lower trait anxiety levels in normal human volunteers.[50] This kind of work has shown that the pathway from the mPFC normally exerts inhibitory control over the amygdala in humans; the more recently evolved brain region, responsible for reason and logic, can suppress the more primitive emotional reactions generated by the amygdala. Note that *trait anxiety* refers to the ongoing level of fear and worry an individual has, as opposed to *state anxiety*, which refers to the more immediate response to a threatening situation. Thus, the strength of the mPFC to amygdala connection seems to determine an aspect of a person's basic personality structure. LeDoux noted in a *New York Times* editorial that there is remarkable variation in both rats and humans in the strength of the fear response: "A vivid example of freezing was captured in a video of the Centennial Olympic Park bombing during the 1996 Summer Olympics in Atlanta. After the bomb went off, many people froze. Then, some began to try to escape (run), while others were slower on the uptake. This variation in response is typical."[51] One factor that differentiates those who run from those who remain frozen appears to be the ability to apply reason to the situation and exert prefrontal cortical control over the amygdala.

The next question to ask is whether there is evidence that people with fear-based psychiatric illnesses, like anxiety disorders, PTSD, and depression, have abnormalities in any of these connections. Indeed, innumerable studies have consistently shown hyperactivity in the amygdala and/or disrupted mPFC to amygdala connections in a wide variety of psychiatric illnesses including major depression, bipolar disorder, generalized anxiety disorder, and PTSD. These studies show that even young children with depression already manifest these abnormalities. As children mature through adolescence and adulthood, control of limbic and other "subcortical" brain structures by the prefrontal cortex strengthens.[52] Children exposed to abuse, maltreatment, orphanage rearing, or compromised paternal care, however, have enlarged amygdala volumes without a corresponding increase in other brain regions like the hippocampus, again suggesting disruption in the normal relationships among brain structures that control emotion.[53] Brain imaging of newborn infants shows that

[50] Kim MJ, Whalen PJ: The structural integrity of an amygdala-prefrontal pathway predicts trait anxiety. *J Neurosci* 2009;29:11614–11618.

[51] LeDoux J: "Run, hide, fight' is not how our brains work. *New York Times*, December 18, 2015.

[52] Hwang K Velanova K, Luna B: Strengthening of top-down frontal cognitive control networks underlying the developing of inhibitory control: a functional magnetic resonance imaging effective connectivity study. *J Neurosci* 2010;30:15535–15545.

[53] Lupien SJ, Parent S, Evans AC, et al.: Larger amygdala but no change in hippocampal volume in 10-year-old children exposed to maternal depressive symptomatology since birth. *Proc Natl Acad Sci USA* 2011 Aug 23;108(34):14324–14329.

decreased connectivity between the amygdala and other brain regions is associated with depressive and anxiety symptoms at 2 years of age.[54]

The biggest increase in brain connectivity occurs in our teenage years.[55] This normal developmental phenomenon is disrupted in people who develop mood and anxiety disorders in which exaggerated fearfulness plays a prominent role. A group of Norwegian investigators showed that a failure of the functional connectome to display normal stabilization and individualization is associated with higher scores on measures of psychiatric symptoms.[56] The authors note that "individuality of brain development in genetically identical mice directly relates to the level of experience that mice were exposed to during development. Although speculative, our results [in humans] may therefore provide a neural perspective on the known gene–environment interactions in mental health" (p. 514). A key finding in patients with anxiety disorders is a reduction in prefrontal cortical activation during fear conditioning.[57] In some studies, psychotherapy and antidepressant medications that improve these conditions also result in normalization of activity in the fear-related brain network.[58,59]

These findings extend to patients with depression, many, but not all, of whom suffer from a host of irrational and exaggerated fears. A group of investigators from multiple universities, including Eric Nestler from Mount Sinai School of Medicine in New York City and Karl Deisseroth from Stamford, obtained tissue from the prefrontal cortex of people who had a history of depression before their deaths. They showed that, compared to normal brains, there was a decrease in the expression patterns of several genes in the depressed patients' brains.[60] They then subjected mice to a chronic form of stress called *social defeat stress*, which produces depression-like behaviors, and showed that this caused a reduction in expression of the same genes in the mouse prefrontal cortex. They also showed that stimulating mouse prefrontal cortex using the optogenetic technique had an antidepressant effect on those animals that had been exposed to social defeat stress.

[54] Rogers CE, Sylvester CM, Mintz C, Kenley JK, Shimony JS, Barch D, Smyser CD: Neonatal amygdala functional connectivity at rest in health and preterm infants and early internalizing symptoms. *J Am Acad Child Adolesc Psychiatry* 2017;56:157–186.

[55] Galvan A: Adolescence, brain maturation and mental health. *Nature Neurosci* 2017;20:503–504.

[56] Kaufmann T, Alnaes D, Doan NT, Brandt CL, Andreassen OA, Westlye L: Delayed stabilization and individualization in connectome development are related to psychiatric disorders. *Nat Neurosci* 2017;20:513–515.

[57] Marin M-F, Zsido RG, Song H, et al.: Skin conductance responses and neural activations during fear conditioning and extinction recall across anxiety disorders. *JAMA Psychiatry* 2017;74:622–631.

[58] Gorman and Nathan, *A Guide To Treatments That Work*, for a review of these studies and complete citations.

[59] Mansson KN, Salami A, Frick A, Carlbring P, Andersson G, Fumark T, Boraxbekk CJ: Neuroplasticity in response to cognitive behavior therapy for social anxiety disorder. *Transl Psychiatry* 2016;6:e727.; Liebscher C, Wittmann A, Gechter J, et al.: Facing the fear—clinical and neural effects of cognitive behavioural and pharmacotherapy in panic disorder and agoraphobia. *Eur Neuropsycopharmacol* 2016;26:431–444.

[60] Covington HE, Lobo MK, Maze I, et al.: Antidepressant effect of optogenetic stimulation of the medial prefrontal cortex. *J Neurosci* 2010;30:16082–16090.

Imaging studies show that, compared to healthy control subjects and to patients with remitted depression, currently depressed patients have reduced amygdala activation when asked to recall positive memories and increased amygdala activation when recalling negative memories.[61] Suppressing memories of negative events is accompanied by decreased amygdala activation.[62] Increased bilateral amygdala responses to viewing sad faces were abolished in depressed patients after treatment with the antidepressant medication citalopram.[63] Women with depression showed reduced connectivity between the amygdala and the mPFC.[64] Once again, a pattern of reduced prefrontal cortex and increased amygdala activity emerges in patients with depression, abnormalities that seem responsive to antidepressant medication.

Children with PTSD also have weaker connections between the amygdala and the mPFC than do normal children.[65] A 5-year follow-up study of adult patients with PTSD showed that recovery was associated with strengthening of the connections between the amygdala and the PFC and normalization of connections between amygdala and several other brain regions as well.[66] Areas of the brain can be directly stimulated with a technique called *transcranial direct current stimulation* (tDCS). When investigators used tDCS to stimulate a part of the prefrontal cortex, they found that it reduced vigilance to threatening stimuli in a group of healthy volunteers.[67] The scientists who did the experiment noted that the effect of stimulating the prefrontal cortex is similar to what is seen when patients are given anti-anxiety drugs.

One interesting complication in painting the picture of amygdala abnormalities in humans with anxiety disorders came with the surprising finding from a group of investigators at the University of Iowa when they showed they could induce panic attacks in patients with Urbach-Wiethe disease, the condition mentioned earlier that causes severe damage to the amygdala on both sides of the brain, by having them

[61] Young KD, Siegle GJ, Bodurka J, Drevets WC: Amygdala activity during autobiographical memory recall in depressed and vulnerable individuals: association with symptom severity and autobiographical overgenerality. *Am J Psychiatry* 2016;173:78–89.

[62] Dolcos S, Katsumi Y: Suppress to feel and remember less: Neural correlates of explicit and impact emotional suppression on perception and memory. *Neuropsychologia* 2018;Epub ahead of print. doi:10.1016

[63] Arnone D, McKie S, Elliot R, et al.: Increased amygdala responses to sad but not fearful faces in major depression: relation to mood state and pharmacological treatment. *Am J Psychiatry* 2012;169:841–850.

[64] Satterhwaite TD, Cook PA, Bruce SE, et al.: Dimensional depression severity in women with major depression and post-traumatic stress disorder correlates with fronto-amygdalar hypoconnectivity. *Mol Psychiatr* 2016;21:894–902.

[65] Wolf RC, Herringa RJ: Prefrontal-amygdala dysregulation to threat in pediatric posttraumatic stress disorder. *Neuropsychopharmacology* 2016;41:822–831.

[66] Yoon S, Kim JE, Hwang J, et al.: Recovery from posttraumatic stress requires dynamic and sequential shifts in amygdalar connectivities. *Neuropsychopharmacology* 2016;42:454–461.

[67] Ironside M, O'Shea J, Cowen PJ, Harmer CJ: Frontal cortex stimulation reduces vigilance to threat: implications for the treatment of depression and anxiety. *Biol Psychiatry* 2016;79:823–830.

breathe carbon dioxide.[68] My lab and others had shown over the course of many years that patients with panic disorder, but not people without panic disorder, have panic attacks when asked to breathe small concentrations of carbon dioxide mixed in room air for short periods of time. We found that there is nothing intrinsically abnormal with the respiratory system in patients with panic disorder, and therefore we speculated that because breathing carbon dioxide creates a feeling of air hunger and increases the depth of breathing that it reminded panic disorder patients of prior panic attacks and, through a kind of conditioned fear mechanism, triggered an acute panic attack.[69] Because this mechanism involves fear memory, we further speculated that panic disorder patients might have an abnormally sensitive amygdala. But the finding that panic attacks could be induced without a functioning amygdala seemed to contradict that hypothesis.

There are, of course, many ways to understand this finding. It is unclear, for example, if patients with Urbach-Wiethe disease, who have a genetic disease that also affects the skin, are comparable to people with panic disorder. It could also be that there may be several different brain circuits capable of triggering panic attacks when stimulated, so that when the amygdala is damaged another panic mechanism is still intact. Perhaps, as some have suggested, the abnormality in panic disorder is not in the amygdala itself but rather in the BNST, part of what is sometimes called the "extended amygdala," or in yet another brain structure that has been linked to fearful behavior, an area called the *anterior insula*. In another brain imaging study, we found that increased activity in a part of the prefrontal cortex called the *orbitofrontal cortex* just before receiving an injection of another respiratory stimulant, doxapram, predicted which patients with panic disorder would actually have a panic attack.[70] Nevertheless, the finding that panic attacks can be induced without a working amygdala is a caution that we proceed carefully whenever we attempt to make the leap from rodent to human.

Although not every patient with a mood or anxiety disorder, then, has something wrong with the strength of connections in this network, and this network alone does not account for every aspect of depression and anxiety disorders, there is little doubt at this point that amygdala, mPFC, and other fear network structures are involved in human fear. Despite differences among studies, the authors of a systematic review of imaging studies concluded that "The amygdala is involved in the generation of affective responses and emotional memories. Dysregulation in this region is consistently observed in patients with MDD [major depressive disorder] or anxiety, and it tends

[68] Feinstein JS, Buzza C, Hurlemann R, et al.: Fear and panic in humans with bilateral amygdala damage. *Nat Neurosci* 2013;16:270–272.
[69] Gorman JM, Kent J, Martinez J, Browne S, Coplan J, Papp LA: Physiological changes during carbon dioxide inhalation in patients with panic disorder, major depression, and premenstrual dysphoric disorder: evidence for a central fear mechanism. *Arch Gen Psychiatry* 2001;58:125–131.
[70] Kent JM, Coplan JD, Mawlawi O, et al.: Prediction of panic response to a respiratory stimulant by reduced orbitofrontal cerebral blood flow in panic disorder. *Am J Psychiatry* 2005;162:1379–1381.

to normalize with successful treatment" (p. 399).[71] Neuroimaging studies suggest that the loss of prefrontal cortical control over the limbic brain may even be part of the problem in patients with schizophrenia who suffer with the most extreme form of irrational fear, paranoid delusions.[72] Very few areas of neuroscience have seen this robust a convergence of data from animal research and brain imaging studies in humans.

How do abnormalities in brain connectivity that are associated with psychiatric illnesses arise? There is little doubt that part of what determines our individual brain connectome "fingerprint" is genetic and inherited. But there are also data that adverse life experiences disrupt the development of normal brain connections. For example, poverty among children aged 3–5 was associated with both greater negative mood and depression at school age and with reduced connectivity between amygdala and hippocampus and other brain regions, including the frontal cortex.[73] We noted earlier a study in which children exposed to early life abuse have enlarged amygdalas. We can model the effects of early life stress on regional brain connectivity in laboratory animals. Rats exposed to early life stress show life-long abnormalities in connectivity in multiple brain networks and in brain structures like the hippocampus and nucleus accumbens, a part of the striatum.[74] In earlier chapters, we have detailed the profound effects that early life stress have on molecules and cells in the brain, making it unsurprising that this phenomenon is also appreciated at the level of brain connections.

We have emphasized the fear network in this chapter to illustrate how connected regions of the brain function in the expression of complex emotions and behaviors, but there are, of course, many other networks in the animal and human brain. Scientists often speak about the "default mode network," for example, which is active when we are not engaged in any specific task but instead are thinking about ourselves or daydreaming. Included in this network are brain regions we have not mentioned so far, like the posterior cingulate and precuneus, and some we have mentioned, like the mPFC and hippocampus. This highlights the fact that a brain region may be part of more than one network; what counts is not what it does by itself but how it interacts with our brain regions.

There is also an executive network that is involved with higher cognitive processes like decision-making and calculations, and a salience network, responsible for focusing our attention on important stimuli. Advanced imaging techniques show us that these networks collaborate with each other in a multitude of different ways. For example, as we are increasingly aroused by a stimulus, the salience and executive networks act together to focus our attention and enable us to make appropriate decisions. But if

[71] Chakrabarty T, Ogrodniczuk J, Hadjipavlou G: Predictive neuroimaging markers of psychotherapy response: a systematic review. *Harvard Rev Psychiatry* 2016;24:396–405.

[72] Park S, Thakkar KN: "Splitting of the mind" revisited: recent neuroimaging evidence for functional disconnection in schizophrenia and its relation to symptoms. *Am J Psychiatry* 2010;167:366–368.

[73] Barch D, Pagliaccio D, Belden A, et al.: Effect of hippocampal and amygdala connectivity on the relationship between preschool poverty and school-age depression. *Am J Psychiatry* 2016;173:625–634.

[74] Nephew BC, Huang W, Poirier GL, Payne L, King JA: Altered neural connectivity in adult female rats exposed to early life social stress. *Behav Brain Res* 2017;316:225–233.

stimulation exceeds a threshold, as when, for example, we are overdoing it with multi-tasking, the two networks disengage and our decision-making capacities become un-focused and less efficient.[75] One fMRI study showed that patients with depression demonstrate uncoupling of the amygdala from the salience network and, at the same time, increased connectivity within the default mode network.[76] This fits with what we observe in patients with depression clinically: irrational fears reflected in the di-vorce of the fear-inducing parts of the brain, like the amygdala, from regions of the brain that allow us to focus our attention on what is really going on in the world (the salience network), plus a tendency to excessive self-rumination that is mirrored by increased activity in the default mode network.

Every day, from the moment we are born, our brains take in what we see and hear, what moves us and what disturbs us, whom we meet and what we do, and translates these experiences into the language of molecules, cells, and networks. Genes in our billions of neurons are constantly activated and silenced, new proteins made and destroyed, and dendritic trees expanded and retracted to form and rescind new synapses. Axons joined together in white matter tracts connect brain regions into mul-tiple networks and conduct neural signals at varying speeds depending on the status of all those molecules and cells. It is far from a simple assembly. In fact, it is hard to imagine anything more complicated. Anyone who insists that neuroscience and brain imaging is reducing the mind to simple terms simply hasn't delved into the brain in any detail. I am aware with every word I write in this book that my attempts to explain what goes on in the brain as we experience life of necessity simplifies what the brain is actually doing. That cannot be helped, but I hope that our extended tour through the biology of one emotion—fear—adequately conveyed two basic messages about the brain simultaneously: first, that it is very complicated and, second, that it is possible to combine the preclinical studies in laboratory animals with modern brain imaging technology in humans to gain increasingly greater understanding of how it works. I be-lieve this has worked remarkably well in the exploration of fear biology and that, in-creasingly, this strategy will prove successful in elucidating the underpinnings of many other emotions and behaviors.

In the next chapter, we will focus on another brain network, one that drives perhaps the most precious of all human endeavors: how we love and connect with each other.

[75] Young CB, Raz G, Everaerd D, Beckmann CF, Tendolkar I, Hendler T, Fernandez G, Hermans EJ: Dynamic shifts in large-scale brain network balance as a function of arousal. *J Neurosci* 2017;37:281–290.
[76] Jacobs RH, Barba A, Gowins JR, et al.: Decoupling of the amygdala to other salience network regions in adolescent-onset recurrent major depressive disorder. *Psychol Med* 2016;46:1055–1067.

# 7

# Love, Reward, and Social Connections

The basic fact is that humanity survives through kindness, love and compassion. That human beings can develop these qualities is their real blessing.
—The 14th Dalai Lama

Finding out how the brain works in order to develop treatments for illnesses like depression and schizophrenia is the raison d'être for public funding of biomedical research, including neuroscience. That means we tend to focus our research on what can go wrong with brain function. We used the generation of fear in the preceding chapter to illustrate how brain networks and connections between brain regions work to support a complex emotion, one that is the basis of many forms of mental illness. We are particularly interested in the way that stressful life events alter the normal function of fear-related networks in the brain and make us vulnerable to depression, anxiety disorders, and many other psychiatric problems.

But, of course, brain networks and connections also serve many positive emotions and behaviors, and we are beginning to learn more about these as well, once again by combining laboratory studies using animal models and brain imaging studies on humans. We can now ask questions like: How does a parent overcome normal fear to protect her child? What brain regions are involved in romantic love? Why is it so much fun for most people to be part of a group? And, what parts of the brain are involved in our remarkable penchant for empathy and altruism? As we approach brain systems that underlie positive emotions, we will, of course, again find that abnormalities in them can be associated with aberrant behavior and unpleasant emotions.

We cannot escape the basic fact that emotions and behaviors like love, social connections, empathy, and enjoyment all have a neural basis. That is, special things occur in the brain when we learn to like ice cream, become attached to a specific sports team, help a person in need, or fall in love. These same brain events can help us understand why some people become addicted to alcohol or opioids, are unable to empathize with someone else's needs, or live withdrawn and lonely lives. Substance use disorders and sociopathy represent in part problems in the neural systems responsible for reward and social behavior, respectively. Autism may also involve changes in neural systems responsible for social connections, although this is currently not as firmly established. Thus, even when we study the neuroscience of positive emotions and behaviors, we may be making contributions to understanding abnormalities and disorders.

These assertions will no doubt trigger the familiar objection dealt with throughout this book that they are an attempt to reduce complex human traits to chemicals and synapses. How dare I say that we can explain so beautiful a phenomenon as love by reference to neuronal genes, dendrites, and brain connections? But there is nothing reductionistic about explaining how emotions and behaviors are based on brain function. This does not mean that love is "simply" a matter of electrical impulses whizzing around the brain. It is true that we do not yet know enough about the brain to be able to describe every aspect of a complex emotion like love, but that doesn't mean it is an emotion with no basis in the brain or that there is some mysterious "soul-like" entity that is responsible for love.

Of course, it is extremely important to keep in mind how we gain insights into brain function when it concerns complex behaviors and emotions and where our current limitations lay. When a person is in love, a specific set of brain regions and their associated hormones and neurotransmitters are activated while others are suppressed. Some of these will be very similar from one person to the next, but each individual will also have his or her own, unique pattern of brain activation. It is tough to capture all of this with a magnetic resonance imaging (MRI) or positron emission tomography (PET) scan for several reasons. For example, the emotion itself differs from one person to the next. Science operates by eliminating variability to find definitive patterns and predictions. So, we may develop a scale to "rate" love or a task that evokes an emotion that is consistent among individuals and seems akin to "love." That is the only way, given how our current brain imaging technologies work, that we can hope to find any specific brain systems that seem to be activated by "love." We must acknowledge that this approach definitely blurs individual differences among people.

Another limitation is that brain imaging can only show us the activity of relatively large swathes of the brain, even though this is now measured in millimeters. Remember that MRI scans reconstruct a brain in anatomical units called voxels, three-dimensional boxes that can be as small as 1 millimeter on each of the three sides. But even in a space as small as a voxel there can be more than a million neurons. Brain imaging cannot tell us what individual neurons are doing in a human brain, let alone dendrites, axons, neurotransmitters, and genes.

We can overcome some of the limitations of our brain imaging technologies by examining animal models of social behaviors, but these are only approximations of what humans think and feel. As we will see shortly, we can model parental attachment and even monogamous bonding in animals, and these have led to important insights into human experience. But we will never know if rats or even chimpanzees love each other the way a romantic human couple does. Hence, it is important to keep in mind throughout this chapter the limitations imposed by current brain imaging methods and our use of animal models.

As our technologies become more sophisticated, more and more of the details will be worked out. Hopefully, as this happens, we will lose our fear that knowing how the brain operates to allow us to fall in love or donate to a charity will somehow diminish those activities. Love and generosity will still be wonderful things, but we will have the additional pleasure of knowing their neural basis and perhaps someday of helping people who have trouble experiencing them.

In this chapter, we will spend most of our time on two systems, one that involves the hormone oxytocin and the other a pathway centered in a part of the brain called the ventral striatum. Many, many other chemicals and structures in the brain are involved in social connections, but what is known about these two systems can already tell us some very interesting things. And they are connected to each other, which makes things even more interesting.

## BRAIN HORMONES AND SOCIAL CONNECTIONS

Having acknowledged our limitations and addressed the "reductionist" charge, we can move on to discussing what we do know about the neural basis for love and social connection. A key player in this is the hormone oxytocin, which has been incorrectly referred to as the "love hormone." It is more correct to say that oxytocin is one part of the story behind specific types of social affiliation. Some of these roles for oxytocin have been worked out in substantial detail in animals and to some degree in humans, including parental attachment to offspring and monogamous pair bonding.

We discussed at some length in Chapter 6 the biology of classical fear conditioning, in which a mouse or rat is trained to freeze to a previously innocuous cue, like a tone or odor, after the cue has been paired with an aversive stimulus, like a mild electrical shock. Indeed, freezing can be an adaptive response to threat under many conditions. If you have ever watched one of those incredible documentaries about wild animals in which you wonder where in the world the camera could possibly be to capture so much detail, you may have seen one in which a gazelle is being stalked by a lion. The lion is expert at this and remains hidden from the gazelle's view as it plans its attack, but, at some point, the gazelle senses the presence of the predator. It doesn't know exactly where the lion is, so if it runs it might go right into the lion's grasp. Instead, the gazelle freezes in place and all that moves are its ears, eyes, and nose as it attempts to use its senses to determine the exact location of the threat. Humans freeze under threatening conditions as well, as anyone knows who has been a driver in a car crash and later wondered why he didn't swerve to avoid the inevitable collision.

Animals also flee from threat when that is their best defense. Although black bears are much bigger and stronger than humans, most of them will run away when they spot one of us (not true, I am told, of grizzly bears). We behave similarly: if you are hiking in the woods and see a snake, you are not likely to attack it.

But under one circumstance, despite the presence of threat, animals and humans do not freeze or flee but rather take aggressive action—to protect their young. The same black bear that runs away when it sees a human will attack the human if it comes close to its cubs. In a remarkable recent experiment, scientists paired an electric shock, which makes rats freeze in place, with a previously innocuous odor and trained rats to freeze whenever the odor alone was presented. They then showed that these fear-conditioned rats do not freeze if their pups are present. Rather, the rat mothers (in the case of rats, this kind of thing only works with mothers) rush to gather in their pups and may even try to attack the source from which the odor is emanating. This aggressive, offspring-protecting behavior was then completely blocked by inhibiting the ability of oxytocin to reach the amygdala.[1] Without oxytocin activity in the amygdala, rat mothers freeze in the presence of the conditioned stimulus even when their pups are present. Notice that oxytocin, in promoting rat maternal behavior, does not seem to make the rat mother more "loving" as it attempts to rip apart the source of the odor. Rather, oxytocin makes mother rats more aggressive. Experiments like this demonstrate that oxytocin is not exactly a "love hormone," but rather promotes behaviors necessary for social connections: in this case, the maternal attachment to her offspring.

Human parents generally mate for long periods of time, an adaptation thought to have evolved to accommodate the uniquely long period of maturation necessary for human children. Despite high rates of divorce and infidelity, it is generally recognized that humans form long-term monogamous pair bonds in part to rear their offspring. In this way, we are unusual. Most other species, including our nearest genetic neighbors, the chimpanzees, come together only to copulate and then have little to do with each other again. Chimpanzee and rat fathers take very little interest in their children or in the mothers of their children. In fact, only about 5% of mammalian species mate for life and share offspring-rearing responsibilities.

One of those exceptions is a tiny animal called the prairie vole (Figure 7.1). Unlike most mammalian species, and even its own very close cousins the montane vole and the meadow vole, prairie vole males and females mate for extended periods after copulating, often for life. They rear their offspring together, and the male aggressively fights off intruders. Just as in humans, when the male partner of a prairie vole couple imbibes alcohol without his mate, the relationship is seriously disrupted.[2] Because the prairie vole is monogamous, but its close genetic relatives are not, it presented a perfect experiment in nature for neuroscientist and former head of the National Institute of Mental Health (NIMH) Thomas Insel to investigate. I first met Tom Insel when he was still doing clinical research on human patients with obsessive compulsive disorder at the NIMH. But he moved on to a series of pioneering basic science studies at the Yerkes Primate Center in Atlanta, Georgia, in which he elucidated the biology of pairwise bonding in the prairie vole.

It turns out that prairie voles' tendency to form permanent bonds depends on the action of two hormones that are produced in the brain, oxytocin (primarily in females but also to some degree in males) and vasopressin (in males). Shortly after mating, the expression of genes for oxytocin and vasopressin receptors in key brain areas increases.[3]

[1] Rickenbacher E, Perry RE, Sulivan RM, Moita MA: Freezing suppression by oxytocin in central amygdala allows alternate defensive behaviours and mother-pup interactions. *eLife* 2017; doi:10.7554/eLife.24080.
[2] Walcott AT, Ryabinin AE: Alcohol's effects on pair-bond maintenance in male prairie voles. *Front Psychiatry* November 17, 2017.
[3] Wang H, Duciot F, Liu Y, Wang Z, Kabbaj M: Histone deacetylase inhibitors facilitate partner preference formation in female prairie voles. *Nat Neuroscience* 2013;16:919–924.

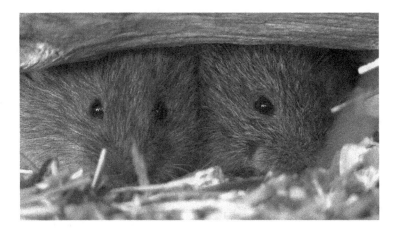

**Figure 7.1** Male and female prairie voles form lifelong bonds after mating.
http://ak5.picdn.net/shutterstock/videos/6488375/thumb/1.jpg

No such increase in receptor density for oxytocin or vasopressin is found in brains of polygamous montane voles after mating.[4] Studies subsequently showed that injecting oxytocin or vasopressin into brains of the polygamous vole species induced bonding behavior, whereas inhibiting these hormones in the prairie vole disrupts their normal bonding patterns. Although our attention will be mainly on oxytocin in this chapter, it is worth noting that the effects of vasopressin are highly complex. In humans, for example, inhaling vasopressin decreases men's emotional recognition abilities,[5] which seems exactly the opposite of what is observed in male prairie voles. Drugs that block the ability of vasopressin to bind to its brain receptors are even being looked at as possible antianxiety and antidepressant agents.

Oxytocin also has profound effects on nurturing behavior of female prairie voles and other rodents toward their pups. The denser the concentration of oxytocin receptors in prairie vole mothers' brains, the more extensive is their maternal behavior. Once again, inhibiting oxytocin in female prairie voles also disrupts maternal behavior.[6] Ordinarily, virgin female mice show very little maternal behavior, but Robert Froemke and colleagues at New York University have shown that injecting their brains with oxytocin makes them act like mothers, including picking up the pups of other females with their mouths. The NYU group showed that oxytocin activated

[4] Insel TR, Shapiro LE: Oxytocin receptor distribution reflects social organization in monogamous and polygamous voles. *Proc Natl Acad Sci USA* 1992;89:5981–5985; Winslow JT, Hastings N, Carter CS, Harbaugh CR, Insel TR: A role for central vasopressin in pair bonding in monogamous prairie voles *Nature* 1993;365:545–548.

[5] Uyzefovsky F, Shalev I, Israel S, Knafo A, Ebstein RF: Vasopressin selectively impairs emotion recognition in men. *Psychoneuroendocrinology* 2012;37:576–580.

[6] McGraw LA, Young LJ: The prairie vole: an emerging model organism for understanding the social brain. *Trends Neuroscience* 2010;33:103–115.

neural responses to the pups' calls in these virgin females, turning indifference into mothering behavior.[7]

In previous chapters, it was pointed out that another brain hormone, corticotropin releasing hormone (CRH), is released during stress and causes fear and avoidance responses when administered to animals. Oxytocin may have an opposite effect. The group of scientists at SUNY Downstate with whom I worked, led by Leonard Rosenblum and Jeremy Coplan, observed this when we compared two species of monkeys that belong to the same genus, the bonnet (*Macaca radiata*) and pigtail macaques (*Macaca nemestrina*). The bonnet macaque is a gregarious and affiliative animal, whereas pigtails are volatile and socially aloof. We measured these hormones in the cerebrospinal fluid (CSF) of adults of both species and, as predicted, found that bonnets had lower CRH and higher oxytocin levels than pigtails.[8] These hormonal differences correlated strongly with the behavioral differences between bonnets and pigtails. And remember that growling dog that frightened you as a child? Well give that dog oxytocin and it becomes less interested in angry faces and more attentive to smiling faces.[9]

A human study produced results compatible with our observations in monkeys. Scientists gave intranasal oxytocin to 15 health men and showed them fear-inducing pictures while they underwent functional MRI (fMRI) of the brain. Compared to placebo, oxytocin had a marked effect in reducing amygdala activity and amygdala connections to downstream brainstem regions that mediate many of the signs of anxiety, like freezing and increased heart rate (see Chapter 6 for a more complete discussion of the amygdala and its role in fear).[10] Administering oxytocin increases cooperation among men.[11] Other data also suggest that oxytocin has antianxiety effects. Furthermore, oxytocin increases the birth of new neurons (neurogenesis, see Chapter 4) in the hippocampus, an effect seen with most antidepressants drugs.[12]

Furthermore, the level of gene expression for proteins that function in the oxytocin and vasopressin system accounts for some of the differences people show in their levels of social connectedness. One study found that higher expression of a key gene

[7] Martin BJ, Mitre M, D'amour JA, Chao MV, Froemke RC: Oxytocin enables maternal behaviour by balancing cortical inhibition. *Nature* 2015;520:499–504.

[8] Rosenblum LA, Smith EL, Altemus M, et al.: Differing concentrations of corticotropin-releasing factor and oxytocin in the cerebrospinal fluid of bonnet and pigtail macaques. *Psychoneuroendocrinology* 2002;27:651–660.

[9] Somppi S, Tornqvist H, Topal J, Koskela A, Hanninen L, Krause CM, Vainio O: Oxytocin treatment biases dogs' visual attention and emotional response toward positive human facial expressions. *Front Psychology*, published online October 17, 2017. https://www.frontiersin.org/articles/10.3389/fpsyg.2017.01854/full

[10] Kirsch P, Essinger C, Chen Q, et al.: Oxytocin modulates neural circuitry for social cognition and fear in humans. *J Neurosci* 2005;25:11489–11493.

[11] Rilling JK, DeMarco AC, Hackelt PD, et al.: Effects of intranasal oxytocin and vasopressin on cooperative behavior and associated brain activity in men. *Psychoneuroendocrinology* 2012;137:447–461.

[12] Opendak M, Offit L, Monari P, et al.: Lasting adaptions in social behavior produced by social disruption and inhibition of adult neurogenesis. *J Neurosci* 2016;36:7027–7038.

in the oxytocin system, *CD38*, and differences in the nucleotide sequence of a related gene, *CD157*, in young adults are associated with being friendly and more socially adept.[13] Men with a specific form (or allele) of the gene that codes for the oxytocin receptor (OXTR) that is expressed in a brain structure called the *nucleus accumbens* (NAc) have enhanced social attachment.[14] Incidentally, variations in the OXTR gene in dogs mediates some of the differences in their human-directed social behavior.[15] Other studies have shown that variations in the gene for vasopressin correlate with differences in social cognition.

In general, giving oxytocin to humans boosts feelings of trust and generosity. For example, oxytocin administration makes people feel less likely to want to give offenders harsh punishments in an experimental social justice test.[16] One study showed that oxytocin levels are lower in patients with social anxiety disorder (also known as social phobia) than healthy controls after a participating in the Trust Game.[17] Such findings have prompted studies investigating whether oxytocin can improve social cognition in people with autistic spectrum disorders (ASD) or reduce fear in patients with anxiety disorders. So far, unfortunately, the results of these studies are decidedly mixed.

We can conclude, then, that in animals and humans oxytocin promotes social affiliation, parental nurturing behavior, and monogamous pair bonding and seems to have antianxiety effects. On the other hand, merely boosting oxytocin levels may not be sufficient to treat any psychiatric disorder. Still, it is worth reviewing what oxytocin is and does in the brain.

## WHAT IS OXYTOCIN?

Oxytocin was discovered in 1904, and its chemical structure—nine amino acids—was determined in 1952. Most of it is made in a brain structure called the *hypothalamus*, which transports it to the pituitary gland, from which oxytocin is released into the blood stream (see Figure 7.2). Oxytocin levels naturally rise in women during labor, and it is often administered to induce or augment labor. A brand name for oxytocin is Pitocin, and I remember during medical school overhearing obstetricians refer to "pitting the baby out" when they induced labor with oxytocin. It is also necessary for

[13] Chong A, Malavasi F, Israel S, et al.: ADP ribosyl-clyclases (CD38/CD157), social skills and friendship. *Psychoneuroendocrinology* 2017;78:185–192.

[14] King LB, Walum H, Inoue K, Eyrich N, Young LJ: Variation in the oxytocin receptor gene predicts brain region-specific expression and social attachment. *Biol Psychiatry* 2016;80:160–169.

[15] Persson ME, Trottier AJ, Belteky J, Roth LSV, Jensen P: Intranasal oxytocin and a polymorphism in the oxytocin receptor gene are associated with human-directed social behavior in golden retriever dogs. *Horm Behav* 2017;95:85–93.

[16] Stallen M, Rossi F, Heijne A, Smidts A, De Dreu CKW, Sanfey AG: Neurobiological mechanisms of responding to injustice. *J Neuroscience* 2018;38:2944–2954.

[17] Hoge EA, Lawson EA, Metcalf CA, et al.: Plasma oxytocin immunoreactive products and response to trust in patients with social anxiety disorder. *Depress Anxiety* 2012;29:924–930.

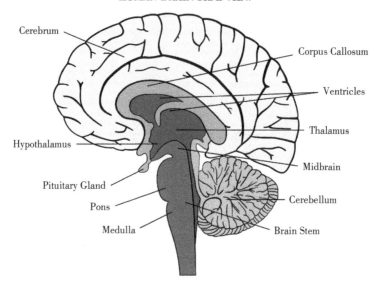

**HUMAN BRAIN-SIDE VIEW**

Cerebrum

Corpus Callosum

Ventricles

Thalamus

Hypothalamus

Midbrain

Pituitary Gland

Cerebellum

Pons

Medulla

Brain Stem

**Figure 7.2** The hypothalamus synthesizes many brain hormones, including oxytocin and corticotropin releasing hormone. Oxytocin is transported to the pituitary gland, which rests right behind the eyes, from which it is released into the bloodstream during labor, delivery, orgasm, and breastfeeding. Another route takes oxytocin from the hypothalamus to other brain regions, including the amygdala, ventral pallidum, and nucleus accumbens.
Shutterstock.

release of milk by the breasts after delivery. Hence, its role in pregnancy, delivery, and breastfeeding was appreciated before its actions in the brain were determined.

Oxytocin has been called the "love hormone" for a variety of reasons, including the fact that it is released during sex and orgasm. Some studies suggest that oxytocin levels increase when people first fall in love. But the characterization of oxytocin in this way oversimplifies its biological purposes, which are many and complex. Because it plays a key role in sex, labor, delivery, and breastfeeding, it is more accurate to say that its real purpose is the preservation of mammalian species, including humans, through enhanced reproductive efficiency.

As always, what seems like straightforward biology in an animal model can get confusing when we approach that biology in humans. For example, although there is evidence that oxytocin is released when people first fall in love and therefore seems to have something to do with promoting relationships in a manner that might be akin to its fostering bonding in animals, other studies have shown that oxytocin is released when humans feel a relationship that they are already in is threatened.[18] Does this

[18] Grebe NM, Kristoffersen AA, Grontvedt TV, Thompson ME, Kennair LEO, Gangestad SW: Oxytocin and vulnerable romantic relationships. *Horm Behav* 2017; 90:64–74. doi:10.1016/j.yhbeh.2017.02.009

serve to soothe someone's despair when he or she senses an impending break-up? Does it make him or her more open to finding new partners? It is also likely that the oxytocin response to a threatened break-up varies considerably among individuals. We know that some people handle romantic upheavals better than others, so the signal to release oxytocin under such circumstances must depend on input from other areas of the brain, areas that evaluate how real the threat of a break-up is and how much it matters to the individuals involved. This kind of emotion is, of course, hard to model in the prairie vole, but it again extends our understanding of how oxytocin functions in social and romantic situations. As always, it does not mean we should throw up our hands and declare that human emotions are somehow "beyond" the realm of neuroscience but rather that we are going to need to do many more experiments and develop better technologies to understand the complexity of the human mind.

We know that human parents differ in their parenting behavior. Some people attach more easily to newborns than others, while mothers and fathers interact with toddlers and school-aged children in many different ways, ranging from abusive to overly attentive and hovering. There is compelling evidence that variations in oxytocin levels determine some of these differences among humans in parenting behaviors. Ruth Feldman at Bar-Ilan University, Israel, for example, has extensively studied oxytocin levels in new mothers and fathers. In one such study, she and her colleagues obtained levels from parents during the first postpartum weeks and again when the infants were 6 months old. They found that oxytocin levels increased in both mothers and fathers across the time frame. Higher oxytocin levels were associated with several positive parenting attributes like affectionate touch by the mothers and tactile stimulation by the fathers.[19] Feldman's group also found that higher oxytocin levels are associated with greater parental care in both parents.[20] Brain imaging studies show higher oxytocin levels and greater response to infant cues of the oxytocin-producing regions of the hypothalamus in new mothers who feel secure in their attachments with other people compared to mothers who are insecure and dismissive.[21] James Rilling and Larry Young of Emory University conclude in their review of parenting behavior that "oxytocin supports sensitive caregiving" in humans.[22]

A caution about these studies, however, is that there is never any way to know whether oxytocin levels measured in human blood reflect those in the brain. Because of the blood–brain barrier (see Chapter 5), we never know how much of what is in the brain is getting into the blood and vice versa. It could also be that people with stronger parental behavior somehow cause oxytocin to be squeezed out of the pituitary gland

[19] Gordon J, Zagoory-Sharon O, Leckman JF, Feldman R: Oxytocin and the development of parenting in humans. *Biol Psychiatry* 2010;15:377–382.

[20] Feldman R, Zagoory-Sharon O, Welsman O, et al.: Sensitive parenting is associated with plasma oxytocin and polymorphisms in the *OXTR and CD38* genes. *Biol Psychiatry* 2012;77:175–181.

[21] Strathearn L, Fonagy P, Amico J, Montague PR: Adult attachment predicts maternal and oxytocin response to infant cues. *Neuropsychopharmacology* 2009;34:2655–2666.

[22] Rilling JK, Young LJ: The biology of mammalian parenting and its effect on offspring social development. *Science* 2014;345:771–776.

into the blood without more being produced in the hypothalamus. In such a case, strong parental behavior would be causing the rise in oxytocin levels and not the other way around. PET scanning allows us to measure the levels of many substances produced in the brain, but as of yet we do not have a PET tracer for oxytocin.

If we could deliver oxytocin directly to a human brain, it might be possible to get a better handle on cause-and-effect relationships, but, of course, this is not possible and because oxytocin when taken orally does not cross the blood–brain barrier, giving it in pill form won't help further that aim either. One approach that may work, however, is intranasal administration. People who use illegal drugs like cocaine and heroin often "snort" them—that is, inhale them through the nose—which results in a rapid "high." It is believed that inhaled drugs have a way of bypassing the blood–brain barrier by traveling along nerves like the olfactory and trigeminal nerves directly into the brain. The extent of this is somewhat controversial, but interesting experiments have been conducted with intranasal administration of oxytocin to human subjects. These have shown that oxytocin increases trust, eye-to-eye contact, and the ability to detect another person's feelings from facial expressions.[23] Intranasal oxytocin also increased positive communication behavior in couples during conflict discussions.[24] A study in monkeys does in fact indicate that intranasally-delivered oxytocin can enter the cerebrospinal fluid (CSF), the fluid that surrounds the brain.[25]

On the other hand, there are compelling data that oxytocin promotes aggression to outsiders and unfamiliar people.[26] In wild chimpanzees, urinary oxytocin levels are highest when a group of animals engages in coordinated action to battle another group.[27] In this case, oxytocin is affecting social bonding—coordinated behavior among a group—in the service of violence. Other evidence supports the idea that oxytocin only increases social connectedness among people within a prespecified group and fosters defensiveness and hostility to those outside of the group. Thus, oxytocin might increase prejudice and decrease empathy to outsiders. Furthermore, one study in mice showed that after a negative social interaction, oxytocin actually promoted avoidance of unfamiliar social encounters in the future.[28] We are learning a lot about the relationship between oxytocin and social bonding in both animals and humans,

[23] Insel TR: The challenge of translation in social neuroscience: a review of oxytocin, vasopressin, and affiliative behavior. *Neuron* 2010;65:768–779.

[24] Ditzen B, Schaer M, Gabriel B, Bonenmann G, Ehlert U, Heinrichs M: Intranasal oxytocin increases positive communication and reduces cortisol levels during couple conflict. *Biol Psychiatry* 2009;65:728–731.

[25] Lee MR, Scheidweiler KB, Diao XX, et al.: Oxytocin by intranasal routeds reaches the cerebrospinal fluid in rhesus macaques: determination using a novel oxytocin assay. *Molecular Psychiatry* 2018;23:115–122.

[26] Miller G: The promise and perils of oxytocin. *Science* 2013;339:267–269.

[27] Samuni L, Preis A, Mundry R, Deschner T, Crockford C, Wittig RM: Oxytocin reactivity during intergroup conflict in wild chimpanzees. *Proc Natl Acad Sci USA* 2016;114:268–273.

[28] Duque-Wilckens N, Steinman MZ, Busnelli M, et al.: Oxytocin receptors in the anteromedial bed nucleus of the stria terminalis promote stress-induced social avoidance in females. *Biol Psychiatry* 2018 Feb 1;83:203–213. doi:10.1016; Epub ahead of print

but we need to be cautious in predicting that it will be a useful treatment for depression, anxiety, abnormal social affiliation, or any other human malady. First, it is hard to get it into the brain. Second, it is only one part of a complex system of checks and balances that control social behavior. Third, it may have many paradoxical effects, especially when dealing with the complexities of human social interactions.

The importance of studying oxytocin is that it isolates one aspect of the biology of attachment, allowing us to see how the release of a hormone by the brain strengthens behaviors and feelings associated with social connectivity and even love. It may turn out that specific abnormalities in the synthesis or actions of oxytocin in the brain are responsible for diagnosable illnesses and maladaptive traits and that administering oxytocin or blocking vasopressin might offer some symptomatic relief. My guess is that things will not work out to be so simple. On the other hand, I do believe that oxytocin might serve as an indicator of an individual's potential for bonding to others. Perhaps abusive parents have diminished release of or response to oxytocin, reflected in its measurable blood level. Then, psychosocial interventions to improve parenting could be monitored by serial measurement of oxytocin levels. In such a case, we would not need to see oxytocin as the only factor in a parent's ability to nurture a child. Instead, we would be taking advantage of a mass of animal and human research to develop an objective marker of the effectiveness of a treatment intervention.

## THE BRAIN'S "REWARD" PATHWAY

In the 1970s, it was discovered that oxytocin produced in the hypothalamus is transported directly to other places in addition to the pituitary gland. One of these is the already mentioned amygdala (see Chapter 6), and there is evidence that this pathway is activated to reduce the effects of stress,[29] perhaps in part by opposing the effects of CRH.

Another important target of hypothalamic oxytocin is the NAc (or NAcc) (Figure 7.3). Just as oxytocin has been somewhat glibly called the "love hormone," the NAc's role has been oversimplified by referring to it as the terminal point of the brain's "reward pathway." What is commonly called the reward pathway begins in the upper portion of the brain stem, the midbrain, in a structure called the *ventral tegmental area* (VTA). The VTA is rich in neurons that synthesize the neurotransmitter dopamine, and its axons release dopamine onto the dendrites of neurons in the NAc. This pathway from VTA to NAc is also referred to as the mesolimbic pathway.

A bit of neuroanatomy terminology may be interesting to some readers to explain just what the NAc is. Deep in the brain resides a major structure called the *basal ganglia* (see Figure 7.4). The basal ganglia are divided into several substructures. One of these is the striatum, which is further divided into the dorsal striatum (composed of the caudate nucleus and putamen) and the ventral striatum, which is mostly the NAc

---

[29] Spengler FB, Schultz J, Scheele D, et al.: Kinetics and dose dependency of intranasal oxytocin effects on amygdala reactivity. *Biol Psychiatry* 2017;82:885–894.

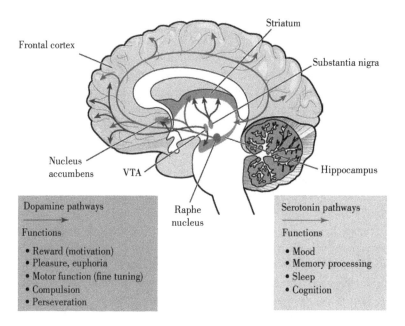

**Figure 7.3** The nucleus accumbens (NAc) is part of the basal ganglia and receives projections from the ventral tegmental area (VTA) in the brainstem that carry the neurotransmitter dopamine. The NAc is part of the ventral striatum. The image also shows pathways that carry the neurotransmitter serotonin.

Shutterstock.

**Basal Ganglia and Related Structures of the Brain**

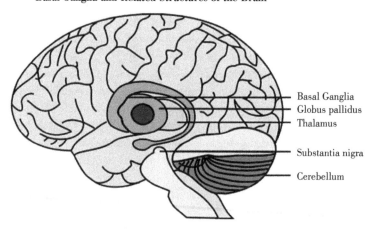

**Figure 7.4** The basal ganglia include the nucleus accumbens (NAc), the globus pallidus, the substantia nigra, and several other structures. It is buried deep in the brain.

From John Henkel, US Food and Drug Administration (image in public domain).

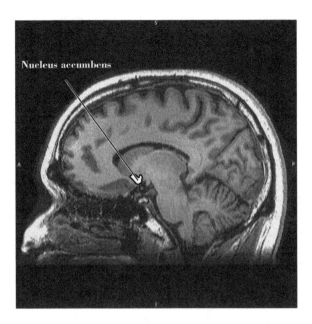

**Figure 7.5** The nucleus accumbens is shown outlined and in white. It is divided into a shell and a core, each with somewhat different functions. Despite being a very small structure, it receives inputs and sends outputs to many other important parts of the brain and is critically involved in motivation and reward. Image in public domain.

(plus something called the olfactory tubercle). The dorsal striatum is involved in the control of physical motion and in decision-making; the ventral striatum regulates our perception of rewarding and pleasurable stimuli.[30] The basal ganglia also include the globus pallidus, which we won't be discussing much in this book; the ventral pallidum, to which the hypothalamus sends vasopressin and also plays a role in reward perception; the substantia nigra, which is affected by Parkinson's disease; and the subthalamic nucleus, which we also won't be saying much more about.

I apologize for all the neuroanatomy and barrage of brain regions. For some, it is important to square away all of these terms because they are often used interchangeably in the scientific literature. For example, the NAc and the ventral striatum are sometimes considered the same thing, even though technically the NAc is a part of the ventral striatum. Some authors only use the term "striatum" when they really mean the NAc. And the VTA-to-NAc pathway is called the reward pathway, the dopaminergic pathway, and the mesolimbic pathway.

But, for now, let's get back to the NAc, even though it is tiny (Figure 7.5). The nucleus accumbens is divided into its core and shell, each with slightly different functions but both critical to mediating motivation and reward. Recordings using electrodes buried in the NAc of animals show that they learn to anticipate positive reinforcement

[30] Flanigan M, LeClair K: Shared motivation functions of ventral striatum D1 and D2 medium spiny neurons. *J Neurosci* 2017;37:6177–6179.

because of activity in the NAc. This behavior can be abolished by injecting drugs that block the ability of dopamine to bind to its receptors in the NAc, proving that it is the VTA-to-NAc dopamine pathway that is necessary for the reinforcement of reward learning.

The way this works is a bit complicated and not simply, as some think, that dopamine levels go up every time the animal is rewarded. Rather, dopamine levels in the NAc go up whenever an outcome is better than expected, dopamine levels are unchanged if the outcome is the same as expected, and dopamine levels decrease below baseline if the outcome is worse than expected.[31] Through the detection of prediction error—instances in which the outcome is different from expectation—animals learn to anticipate reward and avoid danger. Scientists have worked out the complex mathematical computations that even a rat brain uses to perform this kind of learning by trial and error. We can simplify this without distorting reality too grievously by saying that increased activity of dopamine neurons in the VTA-to-NAc pathway is necessary for animals to learn about and anticipate reward. Indeed, now that scientists can precisely stimulate specific neurons in the animal brain using optogenetics, it is clear that rats like having the NAc stimulated and doing so motivates them to learn faster.[32] It is also important to note that stress downregulates activity in VTA dopamine neurons—and in serotonin pathways as well (see Figure 7.3)—making the reward response less robust.[33] This seems like analogous to what might happen in people who respond to high levels of stress by becoming depressed.

In human imaging studies, NAc activity increases during the anticipation of pleasurable stimuli; whenever we eat food that we like (especially sugary and high-fat foods), have sex, or exercise, neurons in the VTA synthesize dopamine, which then travels along axons, traverses synapses, and binds to receptors on dendrites in our NAc. Neuroscientist Richard Davidson and his group at the University of Wisconsin, Madison, showed that the ability to keep the NAc engaged in a task involving reward responses during fMRI scanning predicted long-term real-world positive emotional responses.[34] In other words, people whose NAc sustains an appreciation for pleasurable stimuli are the most able to maintain a positive attitude. People who are intensely in love have specifically increased activity in the dopamine pathway from the VTA to the striatum.[35] So far, then, stimulating the VTA-to-NAc pathway seems linked to a

---

[31] Eshel N: Trial and error: Optongenetic techniques offer insight into the dopamine circuit underlying learning. *Science* 2016;354:1108–1109.

[32] Tsai HC, Zhang F, Adamantidis A, et al.: Phasic firing in dopaminergic neurons is sufficient for behavioral conditioning. *Science* 2009;324:1080–1084.

[33] Zhong W, Li Y, Feng Q, Luo M: Learning and stress shape the reward response patterns of serotonin neurons. *J Neuroscience* 2017;37:8863–8875.

[34] Heller AS, Fox AS, Wing EK, McQuisition KM, Vack NJ, Davidson RJ: The neurodynamics of affect in the laboratory predicts persistence of real-world emotional responses. *J Neurosci* 2015;35:1503–10509.

[35] Fisher H, Aron A, Brown LL: Romantic love: an fMRI study of a neural mechanism for mate choice. *J Comparative Neurol* 2005;493:58–62.

bevy of positive feelings and emotions. Like any other human brain system, however, there are unfortunately many things that can go wrong.

Activation of the VTA-to-NAc pathway also plays an important role in parental behavior, and here it often interacts with the oxytocin system. In multiple studies on mammals and other species, both activation of the VTA and oxytocin release are necessary for the initiation of maternal behavior.[36] In humans, imaging studies show activation of the VTA and NAc as parents view pictures of their children, with fathers who are the most involved in caregiving showing the most VTA activation.[37] In animals, oxytocin activates the VTA-to-NAc pathway to motivate mothers to approach infants in need, and, in humans, the level of oxytocin in blood correlates with activation of the NAc when parents are shown pictures or videos of their own children.

It may also be the case that people who naturally have higher levels of response by the ventral striatum to positive feedback are better able to fend off the effects of stressful life events. A Duke University study of 200 people who were not psychiatric patients measured "positive affect"—essentially a good mood—during fMRI scanning. Those with a combination of lower levels of ventral striatum reactivity to positive feedback and recent life stress experienced lower levels of positive affect compared to people with higher levels of ventral striatum reactivity and no recent life stress.[38] The authors of the study concluded that it provided "empirical evidence for the potentially protective role of robust reward-related neural responsiveness against reduction in PA [positive affect] that may occur in the wake of life stress." (p. 157). A study like this has too many variables to tease apart what is causing what, of course. Does life stress lower ventral striatum reactivity? Is there another factor that makes some people's ventral striatum react more strongly to positive feedback? Or does inherently low ventral striatum reactivity to positive feedback make a person more vulnerable to stressful life events?

For some people, the 2016 U.S. presidential election was a stressful life event. Psychologists at UCLA recruited people who felt distressed by the election results. Those who had no symptoms of depression had either strong family support or increased activation in two specific brain regions, one of which was the NAc.[39]

These are obviously important questions because, if the latter is true, we might have a clue to why some people are more prone to depressed moods following a significantly stressful life event. Such people might lose the ability to respond to praise and success, certainly a characteristic of people suffering with depression. Indeed, the tendency to ignore positive feedback and only attend to negative feedback is a target of

[36] Dulac C, O'Connell LA, Wu Z: Neural control of maternal and paternal behaviors. *Science* 2014;345:765–770.

[37] Rilling JK, Young LJ: The biology of mammalian parenting and its effect on offspring social development. *Science* 2014;345:771–776.

[38] Nikolova YS, Bogdan R, Brigidi R, Hariri AR: Ventral striatum reactivity to reward and recent life stress interact to predict positive affect. *Biol Psychiatry* 2012;72:157–163.

[39] Tashjian SM, Galvan A: The role of mesolimbic circuitry in buffering election-related distress. *J Neuroscience* 2018;38:2887–2898.

cognitive behavioral therapy (CBT) for depression. What an imaging study like this does tell us is that there is an interesting interaction among stress, ventral striatum re-activity to positive feedback, and mood.

Therapists cannot prevent people from experiencing stressful life events, but there are many ways to approach a person suffering with depression who has recently faced a major life setback. Antidepressant medications are, of course, one approach. Psychotherapies are also effective for depressed people, but some of them encourage the patient to recall and "process" the stressful event, others to put it behind him, and still others to see it only as a reminder of earlier life traumas. Understanding how stressful life events affect the responsivity of the ventral striatum to positive and negative stimuli could help us figure out which approach is best for which patient.

On a broader level, activation of the NAc and ventral striatum is involved in reinforcing the satisfaction we derive from belonging to a social group. In experiments in which people are asked to give rewards to other people, there is greater ventral striatum activity when those rewards are given to members of the subject's own group as opposed to another, so-called out-group.[40] When donating money, the ventral striatum is most active when other people are watching and there is the expectation of social approval.[41] On the other hand, not helping a member of the out-group is also accompanied by activation of the NAc.[42] And we get more ventral striatum excitement when we receive a reward that is bigger than someone else's.[43] The dopamine pathways in our brains may even explain why we become and remain fans of a specific football team.[44] The NAc/ventral striatum thus mediates important aspects of social behavior, making us feel best when we are in a group and doing better than competitors.

## THE REWARD PATHWAY IS HIJACKED BY ADDICTIONS

As is the case for oxytocin's effects, there are two sides of what NAc activity can do for us. On the positive side, it makes us feel secure belonging to a group, but, on the negative side, it makes us feel good when outsiders get punished.

Another downside to NAc activity is its critical role in addiction. It is now known, thanks in part to the brilliant work of Mount Sinai School of Medicine neuroscientist

[40] Molenberghs P, Bosworth R, Nott, Z, et al.: The influence of group membership and individual differences in psychopathy and perspective taking on neural responses when punishing and rewarding others. *Hum Brain Mapp* 2014;35:4989–4999.

[41] Izuma K, Saito D, Sadato N: Processing of the incentive for social approval in the ventral striatum during charitable donations. *J Cognitive Neuroscience* 2010;22:621–631.

[42] Hein G, Silani G, Preuschoff K, Batson CD, Singer T: Neural responses to ingroup and outgroup members' suffering predict individual differences in costly helping. *Neuron* 2010;68:149–160.

[43] Fliessbach K, Weber B, Trautner P, Dohmen T, Sunde U, Elger CE, Falk A: Social comparison affects reward-related brain activity in the human ventral striatum. *Science* 2007;318:1305–1308.

[44] Duarte I, Afonso S, Jorge H, Cayolla R, Ferreira C, Castelo-Branco M: Tribal love: the neural correlates of passionate engagement in football fans. *Soc Cogn Affect Neurosci* 2017;12:718–728.

Eric Nestler and his team, that dopamine binding activates a gene in the nucleus accumbens called ∆FosB. Activation of the ∆FosB gene is necessary for many aspects of our ability to experience reward and pleasure.[45] Blocking the gene's expression interferes with the reinforcement of rewarding behaviors. Just like blocking dopamine receptors, blocking ∆FosB gene activation inhibits a rat's ability to figure out when to anticipate a reward and when to predict something aversive will occur.

Unfortunately, this is also exactly what happens when we consume "recreational" drugs like cocaine, heroin, amphetamines, and alcohol. These abusable substances can hijack the VTA-to-NAc pathway because they are among the most powerful stimulants of dopamine activity. So strong is this effect that some people start to crave the rewarding feelings they get from stimulation of the nucleus accumbens, and they crave drugs and alcohol in between actually taking them. For many addicts, it takes more and more drug to get the same amount of dopamine release, leading to the sad state of needing to spend most of the time acquiring ever-increasing supplies. Nestler and others discovered that increasing the expression of ∆FosB can mimic the effects of giving cocaine and other abusable drugs to laboratory animals.[46] This has opened an important area of research attempting to find medications that block ∆FosB expression to reduce craving in drug addicts. There is already evidence that an experimental drug to reduce craving in alcoholics may work by decreasing activity in the NAc and other parts of the striatum.[47]

The VTA–NAc also fires away in anticipation of foods we like to eat, especially those that contain a lot of fat and sugar.[48] When obesity-susceptible rats eat junk food, there is a rapid and long-lasting increase in activity of a group of neurons in the NAc.[49] For some people, the prefrontal cortex reminds them that eating a lot of junk food makes you fat, and those lucky few can restrict the number of French fries and bowls of ice cream they eat. For unclear reasons, however, other peoples' NAc so enjoy fatty, sweet foods that its enhanced activity overwhelms any good sense coming from the prefrontal cortex. Scientists are, of course, struggling to figure out how to turn down the NAc as one of the strategies to treat our obesity epidemic, but so far nothing is available for clinical use. These are powerful brain systems that resist manipulation.

In addition to the fact that it is involved in drug addiction, there are other reasons to be circumspect in referring to the VTA-to-NAc pathway as *the* reward pathway or

[45] Robinson AJ, Nestler EJ: Transcriptional and epigenetic mechanisms of addiction. *Nat Rev Neurosci* 2011;12:623–637.

[46] Hyman SE, Malenka RC, Nestler EJ: Neural mechanisms of addiction: the role of reward-related learning and memory. *Ann Rev Neurosci* 2006;29:565–598.

[47] Quelch DR, Mick I, McGonigle J, et al.: Nalmefene reduces reward anticipation in alcohol dependence: an experimental functional magnetic resonance imaging study. *Biol Psychiatry* 2017;81:941–948.

[48] Jabr F: That craving for dessert. *Sci Am* January, 2016, 23–24.

[49] Oginsky MF, Goforth PB, Nobile CW, Lopez-Santiago LF, Ferrano CR: Eating "junk food" produces rapid and long-lasting increase in NAc CP-AMPA receptors: implications for enhanced cue-induced motivation and food addiction. *Neuropsychopharmacology* 2016;43:2977–2986.

to the NAc as *the* reward center of the brain. As we have seen repeatedly in this book, many other pathways converge on the NAc, and some of them are also involved in reward and pleasure. For example, the VTA also projects directly to the prefrontal cortex via a route called the *mesocortical pathway*. In turn, the dopamine neurons in the prefrontal cortex project to the NAc, regulating how we perceive rewarding stimuli.[50] Just as the prefrontal cortex exerts control over the amygdala and modulates our fear responses, the prefrontal cortex can affect how we respond to what feels pleasurable. One study in mice suggested that antidepressants work in part by strengthening the prefrontal cortex-to-NAc pathway.[51] This might mean that antidepressants enable a depressed person to overcome the inability to respond to positive events and to experience pleasure by strengthening the connection between the brain's "reward center" and the part of the brain that interprets the meaning of rewarding experiences.

This pathway from the prefrontal cortex to the NAc also affects the monogamous bonding behavior of the prairie vole. Following in the footsteps of Tom Insel, a research group at Emory University is pursuing this model of social affiliation. They recently showed that the strength of the prefrontal cortex-to-NAc pathway predicts how quickly a female prairie vole will begin to cuddle with its partner after a first mating encounter.[52]

We saw in Chapter 6 that the prefrontal cortex has powerful abilities to modify and even suppress automatic fear responses. Here, we see its ability to bias an animal in favor of "marrying" a specific partner. We can assume that this same pathway plays a role in human social bonds as well, but for us it will obviously be more complex because our prefrontal cortex is many times more sophisticated than that of a prairie vole. The decisions we make about whom to marry are going to involve the same VTA-to-NAc pathways as are found in prairie voles, but also our much more powerful prefrontal cortex-to-NAc pathway.

And, while we are on the subject of that famous rodent the prairie vole, it is important to note that oxytocin, the hormone that is crucial to its unique monogamous behavior, also exerts a powerful effect on the NAc by binding to oxytocin receptors (designated as OXTR) on neurons in the VTA. Stimulating the OXTR in the VTA increases dopamine release into the NAc, thus reinforcing behavior. One elegant study showed that this pathway determines how sociable a male mouse will be with an unknown juvenile mouse. Knocking out the OXTR in the VTA reduced the amount of time male mice will spend in a chamber with an unknown mouse.[53]

[50] Jenni NL, Larkin JD, Floresco SB: Prefrontal dopamine D1 and D2 receptors regulate dissociable aspects of decision making via distinct ventral striatal and amygdalar circuits. *J Neurosci* 2017;37:6200–6213.

[51] Chang CH, Chen MC, Lu J: Effect of antidepressant drugs on the vmPFC-limbic circuitry. *Neuropharmacology* 2015;92C:116–124.

[52] Amadel EA, Johnson ZV, Kwon YJ, et al.: Dynamic corticostriatal activity biases social bonding in monogamous female prairie voles. *Nature* 2017;546:297–301. doi:10.1038

[53] Hung LW, Neuner S, Polepalli JS, et al.: Gating of social reward by oxytocin in the ventral tegmental area. *Science* 2017;357:1406–1411.

Clearly, there are other pathways than the mesolimbic pathway that serve reward behavior. If you review the literature on this area you will encounter brain structures such as the ventral pallidum, insula, and orbitofrontal cortex, all playing a role in what we interpret as rewarding. There are also many other neurotransmitters besides dopamine and oxytocin involved, including naturally occurring opioids, serotonin, gamma aminobutyric acid (GABA), and glutamate. So, the VTA–NAc pathway and dopamine are not the only parts of the story.

We should mention one of these other systems here. Recall that the NAc plays a critical role in drug addiction regardless of the type of drug involved. One of those classes of abusable substances is, of course, opioids, both illegal ones like heroin and those prescribed for pain management with brand names like OxyContin, Vicodin, and Percodan. Right now, the United States is in the midst of a terrible epidemic of opioid abuse and overdose, with deaths from these drugs skyrocketing in this century. In addition to triggering the VTA-to-NAc dopamine reward pathway, these substances also bind to receptors for opioids that are naturally produced in the brain. These endogenous opioids, referred to as endorphins and enkephalins, were discovered in 1974 and are synthesized by the brain and released when we feel pain. They also are released during vigorous exercise and may account for the experience some long-distance runners get called "runner's high" (my endorphin system must be defective as I rarely feel anything close to a "high" when running).

It is possible to label the brain's opioid receptors with a radioactive tracer and use PET scanning to measure the concentration of endorphins released during an experimental session. Using this technique, researchers in England and Finland showed that social laughter causes pleasurable feelings and increases release of endorphins in several brain regions.[54] People with the most opioid receptors at baseline laugh the most when they watch films of people laughing. Interestingly, social laughter also made them more tolerant of painful stimuli.

Another reason to be careful ascribing everything about reward to the VTA-to-NAc pathway is that the NAc itself is not just involved in mediating the response to pleasurable stimuli. We obviously learn about many associations besides those that involve pleasure and reward, and it turns out that the NAc is involved in those, too, even when the stimuli are aversive. As neuroscientist Mark Humphries of the University of Manchester put it "[dopamine] signals the error between what you predicted and what you got. That error can be positive, negative, or zero."[55] Thus, it is more accurate to say that the NAc is critical to our learning how what we expect to happen matches up with our experience of what really happens. The neurons in the NAc that receive dopamine from the VTA fire in accordance with the agreement between anticipation and reality.

[54] Manninen S, Tuominen L, Dunbar R, et al.: Social laughter triggers endogenous opioid release in humans. *J Neurosci* 2017; Epub ahead of print
[55] Humphries M: The crimes against dopamine: For they may be many and grievous. *Medium* March 13, 2017, https://medium.com/the-spike/the-crimes-against-dopamine-b82b082d5f3d

This helps to explain the critical role the NAc plays in risky decision-making. Even though we think of the NAc as being central to the reward pathway, it actually prevents laboratory animals from taking risks. Karl Deisseroth of Stanford University, credited with the development of the remarkable technique called optogenetics that allows scientists to stimulate discrete brain areas, showed that risk-preferring rats could be "instantaneously converted to risk-averse rats" by stimulating dopamine neurons in the NAc.[56] This occurs because the NAc neurons are always comparing expectation with outcome, learning what will be rewarding and what will be aversive.

It is obvious that humans, like rats, vary in how much risk with which they feel comfortable. Some amount of daring results in a fuller life. If you always read biographies, perhaps taking the risk of reading a novel occasionally will prove satisfying. In that case, you might at first anticipate being bored, but when the novel grips your attention, you get a nice burst of dopamine activity in your NAc signaling that the outcome was better than your expectation. From this, you learn to enjoy the occasional fiction. On the other hand, anyone who gambles in a casino and expects to make money will soon find that expectation and outcome do not match. Pathological gamblers seem to get a dopamine rush from the thrill of gambling that is not based on outcome; patients with Parkinson's disease who are given drugs that stimulate dopamine release in the brain sometimes develop abnormal gambling behavior. We suspect that something is wrong with the risk prediction system in gamblers that prevents them from learning from experience and causes them to become addicted to the thrill of the chase. We can see how the "reward pathway" indeed rewards us for some degree of daring, cautions us against risk, and severely misleads us when it is hijacked by addictive behaviors.

## IS THERE A BIOLOGY FOR EMPATHY?

I opened this chapter promising to discuss brain pathways involved in some positive aspects of human existence. Thus, oxytocin is critical to monogamous pair bonding, surges during happy events like childbirth and orgasm, and is associated with parental nurturing, trust, and social connectedness. Similarly, the VTA-to-NAc pathway fires when we anticipate pleasure and reward, helps protect us from the effects of stress, and makes us better parents. At the same time, to avoid the criticism of oversimplification, I have shown that the "love hormone" can promote bigotry and make us fight, and the "reward pathway" centered in the nucleus accumbens can turn us into drug and food addicts and gamblers.

While all this is true, another way to look at things is to remember that *without* oxytocin and the nucleus accumbens we would be far less able to love, join and enjoy social groups, and derive pleasure from the world. So, let's put aside the negative aspects of these brain systems for a moment and see if there is a convergence of animal studies

---

[56] Zalocusky KA, Ramakrishnan C, Lerner TN, Davidson TJ, Knutson B, Deisseroth K: Nucleus accumbens D2R cells signal prior outcomes and control risky decision-making. *Nature* 2016;531:642–646, 646.

in the laboratory and brain imaging studies in humans that can tell us a story of how the brain works to allow us to be loving, nurturing, caring, and happy people. To do so, I will take a big risk (there goes my NAc warning me) and consider if we know anything about the biology of a really complicated human emotion, empathy.

One of the traits critical to the survival of human relationships and societies is empathy. We are taught from an early age to "put yourself in his or her place," that is, to try to feel and comprehend another person's experiences and feelings. Human culture also puts great value on a related behavior, altruism, or the ability to give to others without any expectation of personal reward. Human societies flourish based on these ideals. It is easy to point to all the instances in which empathy and altruism break down and fashionable for each generation to accuse itself of being self-centered, selfish, and narcissistic. Some, like Paul Bloom in his book *Against Empathy*[57] even argue that empathy is a bad thing because we tend to empathize most with people who are like us and therefore become bigots.

And there are legitimate arguments about whether empathy is confined to humans. Recent studies, for example, show that chimpanzees are capable of truly altruistic behaviors. In one study, chimpanzees rewarded other chimpanzees who made sacrifices to help others acquire food.[58] Another study showed that male chimpanzees participate in dangerous scouting missions to protect other chimps' wives and children, even when there was no penalty for instead sitting out the missions.[59]

But no matter how much we deny that empathy and altruism are uniquely human, that they are widely enough practiced, or even that they represent positive virtues, it is hard to imagine how human society could function merely on the basis of self-interest. We have very little neurobiology on empathy and altruism drawn from laboratory animals; such features are very hard to identify in mice and rats and have only fairly recently come to light even in apes. But we can read stories of human distress to human volunteers, as scientists from the University of Colorado, Boulder, did, and determine the emotional reactions these volunteers have. The study subjects then listened to the same stories of human distress while undergoing brain imaging and showed remarkable consistency in brain activation patterns among them. When the subjects experienced feelings of empathic "care," brain imaging showed strikingly consistent activation across subjects in the nucleus accumbens and a part of the prefrontal cortex called the orbitofrontal cortex.[60]

This study had two other very interesting findings. First, the extent of empathic care feelings predicted how large a charitable donation the subjects were subsequently willing to make. Second, empathic care could be dissociated from a sense of empathic

[57] Bloom P: *Against Empathy: The Case for Rational Compassion*. New York, HarperCollins, 2016.
[58] Schmelz M, Grueneisen S, Kabalak A, Jost J, Tomasello M: Chimpanzees return favors at a personal cost. *Proc Natl Acad Med USA* 2017;114:7462–7467. doi:10.1073
[59] Langergraber K, Watts DP, Vigilant L, Mitani JC: Group augmentation, collective action, and territorial boundary patrols by male chimpanzees. *Proc Natl Acad Sci USA* 2017;114:7337–7342.
[60] Ashar YK, Andrews-Hanna JR, Dimidjian S, Wager RD: Empathic care and distress: predictive brain markers and dissociable brain systems. *Neuron* 2017;94:1263–1273.

"distress," which, unlike empathic care, was a wholly negative emotion and triggered a different set of brain regions. Thus, the NAc and associated brain regions serve to make us feel rewarded when we experience caring feelings for people in distress and motivation to help them. It would be interesting to see if people with sociopathic and narcissistic traits show less activation of the NAc and orbitofrontal cortex in response to hearing stories of human distress.

In another study, scientists found that when people are deciding to be generous, they activate a brain area called the temporoparietal junction.[61] This projects to the ventral striatum, and the stronger the response of the ventral striatum, the happier the subjects felt with their decisions to be generous. Here again, the "reward center" of the brain is implicated by this experiment in reinforcing altruistic behavior. Similarly, people with a more robust ability for moral reasoning showed greater activity in the ventral striatum compared to those with lower levels of moral reasoning.[62] Virtuous behavior, then, can be highly pleasurable and rewarding, at least for some people.

Once again, when we mention the NAc, oxytocin also crops up. Individuals with medical conditions that cause a reduction in oxytocin appear to have fewer empathy-related behaviors, according to researchers from the University of Cardiff, Wales.[63]

Why did I identify this discussion of empathy as risky? It is hard to think of an emotion that is harder to define and measure. Are we empathic because it makes us feel good about ourselves, or because we are truly selfless? Does it matter? What is meant by "more" or "less" empathic? Is an action necessary to demonstrate empathy, or is the feeling sufficient? Isn't empathy a product of culture and modeling? Imagine, for example, that you see a news report about a person suffering from a life-threatening disease. You feel something because that is a very sad and unpleasant image. When does that feeling become empathy? The dictionary definition would say it is when we feel as if we ourselves were suffering from the same life-threatening disease. Is that when the hypothalamus starts making more oxytocin and the VTA starts sending signals to its axon terminals to release dopamine onto NAc neurons?

Now consider that you are a person of deep religious upbringing who has been taught to live a life of deep caring for the plights of those less fortunate. Have you been secreting more oxytocin and manifesting more NAc activity your whole life? Isn't it a bit crass to reduce great religious and ethical principles to such fundamental, physical processes?

Of course, I can—and will—remind you that I have been very clear throughout this chapter that oxytocin and the nucleus accumbens are only two examples of the

---

[61] Park, SQ, Kahnt T, Dogan A, Strang S, Fehr E, Tobler PN: A neural link between generosity and happiness. *Nat Commun* July 11, 2017.

[62] Fang Z, Jung WH, Korczykowski, et al.: Post-conventional moral reasoning is associated with increased ventral striatal activity at rest and during task. *Sci Rep* August 2, 2017. https://www.nature.com/articles/s41598-017-07115-w

[63] Daughers K, Manstead A, Rees A: Hypopituitarism is associated with decreased oxytocin concentrations and reduced empathic ability. Presented at Society for Endocrinology, November 7-9, 2016, Brighton, UK. Abstract 142.

complex way the brain functions when we experience emotions like love and caring. Still, we somehow want empathy to be above all that, to be a shining example of humanity at its best.

And yet, we cannot escape the fact that to the extent anyone can define or feel something like empathy, it does seem to provoke systems in the brain that are known throughout the animal kingdom to be associated with social connectedness and rewarded behavior. That means we can expect that, in some instances, clear deficits in the ability to feel or express empathy, as occur in people prone to narcissistic and sociopathic behavior, may be accompanied by abnormalities in these pathways.

I do not believe the purpose of this research is to allow us to scan the general population to see who is truly empathic and who is just acting that way to garner social approval or reward. Nor do I think brain imaging is anywhere near sophisticated enough to diagnose sociopathy or determine which criminal acted out of brazen self-interest and which for some other reason. Rather, I hold out hope that just as our experiences shape how cells and regions in our brains connect to each other, new experiences might be able to fix those connections that get hijacked or detoured. In the next chapter, I will try to explore if there is a biology to one type of human experience that attempts to accomplish just that goal—the experience of being in psychotherapy.

# 8

# Is There a Science of Psychotherapy?

The past is never dead. It is not even past.
—William Faulkner, *Requiem for a Nun*

Many, but fortunately not all, psychotherapists seem to see neuroscience as a threat. At some point, in that way of thinking, neuroscience became an arm of psychopharmacology (the treatment of psychiatric illness with medications). According to this view, neuroscience evolved to consider only the "brain" and not the "mind" and adopted a simplistic version of emotion and behavior that is based solely on a few chemical neurotransmitters. Throughout this literature we see complaints that neuroscience is attempting to "reduce" the mind to physiological processes and thereby demean the complexities of the human intellect. It is also charged that neuroscience obfuscates an appreciation of the uniqueness of each individual human in favor of a faceless typology based on an invariant biology.

There are, of course, many exceptions among psychotherapists to this characterization of neuroscience. Some cognitive behavioral psychologists have published impressive work using brain imaging to identify changes in the brain that accompany successful therapy. Others have capitalized on what basic neuroscience has learned about conditioned fear to experiment with drugs that might enhance cognitive behavioral therapy (CBT). A discipline called *neuropsychoanalysis* emerged several years ago that purports to link neuroscience with psychoanalytic theory and practice. We will have much more to say about each of these developments later in this chapter.

Throughout this book, I have tried to assuage the fear that neuroscience is a challenge to psychotherapy while at the same time arguing against the view that there is a "mind" separate from the brain. I wish to pursue this line of argument in this chapter by exploring whether neuroscience has anything to contribute to psychotherapy and vice versa.

There are countless varieties of psychotherapy. In this chapter, I will focus on two of them, CBT and psychoanalytic psychotherapy. I choose CBT because it is among the best studied form of psychotherapy, with abundant evidence from well-designed clinical trials showing that it is effective for a wide range of psychiatric disorders. There is much less evidence supporting the effectiveness of any form of psychoanalytic psychotherapy, including psychoanalysis itself. Nevertheless, this is one of the oldest forms of psychotherapy, based on a theory and techniques that have influenced generations of psychotherapists and that have been applied to millions of patients around the world. Despite the fact that we constantly read articles declaring that psychoanalysis is dead, its principles are very much alive in the minds and work of many, if not most, psychotherapists.

## PSYCHOTHERAPY IS A FORM OF LIFE EXPERIENCE

My argument for the relevance of neuroscience and psychotherapy to each other begins with a seemingly simple assertion: all types of psychotherapy are forms of lived experience. Although that statement may seem benign and perhaps even trivial, I doubt it will meet with universal acceptance among psychotherapists. The idea that psychotherapy is an experience implies that it is something in addition to the application of specific techniques in accordance with a particular set of rules and traditions. But I am adamant about this point: regardless of the kind of psychotherapy involved, a patient lives through the experience of *being* in therapy, of interacting with a therapist over time. Like every experience, then, psychotherapy must change the brain.

Remember that everything we experience activates genes in neurons, causes dendrites to expand or retract, and stimulates (or inhibits) the propagation of electrical impulses that stream from one neuron to the next. In some cases, those impulses remain local, while in others they travel long distances to connect far-flung regions of the brain. Sometimes these changes in brain anatomy and physiology are fleeting, but others are enduring, as when a new memory becomes a long-term memory, something we can summon up years or decades later. The process by which the connections between neurons—called synaptic connections—become stronger when we experience something repeatedly and it becomes consolidated in long-term memory is called long-term potentiation (LTP) and its biochemical features have been extensively elucidated by neuroscientists. Memories can also be diminished by a process that weakens synaptic connections, called long-term depression (LTD). My contention is that psychotherapy, like all experiences, is a constant strengthening and weakening of synaptic connections, of LTP and LTD, involving a complex and highly organized series of physical events in the brain.

If psychotherapy is to be successful, then it must be an experience capable of inducing long-lived changes in the brain, changes that reverse whatever has been causing the problem in the first place. Different types of psychotherapy may cause different changes or different magnitudes of change. Alternatively, different forms of therapy applied successfully to the same illness might instead produce exactly the same changes. Such changes will differ from one individual in therapy to another, just as no two people have exactly the same set of symptoms.

An important determinant of what happens in psychotherapy is the relationship between patient and therapist. William R. Miller, the brilliant psychologist who developed a successful treatment approach called motivational interviewing, has often pointed out that the strength of this relationship is more important in determining whether a therapy is effective than the specific type of therapy being applied.[1] How

[1] Miller WR, Moyers TB: The forest and the trees: relational factors in addiction treatment. *Addiction* 2014;110:401–413.

a person experiences psychotherapy is clearly a fundamental ingredient in whether it works, and everything we experience changes our brains. None of this should strike anyone as particularly radical.

If you accept this idea that psychotherapy is a form of experience that, like any experience, changes the brain, then it should ultimately be possible to reveal those changes. Unfortunately, we are only at the beginning of being able to do so. That is because both the problems that psychotherapies treat and the psychotherapies themselves are highly complex. If we ask 100 people undergoing a functional magnetic resonance imaging (fMRI) scan to move their right index finger, we will see in most of them an increase in activity in a small region called the motor strip in the left side of their brains. Similarly, if we ask those 100 people to look at a picture while they are in the scanner, a region in the back of the brain in the occipital lobe will light up. We have known the pathways that functions like movement and vision travel over for a long time.

For some emotions, the fMRI results are also somewhat predictable. Showing a person a picture that frightens him will usually activate the amygdala, a picture that disgusts him will ignite the insula, and a picture of someone he recognizes will stimulate a brain region called the fusiform gyrus. But a scan of people in love will be far less predictable because love is a complicated emotion that means different things to different people. Hate is another such emotion. And when we get to psychiatric illnesses, the picture becomes even more difficult. Although mental health professionals have criteria for making diagnoses, it is also true that no two cases of depression, schizophrenia, or bipolar disorder are exactly the same. There is as yet no way that an fMRI or any other brain imaging device can be used to help diagnose those conditions in the way an X-ray can prove a bone is broken or a computed axial tomography (CAT) scan can identify a stroke.

So, if we do not know the precise brain signature of any psychiatric disorder, how can we tell if psychotherapy causes changes in the brain? If we had animal models for psychotherapy, our job might be made much easier. Then we could perform all kinds of in-depth studies using sophisticated recording and genetic techniques and figure out what was changing. But the idea of psychotherapy for an animal seems absurd.

Or is it? No, we cannot put mice and rats on the analyst's couch and ask them to talk about their mothers and fathers. But it turns out there are a lot of other things we can do in the basic neuroscience laboratory that can help us understand some aspects of psychotherapy. Strikingly, laboratory experiments that explore the kinds of things psychotherapy concerns itself with show that the whole idea that neuroscience is an enterprise designed to discover more and better medications is incorrect. Although it is possible that neuroscience will someday locate such medicines, so far, all that has been accomplished in that field is working out how to make some adjustments to drugs discovered by accident many years ago. For example, the new antidepressants that are sometimes called "second generation" and include drugs like Prozac, Celexa, and Effexor, are just variants of "first-generation" antidepressants, called *tricyclics*, that were discovered by serendipity in the 1960s.

No new antidepressant that actually works has yet been discovered solely by neuroscientific exploration. It is possible that we will soon get there—ketamine, a drug that blocks a type of receptor for the very abundant neurotransmitter glutamate—could be the first such antidepressant generated by basic science. Unfortunately, however, none of the drugs we use today to treat depression, schizophrenia, anxiety disorders, or bipolar disorder is the result of basic science theory-guided laboratory work.

On the other hand, what basic neuroscience has taught us about learning, memory, behavior, and emotion is more directly related to what happens in psychotherapy. As I will explain, when scientists condition a rat to freeze when hearing a tone that was previously paired with a shock and then extinguish that fear response by presenting the tone over and over again without any shocks, they are performing a very basic form of psychotherapy. When they then tell us exactly what genes, proteins, brain regions, and pathways are involved in both the acquisition and extinction of conditioned fear, they are giving us some insight into how a very straightforward form of psychotherapy might work in humans.

Throughout this book, I have tried to emphasize work done showing the impact of early life experiences on the brain's enduring structure and function. Using rats, mice, prairie voles, and other species seemingly a million miles away from humans, scientists have also discovered ways of blocking those changes with techniques like enriching the environment and providing more physical exercise. This has again enabled them to tell us exactly what changes at very basic levels of brain structure and function those interventions produce.

Knowing where to look from animal studies sharpens our ability to use brain imaging technologies to figure out what aspects of brain physiology psychotherapy alters. The work here is slow going. Brain researchers envy our colleagues who study hearts and livers. You can occlude a dog's coronary artery, see that it leads to infarction of muscle tissue in the heart, then run a catheter into the coronary artery of a person having a heart attack and find out that a blockage is doing exactly the same thing. The anatomy and physiology between dog and human hearts are almost identical, and you can use all kinds of precise tools to image the heart in a living human. But although many animal species do seem capable of exhibiting behaviors that resemble depression, we can't ask them how they feel or figure out if the molecular changes in their brains are seen in humans. Not yet at least.

But the neuroscience of experience has advanced far enough at this point that we can make statements about psychotherapy that are compatible with laboratory evidence, are reasonable, and, most important, are helpful in guiding us where to look and what experiments to do next. What follows in this chapter will necessarily be speculative, and I will try very hard not to become overly enthusiastic and pass off theories as evidence. At the same time, I hope to make the case that neuroscience has a lot to contribute to our understanding of how psychotherapy works and that neuroscience will ultimately contribute much more to developing better psychotherapies than it will to discovering new psychoactive medications.

# CBT AND CONDITIONED FEAR

A quick review of some of the material discussed in Chapter 6 will be helpful at this point. You will remember that in a standard conditioned fear experiment, mice or rats are presented with a benign stimulus, like a loud tone, to which they are largely indifferent. Then the tone is paired with an aversive stimulus, like a mild electric shock, which causes the animal to freeze in place and manifest signs of nervous system and hormonal activation. After this, presentation of the previously benign stimulus alone, called the conditioned stimulus (CS), is sufficient to cause freezing and activation of the nervous system. The neural pathways, genes, and proteins that are required for conditioned fear to occur and to be consolidated into long-term memory have all been well worked out in rodents, and brain imaging experiments indicate that the same pathways are involved in some types of fear-learning in humans as well.

If the CS is next presented over and over again to the animal without any shocks, it now learns that there is no connection between tones and shocks and stops freezing to the tone. This is called *extinction*. It turns out that extinction does not erase the conditioned fear memory, but is a new memory that exists side by side and dominates it, at least for some time. The fear response can easily be reinstated or reactivated, as we shall see a bit later. The neural pathways, genes, and proteins involved in extinction have some overlap with conditioned fear acquisition but also include some novel elements. Both conditioned fear acquisition and extinction require activation of the amygdala, but only acquisition requires the hippocampus and only extinction requires the medial prefrontal cortex (mPFC).

Scientists have long wondered if phobias in humans have any similarities with this conditioned fear model. Phobias are "irrational" fears of things that are not really dangerous. We have all heard and probably know people who are afraid of heights, speaking in public, or dogs. When these fears get to the point of causing a person actual impairment, we say that they have a phobia that requires clinical attention. The most well-studied and effective treatment for this kind of phobia is called *exposure*, which falls under the broad category of behavior therapies.

Let's consider Sam, who has just gotten a new job at an advertising agency in Chicago. At 30 years old, he has had a good career so far, but the new job promises to put him on a trajectory to much greater success. The only problem is that his new office will be on the 30th floor of a skyscraper and Sam has been afraid of heights for as long as he can remember. Right now, his office is on the second floor, and he is able to work around his fears by walking up the stairs and insisting on a cubicle far away from the window. With the news that he must soon move to the 30th floor, however, he is gripped with terror. Going above the second floor of a building makes him shake and perspire; his heart pounds and he becomes dizzy and faint. Just the thought of it makes Sam want to turn down the new job.

At this point, it is unclear why Sam fears heights. A psychoanalytic therapy might uncover those reasons, buried deep in his unconscious, but Sam needs to get better quickly if he is going to accept the new job. So, he makes an appointment to see a psychologist who specializes in behavior therapy. In their first session, the therapist confirms that Sam has a diagnosis of specific phobia because he is afraid of and avoids a single thing, heights. The therapist also confirms that Sam does not have any other psychiatric diagnoses and is in good general medical health. She then collects detailed information on the history and exact nature of Sam's phobia and recommends a course of "in vivo" exposure.

Over subsequent sessions, the therapist goes with Sam to progressively higher and higher floors of buildings, each time having him remain at the window for about 1 hour or longer. At first, this causes Sam a great deal of distress, but gradually his racing heart slows, he stops perspiring, and the butterflies in his stomach abate. In the next phase of treatment, Sam goes to higher and higher floors without the therapist's presence. After a series of such sessions, he is no longer afraid of heights and happily takes his new job.

The specifics of exposure sessions vary depending on a number of factors, including the kind of phobia, the amount of time the patient has to spend on therapy, and the severity of the problem. But the basic theme is clear: Sam has undergone a procedure that is nearly identical to what is done to extinguish a conditioned fear in a laboratory. Note that in Sam's case we do not have evidence that his phobia was "conditioned." That is, his fear of heights did not specifically arise because of some aversive stimulus or traumatic event that occurred when he was on a high floor of a building. So, there is already an important difference between a specific phobia in a human and conditioned fear in a rat.

Nevertheless, what occurs in Sam's therapy is that he is presented with the fear-inducing stimulus—heights—over and over again until he "learns" that no catastrophes occur when he is above the second floor. He comes to recognize that his pounding heart and labored breathing when he is on a high floor do not result in anything he feared would happen, like passing out or even dying. The connection between heights and disasters has been "unlearned" during the therapy, and, in this sense, his fear of heights has been extinguished.

We know, as described in more detail in Chapter 6, that conditioned fear and fear extinction in rodents require the activity of the amygdala and of a neurotransmitter called glutamate. This knowledge led to two questions: First, is the amygdala involved in phobic fear or avoidance in humans? Second, would manipulation of the glutamate neurotransmission system have any effect on extinguishing a phobia?

The answer to the first question turns out to be most likely yes. Using fMRI, researchers have shown in a number of studies that presenting phobic people with the object of their fears leads to an increase in the activity of the amygdala. For example, if you show a spider phobic a picture of a spider while she is in the scanner, fMRI records a nearly synchronous increase in blood flow to the amygdala, signaling that the neurons there are firing away at an increased rate.[2] I hedged in the first sentence of this paragraph with the phrase "most likely" because although many studies have shown this phenomenon, there are a smaller number that have not. It is fair to say that, at this point, as we also explained in Chapter 6, most scientists agree that fear activates

[2] Etkin A, Wager TD: Functional neuroimaging of anxiety: a meta-analysis of emotional processing in PTSD, social anxiety disorder, and specific phobia. *Am J Psychiatry* 2007;164:1476–1488.

the human amygdala and that patients with phobias—and other anxiety disorders as well—have heightened amygdala activity. Equally interesting are studies that show that successful exposure therapy leads to a significant decrease in amygdala activity, something not seen in phobics who do not respond to treatment.[3,4] Thus, there is evidence that the amygdala is as central to phobic fear in humans as it is to conditioned fear in rodents. We therefore have some basis to translate what we see in the laboratory to what we observe in humans and to infer that one way exposure therapy may be working is to reduce the activity of the amygdala.

How might exposure therapy accomplish this? Once again, we can begin with what we know with certainty about conditioned fear extinction in laboratory studies. As discussed in more detail in Chapter 6, another part of the brain is critical for conditioned fear extinction (but not so much for conditioned fear acquisition and consolidation)—the mPFC. The mPFC and the amygdala have a kind of ying-yang relationship in many instances by inhibiting each other. The mPFC can turn down the amygdala, as it does during fear extinction. But very powerful fear causes a level of amygdala activation that overwhelms the mPFC and disrupts functions like extinction.

## ASSERTING THE PFC

As I also reviewed in Chapter 2, the human prefrontal cortex (PFC) is a uniquely powerful machine that is the basis for our ability to perform the things only humans do, like read and write, tame multiple environments, and produce scientific knowledge. The PFC is active when we learn to place reason over emotion, and therefore it makes sense that "teaching" a person that there is nothing to fear might enable the PFC of someone with a phobia to suppress the amygdala.

To illustrate how this might work, let's consider Susan, a 35-year-old pediatrician, who develops crippling panic attacks when she is in social situations. Like Sam, it is unclear why Susan has this reaction because she cannot recall having had a particular traumatic event in her life that occurred in a public place. She has been shy since adolescence, but her problems in social situations now go way beyond shyness. Even being in the company of another person, let alone going to a party or having to speak up at a meeting, makes her heart start to pound, and she feels as if she cannot breathe. In any of these social situation, her head spins and she is certain that everyone can tell how nervous she is and she will embarrass herself. Susan does everything she can to avoid social contacts. She hasn't been on a date in years and volunteers to work in the emergency room on the night shift, when the fewest other professionals are around. Susan can only relax when she is alone and sometimes resorts to heavy alcohol consumption if she has to go to a party or wedding.

[3] Ipser JC, Singh L, Stein DJ: Meta-analysis of functional brain imaging in specific phobia. *Psychiatry Clin Neurosci* 2013;67:311–322.

[4] Goossens L, Sunaert S, Peeters R, Griez EJ, Schruers KR: Amygdala hyperfunction in phobic fear normalizes after exposure. *Biol Psychiatry* 2007;62:1119–1125.

The official diagnosis for Susan's condition is social anxiety disorder (SAD). It is more complex than a specific phobia but generally responds well to either CBT or antidepressant medications that increase levels of the neurotransmitter serotonin in the synapses between neurons. Susan decides to give CBT a try, the best choice for most people since there are no adverse side effects and it works just as well as medication. One part of this treatment involves exposure that is similar to what is done for people like Sam. Susan's therapist will eventually work on exercises that will take Susan into increasingly anxiety-provoking situations.

In this case, however, even confronting the most minor social situation is too terrifying for Susan at first, and that is where the cognitive component of CBT comes in. Once Susan starts panicking in social situations, she is unable to calm herself or make any reasonable assessment of what is actually going on. But many of her thoughts in these situations are likely to be exaggerations of what is actually happening. After all, are people really staring at her? Does everyone in the room really think she is a boring, unattractive, and unsuccessful person? Is it really impossible to conceive of talking to someone who will actually be nice to her? Susan maintains a set of self-defeating ideas that perpetuate her fear of social interactions. None of them is rational; she is in fact a very talented physician who is admired for her fine work and generous spirit. She is far from "hideously ugly," and many people would be interested to hear about her experiences. Cognitive therapy identifies a patient's dysfunctional thoughts and ideas and, one by one, establishes that there are alternative ways of looking at things. A cognitive process like this clearly demands involvement of the reasoning part of the brain, the PFC. As neuroscientists Steven Maier and Linda Watkins put it, "It is as if when behavioral control is possible the [prefrontal cortex] says 'cool it' to ... other stress-responsive structures" (p. 58).[5]

We would therefore expect that a person with social anxiety disorder might have a weakened connection between the PFC and the amygdala, leaving the amygdala uncontrolled. A successful CBT for social anxiety disorder might strengthen that connection, empowering the PFC to suppress the amygdala. And that is exactly what many brain imaging studies of patients with social anxiety disorder have shown.[6] Successful CBT for social anxiety disorder is associated with fMRI evidence of strengthened PFC activity and diminished amygdala activity, implying that the therapy has enabled the patient to exert rational control via the PFC over irrational fears lodged in the amygdala.[7]

The finding that CBT and similar treatments increase frontal cortical activity is true for other psychiatric conditions. In a series of studies with posttraumatic stress disorder (PTSD) patients, scientists showed that, at baseline, those most likely to

[5] Maier SF, Watkins LR: Role of the medial prefrontal cortex in coping and resilience. *Brain Res* 2010;1355:52–60.

[6] Steiger VR, Bruhl AB, Weidt S, et al.: Pattern of structural brain changes in social anxiety disorder after cognitive behavioral group therapy: a longitudinal multimodal MRI study. *Mol Psychiatr* 2017;22:1164–1171.

[7] Goldin PR, Ziv M, Jazaieri H, Hahn K, Heimberg R, Gross JJ: Impact of cognitive behavioral therapy for social anxiety disorder on the neural dynamics of cognitive reappraisal of negative self-beliefs. *JAMA Psychiatry* 2013;70:1048–1056; Mansson KNT, Salami A, Frick A, et al.: Neuroplasticity in response to cognitive behavior therapy for social anxiety disorder. *Transl Psychiatry* 2016;6:e727.

respond to exposure therapy already had increased prefrontal cortex activity and decreased amygdala activity.[8] Then, after treatment, there was further strengthening of frontal cortical activity.[9] Treatment of patients with obsessive compulsive disorder increased connectivity between the prefrontal cortex and another brain structure, the cerebellum.[10] Dialectical behavior therapy (DBT) is an evidence-based psychotherapy used to decrease self-harm in patients with borderline personality disorder. Patients with the best response to DBT show greater increases in activity in the dorsolateral PFC (dlPFC) than do those with less robust response.[11] Similar findings have been found for CBT in the treatment of depression.[12]

One study pulls together parts of the brain highlighted in Chapters 6 and 7 with the PFC.[13] Duke University investigators identified people "at-risk" for anxiety-related problems by showing a group of 120 undergraduate students pictures of angry or scared faces to activate the amygdala (Chapter 6) and having them play a reward-based guessing game to activate the ventral striatum (where the nucleus accumbens resides, Chapter 7). Students with high levels of amygdala activation to threat and low levels of ventral striatum reaction to reward indeed have a heightened risk of developing anxiety. But there turned out to be an exception to this rule: students in the "at-risk" group who also had high levels of dlPFC activity did not develop anxiety. The Duke scientists conclude that the PFC can "rescue" people with high levels of amygdala activity from developing anxiety.

Recall that in Chapter 6 we described animal and human studies showing that taking an action during a threatening situation reroutes the fear circuitry toward the ventral striatum, resulting in less freezing and reduced fear. Hence, there appear to be two ways to decrease amygdala activity and irrational responses to perceived threat that are characteristic of people with a host of psychiatric disorders: become active, which involves the ventral striatum, and use reason to reappraise the threat and the reaction to it, which involves the PFC. The former is exactly what the behavioral

[8] Fonzo GA, Goodkind MS, Oathese DJ, et al.: PTSD psychotherapy outcome predicted by brain activation during emotional reactivity and regulation. *Am J Psychiatry* 2017; Epub ahead of print

[9] Fonzo GA, Goodkind MS, Oathese DJ: Selective effects of psychotherapy on frontopolar cortical function in PTSD. *Am J Psychiatry* 2017; Epub ahead of print

[10] Moody TD, Morfini F, Cheng G, et al.: Mechanisms of cognitive-behavioral therapy for obsessive-compulsive disorder involve robust and extensive increases in brain network connectivity. *Transl Psychiatry* September 15, 2017.

[11] Ruocco A, Rodrigo AH, McMain SF, Page-Gould E, Ayaz H, Links PS: Predicting treatment outcomes from prefrontal cortex activation for self-harming patients with borderline personality disorder: a preliminary study. *Front Hum Neurosci* 2016;10:220.

[12] Crocker LD, Heller W, Warren SL: Relationships among cognition, emotion, and motivation: implications for intervention and neuroplasticity in psychopathology. *Front Hum Neurosci* 2013;7:261.

[13] Scult MA, Knodt AR, Radtke S, Brigidi BD, Hariri A: Prefrontal executive control rescues risk for anxiety associated with high threat and low reward brain function. *Cereb Cortex* November 17, 2017. doi:10.1093/cercor/bhx304, https://www.ncbi.nlm.nih.gov/pubmed/29161340.

component of CBT does, and the latter is the domain of the cognitive component. Both preclinical and clinical neuroscience provide intriguing insight, then, into how CBT works.

The second question we posed about the relevance of preclinical studies of fear conditioning to the treatment of phobias in humans is whether manipulation of the glutamate neurotransmission system could enhance treatment outcome. In order for a conditioned fear memory to be consolidated into long-term memory, the neurotransmitter glutamate must be able to traverse synapses in the amygdala and the hippocampus and activate glutamate receptors on the surfaces of dendrites of neurons on the receiving end of the synapse. If a drug that blocks glutamate is infused into a rat's amygdala immediately after it has been presented with the pairing of a tone (CS) and a shock (unconditioned stimulus; UCS), the rat will not learn to freeze when the tone alone is subsequently presented. That is, the acquisition of conditioned fear and its consolidation into long-term memory is completely inhibited by glutamate receptor blockers.

Glutamate activity is also essential for extinction learning, and blocking glutamate receptors renders an animal unable to extinguish conditioned fear. Based on this, several researcher groups asked whether boosting the glutamate system could enhance extinction of fear and avoidance in humans with phobias. They indeed were able to show that a compound called D-cycloserine (DCS) that stimulates the glutamate receptor improved response to CBT compared to placebo plus CBT for patients with social phobia and other anxiety disorders.[14]

Unfortunately, not all studies that attempted to use glutamate analogues to enhance CBT worked. It is still unclear why some studies with this strategy showed positive results and other failed. It may be that DCS is not a sufficiently potent glutamate stimulator or that the right dose has yet to be found. It is clear that CBT by itself is very effective for most anxiety disorders, including specific phobias and social anxiety disorder, and therefore there is not a huge need to develop drugs to enhance it. The fact that boosting the glutamate system did enhance extinction learning in humans in some studies suggests that the basic science studies may be applicable to humans, although perhaps not yet in the form of new treatments. Scientists were very encouraged by the initial positive results of these experiments and will undoubtedly continue to pursue the strategy using different glutamate receptor drugs. Given that most psychiatric drugs in use were discovered accidentally or are simply tweaks on those accidental discoveries, this is a rare example of basic science informing human clinical research in psychiatry.

What we see from this example linking conditioned fear in the laboratory to CBT for patients with phobias is that it is indeed possible to apply neuroscience to psychotherapy. Doing so in no way compromises the psychotherapy. No one is using basic neuroscience to change any of the theories about mental function and human

---

[14] Hofmann SG, Meuret AE, Smits JA, et al.: Augmentation of exposure therapy with D-cycloserine for social anxiety disorder. *Arch Gen Psychiatry* 2006;63:298–304.

behavior upon which CBT is based or the way cognitive psychologists practice it. Rather, by applying neuroscience to psychotherapy, scientists are trying to see if they can improve CBT outcomes and get better objective measures of illness and treatment progress. No responsible scientist suggests that we are ready to have all phobic patients routinely undergo fMRI scans before and after treatment. Rather, we are learning that CBT is a therapy that changes the brain, just like any other experience we encounter.

## WAS FREUD RIGHT ALL ALONG?

Imaging studies have confirmed that what basic scientists learned about the anatomy of conditioned fear applies equally to humans and that CBT works in part by interacting with the same pathways in humans that operate during fear and extinction learning in laboratory animals. Some molecular findings have even stimulated treatment research to improve CBT outcomes. Hence, it can fairly be said that basic neuroscience is relevant to some of what goes on in CBT.

A much more difficult task is to see if neuroscience has anything to offer psychoanalysis. Very few treatments in psychiatry and psychology have been more controversial than psychoanalysis, with some commentators even insisting that there is nothing scientific at all about it and it should be abandoned altogether as a theory of the mind and treatment for psychiatric problems. On the other hand, many people claim to have been helped by the various versions of psychoanalytic therapy, and the theory behind it is intriguing. So, let's delve a bit into psychoanalysis and then see if there is anything science has to offer here.

The original version of psychoanalysis was developed by Sigmund Freud. After him, a series of emendations, clarifications, additions, and subtractions were made to both psychoanalytic theory and practice, resulting in a number of different schools and different treatment approaches. To become a psychoanalyst, candidates must themselves have a "training" analysis," attend years of classroom work, and analyze several cases under close supervision by a senior analyst. In the "classic" form of psychoanalysis, patients lie on a couch and free associate; that is, they say whatever comes to mind even if it seems not to be important. Sessions occur multiple times per week for years. A psychoanalyst is expected to be a "neutral" figure, divulging little if any personal information to the patient and interfering with her free associations only sparingly. In theory, any relationship a patient in classical psychoanalysis develops with her analyst is based on fantasies about the analyst, not real information.

But the theory behind psychoanalysis has been used in other, somewhat less intensive approaches. These are usually called *psychodynamic, psychoanalytic,* or *psychodynamic psychotherapy.* In these approaches, the patient generally sits in a chair and the therapist may or may not have had formal training in a psychoanalytic institute. Sessions occur once or twice a week, and therapy can last anywhere from months to years. The therapist is more of a "real" person for the patient.

Despite the fact that people have been conducting psychoanalytic therapies for a century, there is almost no research showing it works. Psychoanalysis grew up before it was customary to demand rigorous controlled clinical trials to determine if a treatment is effective. The current requirement that medical interventions be tested using scientific methods did not really begin until after World War II, by which time psychoanalysis had gripped the psychiatric world. Hence, psychoanalysis did not emerge from a clinical trial tradition. Rather, it is based on an elegant theory, initiated by Freud and built upon by many subsequent theorists, about how the human mind develops and works. Until recently, the leaders of psychoanalysis took the position that the theory is so well-worked out that it doesn't require experimental evaluation. That stance is clearly proving unfortunate, and some psychoanalysts, like Steven P. Roose of Columbia University,[15] have turned their attention to formal psychoanalytic research.

It has been difficult to figure out how to design meaningful studies to test whether psychoanalytic therapies actually work. Even the purpose of psychoanalysis is not agreed upon by all. Although Freud is often quoted as saying that the goal of psychoanalysis is to help people "to love and to work" and turn "neurotic misery into everyday suffering," these quips obviously don't readily lend themselves to the kinds of measurable outcomes that clinical trials require. To make matters worse, some psychoanalyst in the past denied that the treatment had any practical utility, but rather was to help the patient learn about him- or herself. Once again, this is interesting but hardly testable.

Nowadays, it is likely that most practicing psychoanalysts believe that the purpose of treatment is to help patients overcome emotional and behavioral problems. More recently, some psychoanalytic institutes have instituted rigorous diagnostic procedures in order to document what disorder a person is suffering with at the beginning of treatment and have begun to measure outcomes as therapy is carried out. But even if outcomes are measured more exactly in psychoanalytic settings, other aspects of study design are still very challenging. What is the credible control condition to which a multiple-times per week, multiyear treatment can be compared? In standard controlled trial format, patients are randomly assigned to either an active or a control condition, and a "double-blind" is maintained so that neither patient nor provider know to which condition any individual patient has been assigned. This limits the chance for biased assessments. It would seem impossible, however, to keep a patient blind to whether she is receiving a psychoanalytic therapy or some other intervention. And how could you ethically give someone in need of help an inactive control intervention for enough years to match what goes on with psychoanalysis? It is much easier to maintain a double-blind when the choices are an active experimental medication and an identically appearing placebo pill. Even designing control interventions to match a 6-week-long long CBT intervention and having assessment made by independent evaluators who are kept blind to assigned condition is now standard practice. But randomized trials of psychoanalytic therapies are rarely undertaken.

---

[15] Caligor E, Roose SP, Hilsenoth MJ, Rutherford BR: Developing a protocol design for an outcome study of psychoanalysis. *Psychoanal Inq* 2015;35:150–168.

It is no surprise, then, that as data accumulated making it clear that both psychiatric medications and short-term psychotherapies like CBT definitely work, psychoanalysis and psychoanalytic psychotherapy fell out of favor among academic psychiatrists and psychologists. Health insurance companies refused to pay for long-term psychoanalytic therapies. Articles with titles like "Freud Is Dead" became regular features in the media. As George Prochnik wrote in a *New York Times Book Review* article, "Medical authorities have broadly recognized the faulty empirical scaffolding of psychoanalysis and its reliance on outmoded biological models. Mainstream American psychologists moved on decades ago" (p. 1).[16]

It could be, of course, that psychoanalysis is something of a religion, based more on faith than evidence. Some indeed believe that psychoanalytic therapists are modern-day high priests who administer a form of spiritual guidance to adherents. If that makes people feel better, some say, no harm is done—except that we don't really know if it makes people feel any better than not having treatment would or having a much less time-intensive and costly intervention like medication or CBT.

Despite all of this, psychoanalytic therapy hangs on. Psychiatric residents are still taught about it, and psychoanalytic institutes continue to train psychoanalysts. And, despite all the bad press it has received, thousands of people continue to receive psychoanalytically informed psychotherapy. It is important to remember the old adage that "absence of evidence is not evidence of absence." That is, psychoanalysis has never been proved ineffective, and, although many of Freud's concepts now seem entirely absurd to us (things like "penis envy"), there are a number of aspects of psychoanalytic theory, as we will see, that appear to be correct.

There is no question that studies need to be completed that adjudicate the effectiveness of psychoanalytic therapy once and for all. Some are currently under way, despite the methodological challenges. In the meantime, however, our task here is to consider whether there is any neuroscientific basis for psychoanalytic theory and practice. Freud certainly hoped there would be; as many biographers have noted, he started his medical career as a devotee of neurobiology and student of the famous French neurologist Charcot. Among his first forays into studying the mind was his 1895 book *Project for a Scientific Psychology* (often referred to in psychoanalytic circles simply as "the Project") in which, according to some neuroscientists, he anticipated what happens at the level of the neuronal synapse following an event.[17] I remember reading "the Project" during my brief stint in psychoanalytic training at Columbia University's psychoanalytic center. It is a very dense tract that accords nicely with what modern neuroscience has shown happens when a neural impulse travels down the axon of one neuron, crosses a synapse, and excites receptors on the dendrite of an adjoining neuron.

[16] Prochnik G: The Curious Conundrum of Freud's Persistent Influence. New York Times, August 14, 2017. https://www.nytimes.com/2017/08/14/books/review/freud-biography-frederick-crews.html

[17] Centronze D, Siracusano A, Calabresi P, Bernardi G: The Project for a Scientific Psychology (1895): a Freudian anticipation of LTP-memory connection theory *Brain Res Rev* 2004;46:310–314.

One of the problems for Freud in 1895 was what to do with all of these excitatory neural impulses. He could not figure out what happened to all that energy once it had done its work and therefore posited at first that it must get dammed up, needing discharge as either normal or neurotic behavior. His psychological theories later became far more sophisticated, and the "dammed up energy" theories of early Freudian thought are no longer a part of modern psychoanalysis. No one knew at the time, of course, that the brain has its own intrinsic mechanism for balancing out its energy, mainly through the action of the inhibitory neurotransmitter gamma aminobutyric acid (GABA). Freud seems to have recognized how limited he was by what was then the available technologies for investigating the brain, but he never stopped believing that someday science would explain how the brain works to make his theories of the mind reality.

It cannot be emphasized enough that science proceeds by trying to bite off measurable chunks of observations and theories, often resorting to deliberately simplifying things in order to design tractable experiments. We do not try to figure out what causes diabetes in one enormous experiment, but rather examine the problem from many vantage points and in many different laboratories. In that spirit, it is useful to take a few psychoanalytic practices and theories, simplify them (perhaps outrageously so), and see if there is any science that sticks.

In that spirit, let's consider that there are two pillars to psychoanalytic theory, as described by Freud, that may have a basis in physical processes in the brain: the existence of a dynamic unconscious that affects behavior and emotion and the influence of early life experiences on adult emotion.[18] There are two further aspects of psychoanalytic therapy that are of particular interest to neuroscientists: the use of memories to understand a person's mind and the establishment of a particular type of relationship between patient and therapist called *transference*. These four things—the unconscious, early life events, memories, and transference—are a small slice of the complex theory and practice of psychoanalysis, but they are a good place to start. We want to see if Freud was right all along and that science can now begin to explain some of the things he posited a century ago.

## WE ARE MORE UNCONSCIOUS THAN CONSCIOUS

The idea that we have an unconscious mind seems obvious on some levels. After all, we recognize that we know many things but are only thinking about a small subset of them at any given moment. The rest are there, somewhere, stored away and capable of being summoned when needed. You were not thinking about the sixteenth president of the United States until just this moment when I mentioned it, and now you have an image of Abraham Lincoln in your mind's eye. Of course, you have a memory trace of Abraham Lincoln as the sixteenth president since you first learned that fact in

---

[18] It is asserted by some that these ideas are not original with Freud, but that issue is not relevant to our exploration here.

elementary school, but it isn't something you think about all the time. In that sense, most of what you know and experience is stored in your unconscious.

You also know that some of the things in your unconscious are harder to retrieve than others. You've heard and read about Abraham Lincoln many times since grade school, so that one is easy to retrieve. But if I ask you to tell me what you had for lunch on Tuesday last week, it is not going to be so easy. Probably, you will look for associated memories to help. First, you will try to remember what you were doing last Tuesday and will probably quickly summon up something notable. As I am writing this on a Monday, I remember that last Tuesday I attended a concert with my wife, mother-in-law, and two friends at Lincoln Center. I even remember what was on the program (Mozart). Now I can fix last Tuesday and begin the process of trying to retrieve everything I did that day and where I was for lunch. Oh yes, I was at a meeting in Manhattan where lunch was served, and I had a salad. Remembering all that was harder than remembering who the sixteenth president was and involved first summoning associated memories. And yet it only took a few minutes to drag it out of my unconscious.

Now, ask me what my relationship was like with my father when I was 5 years old. For me, that was 60 years ago, and I really can't tell you right away what went on between my Dad and me back then. So much transpired between us in the years since I was 5 that my early memories of him are clearly going to be colored by more recent events that I can more easily remember. Yet, if you give me enough time, I am sure I could remember a few things that transpired between my father and me back then. I won't go through that exercise now because it would take quite a while and not be all that interesting for you who are reading this. These memories are available to my conscious mind only with considerable effort.

Then there are the things that happened to me before I was 3 years old, during the period of life when we have what is known as "infantile amnesia." It is impossible for any adult to ever have a conscious memory of what happened during the first 2 to 3 years of life. People who think they remember things from that time are actually remembering what they have been told at a later age. Psychoanalytic theory posits, however, that even things from this earliest period of life are capable of influencing our behavior and emotions through the rest of our lives. How is it possible that something of which we have absolutely no conscious memory is nevertheless still able to exert a powerful influence? A trace, sometimes called an "engram,"[19] of what happened must be stored somewhere in order for it to have such an influence, but where is it?

The idea that unconscious memories affect conscious life is rather easy to demonstrate in the laboratory, even with human subjects. For example, neuropsychologists have used a procedure called *backward masking* for decades in which a visual stimulus is shown to subjects and then, less than 50 milliseconds (0.05 seconds) later, another visual stimulus is shown. The human brain is incapable of registering a visual stimulus

---

[19] For neuropsychologists and neuroscientists, an "engram" is the trace an external event makes in memory by causing a physical change in the brain. It is not to be confused with the term as it is used by the cult known as Scientology, which has no scientific credibility and is to be avoided at all costs.

that is seen for only 50 milliseconds and, consequently, the second stimulus "masks" the first one; subjects will only remember having seen the second stimulus and have no conscious memory of the first stimulus.

Yet studies show that the first stimulus is capable of having an effect on the subjects' subsequent behavior. For example, imagine an experiment in which people are shown a picture of a house for less than 50 milliseconds while at the same time they receive a mild electric shock to the wrist. The subjects will only be conscious of the shock and have no memory of seeing a picture of a house. Yet if we subsequently show them a picture of a house for more than 50 milliseconds without a shock they will nevertheless jerk their arms away. In this case, the picture of the house is an unconscious CS that is stored in memory, out of awareness and yet clearly remembered and capable of producing a physical reaction. Moreover, studies have shown that when subjects are shown a frightening image for less than 50 millisecond there is activation of one of the brain's fear centers, the amygdala.[20] And the extent of amygdala activation is proportional to how frightening the unconsciously perceived image is; thus, people who have snake phobia respond to masked images of snakes with greater amygdala activation than do people without snake phobia. It is even possible to reduce response to a conditioned fear stimulus and simultaneously reduce amygdala activation without the human subject being aware that he is receiving counterconditioning or even of the purpose of the procedure.[21]

Interestingly, the amygdala is a subcortical structure; that is, a primitive part of the brain located outside of the brain's cortex where all the engines of conscious perception are located. We know that some events are detected by subcortical parts of the brain outside of conscious awareness, stored in memory, and capable of exerting effects on observable behavior. There is evidence that the amygdala is fully developed at birth, whereas cortical structures like the PFC take years to mature. Thus, one theory for infantile amnesia is that that the memories of early traumatic events are stored in the amygdala without at the time having access to the conscious memory centers of the brain, which has yet to develop. What is stored in the amygdala, however, is fully capable of affecting our emotions and behaviors throughout life. Thus, early infantile memories are not lost, but they are not accessible to conscious memory retrieval systems. Our ability to reflect on our memories, called "meta-memory," develops slowly from childhood through adolescence in almost direct relation to the maturation that takes place in our PFC.[22]

We know, therefore, from both animal and human studies, that the unconscious exists and that unconscious memories can exert a conscious influence on behavior. Is

[20] Ohman A, Carlsson K, Lundqvist D, Ingvar M: On the unconscious subcortical origin of human fear. *Physiol Behav* 2007;92:180–185.

[21] Koizumi A, Amano K, Cortese A, et al.: Fear reduction without fear through reinforcement of neural activity that bypasses conscious exposure. *Nature Hum Behav* 2016;1:1–7.

[22] Fandakova Y, Selmeczy D, Leckey S, et al.: Changes in ventromedial prefrontal and insular cortex support the development of metamemory from childhood into adolescence. *Proc Natl Acad Sci USA* 2017;114:7582–7587. doi:10.1073/pnas.1703079114

this what Freud had in mind when he detailed the "dynamic" unconscious? Clearly, Freud went way beyond what preclinical and clinical studies have shown in his creation of an unconscious mind that stores all kinds of drives and conflicts like the well-known Oedipus conflict. Those more elaborate constructs are hard to demonstrate empirically. But Freud is given credit for being among the first to emphasize the power of the unconscious mind, and modern neuroscience has validated that pillar of psychoanalytic theory.

Throughout this book, I have stressed the power of early life experiences to affect lifelong emotion and behavior, and the forgoing discussion of the unconscious mind clearly reinforces this principle, a second tenet of psychoanalytic theory. We certainly have abundant evidence that early life events have permanent behavioral effects on animals. If you look back at Chapter 3 of this book, you will see many examples of this phenomenon. How rat mothers treat their newborn pups or monkey mothers behave when their babies are still infants have been shown to determine many of the behavioral traits of their offspring throughout their adult lives. We also know from these studies how changes in the activity of genes and molecules in the newborns' brains are affected by these differences in maternal behavior and, in turn, determine the infant's lifelong behavioral traits.

We also have abundant evidence from clinical studies, as also discussed in Chapter 3, that early life events are important precursors of most psychiatric illnesses. Children who are abused, neglected, or grow up in poverty have higher adult rates of schizophrenia, depression, anxiety disorders, suicide, and most other psychiatric disorders than those who were raised without these challenges. In a report on a neuroscience symposium on this topic, Judy Cameron of the University of Pittsburgh and co-authors summarized the importance of the work on early life adversity as follows:

as science has delved further into mechanistic studies, the specificity of the impact of early life adversities on brain development is becoming apparent. The nature of the adversity, whether it involves abuse, fear, or neglect, matters and it is likely that as we understand these phenomena better, we will be able to define specific neural circuits that respond to each type of adversity, and differences in sensitivity to long-term alternations in functions. (p. 10787)[23]

In humans and other animals, memories are dependent on a brain structure called the hippocampus. Already, neuroscientists are linking the effects of early life trauma to specific changes in the hippocampus and other brain regions. Neuroscientists Cristina Alberini and Alessio Travaglia of New York University note that:

Recent studies suggested that poor cognitive and academic performance among children living in poverty is at least in part, due to reduction in the

---

[23] Cameron JL, Eagleson KL, Fox NA, Hensch TK, Pevitt P: Social origins of developmental risk for mental and physical illness. *J Neurosci* 2017;37:10783–10791.

size of the hippocampus and frontal and temporal lobes. . . . Similarly, reduced volume of the hippocampal subregions CA3 or dentate gyrus correlates with childhood maltreatment and abuse. (p. 5784)[24]

We thus have a robust neurobiology of the ways in which severe early life events, even those experienced before adults can remember them, profoundly affect our future abilities and behaviors. It is very likely that more subtle traumas, like emotionally distant parents, produce subtler but nevertheless real effects on the human brain. There is no question, then, that a second pillar of psychoanalytic theory is supported by animal and human research. Once again, this does not mean that neuroscience proves every aspect of Freud's theories to be true. He posited that little boys unconsciously want to murder their fathers in order to marry their mothers and, consequently, fear violent reprisals from their fathers. It is the resolution of this so-called Oedipus complex that Freud believed resulted in the acquisition of "normal" psychosexual behavior in men. There are so many obvious problems with this theory that it does not even pay to enumerate them here. For our purposes, it is important to note that no animal experiment could ever adjudicate the existence of the Oedipus complex since fathers are not involved in raising offspring in 95% of mammalian species. Nor can we conceive of an imaging experiment or epidemiological study with humans that could even begin to touch on such a notion. That is a challenge for psychoanalysts to accept; if they cannot validate a theory in the laboratory, then it might be best to reconsider it. What they do have, however, is powerful evidence that early life events, even before conscious memory is formed, are important generators of adult psychology. And this, to my mind, is more than enough to warrant continued interest in and investigation Freud's hypotheses.

## THE PAST IS NOT DEAD

One of the things that analysts and other psychoanalytic psychotherapists do in the course of a psychodynamic therapy is encourage the patient to remember his or her past. Recall Sam, the man with a fear of heights. He successfully overcame his phobia with the help of exposure therapy in time to accept a new job on a high floor of an office building. Sam has now been working successfully at his new job for a year when he and his colleagues suddenly learn that the company for which they work has been acquired by a larger corporation. This international corporation already has a division that does many of the things that Sam has been doing, and he is worried that he will be laid off once the acquisition is completed.

Sam worries day and night about his job security. He has trouble sleeping and starts drinking one, then two stiff scotch and sodas after work every day. He notices that he is also a bit nervous getting on the elevator to go up to his office, and, after a week of this,

---

[24] Alberini CM, Travaglia A: Infantile amnesia: a critical period of learning to learn and remember. *J Neurosci* 2017;37:5783–5795.

he is perspiring profusely as he enters the building for work each morning. Once in his office, he finds he is afraid to go near the window. Sam's fear of heights has returned.

Although behavioral therapy for phobias is highly effective, it is not foolproof. We know from animal studies that extinction of a conditioned fear does not erase the fear memory but instead creates a new safety memory that exists side by side with the fear memory. The original fear memory can be reactivated when a new fear stimulus is presented. In Sam's case, the anxiety produced by job insecurity has reactivated his phobia for heights.

Sam could have another course of exposure therapy, which will likely be successful in restoring his ease at being above the second floor of buildings. But it won't address his understandable fear of being fired. Although this fear may seem at first perfectly rational—who wouldn't worry in a situation like this?—several factors make Sam's worry in fact excessive. Sam is highly capable and talented at what he does. His boss has reassured him several times that, although there is a chance the new owners will eliminate his department, they will still very likely need people with Sam's skills. And if in the unlikely event he does get fired, there are many other job possibilities for him. Lying awake nights and drinking too much scotch are certainly not going to make Sam's job predicament any easier.

Could it be that there are other reasons for Sam's emotional response to his company's acquisition? A psychoanalytically oriented therapist would certainly ask that question and might urge Sam to enter a psychodynamic therapy in order to find out. Sam decides to do this, and, in the course of the treatment, recovers memories of his harsh, unsupportive father. If Same came home with anything less than an A on a test or paper in elementary school, his father warned him that he would never get into college if he didn't do better. When Sam didn't make the basketball team in junior high school, his father told him to forget about sports. Sam learns in therapy that he has incorporated his father's catastrophic way of looking at the world. It is as if his father is buried deep in Sam's unconscious mind, still warning him that every adversity in life means he is doomed. Sam and the therapist are able to "work through" these memories and emotions to the point where Sam understands he can be free of his father's harsh view of life and risk taking a more optimistic stance. After 2 years in therapy, Sam finds himself a much more hopeful person who is better able to handle the slings and arrows of life's fortunes.

Scientists and psychoanalysts have considered and debated endlessly the possibility that biological mechanisms might be called upon to explain how a process like this might work in a case such as Sam's. One interesting possibility is that psychoanalytic exploration works in part by reframing reactivated memories before they are reconsolidated into long-term memory storage. My first exposure to this notion came many years ago from an unlikely source. I was waiting for a presentation to begin that I was to give jointly with Dennis Charney, one of our top psychiatrists and neurobiologists, who is now Dean of the Mount Sinai School of Medicine. We were chatting with a third person (I cannot remember his name) who mentioned the recently discovered finding that reactivated memories are labile and can be manipulated before reconsolidation. Although Dennis is a great scientist, he is not known for being interested in psychoanalysis. Nevertheless, he immediately said "that sounds like what happens in psychoanalysis." Neither of us followed up on the idea, but it stuck with me, and, in 2011, Steve Roose of Columbia University and I published a paper in which we attempted to link this reconsolidation phenomenon with psychoanalysis.[25] I must give Dennis Charney credit for first suggesting this possibility to me.

Because so much is known about the biology of the specific emotional memory represented by conditioned fear, I will once again use this as my example. Bear in mind, however, that conditioned fear memories are not the only kinds of memories subject to extinction, reactivation, and reconsolidation. Studies also show that episodic memory in humans—our memories of events in our lives—are also subject to the reactivation and reconsolidation process.[26,27]

So, let's return to our laboratory rat who has been conditioned to freeze when he hears a loud tone because it had previously been paired with a mild electric shock (Figures 8.1–8.3). The fear conditioning had been done in a box-like conditioning chamber that is painted a specific color and has a specific odor. The animal is returned several days later to an identical chamber, and the tone is presented over and over again. At first, the rat freezes each time it hears the tone, just as it would if it were

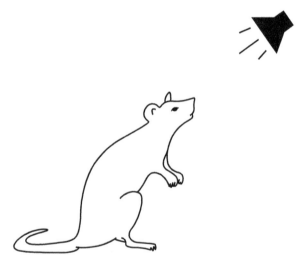

**Figure 8.1** A rat in the conditioning chamber is presented with a loud tone. It looks to see where the tone is coming from, but is not frightened.
Illustration by Catherine DiDesidero.

[25] Gorman JM, Roose SP: The neurobiology of fear memory consolidation and psychoanalysis. *J Am Psychoanal Assoc* 2011;59:1202–1220.

[26] Chan JC, LaPaglia JA: Impairing existing declarative memory in humans. *Proc Natl Acad Sci USA* 2013;110:9309–9313.

[27] Huppbach A, Gomez R, Hardt O, Nadel L: Reconsolidation of episodic memories: a subtle reminder triggers integration of new information. *Learn Mem* 2007;141:47–53.

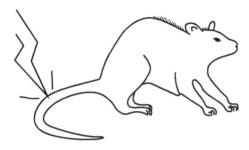

**Figure 8.2** This time, the loud tone is terminated by a brief, mild electric shock. The rat is frightened and freezes in place for several seconds.
Illustration by Catherine DiDesidero.

receiving a shock. But after several of these tones unpaired with shocks are presented, the rat starts freezing for shorter and shorter periods of time until eventually it stops freezing altogether. We say that the conditioned fear memory has been extinguished.

But not forgotten. There are at least three ways that a previously extinguished conditioned fear memory can be reactivated. The first is called "spontaneous recovery," in which after the passage of time, and for unclear reasons, if you play the tone the animal will once again freeze. Evidently, extinction memory can only dominate fear memory

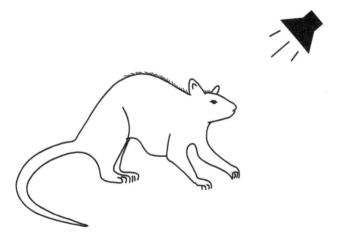

**Figure 8.3** From now on, whenever the tone alone is presented in the same chamber, even without any shock, the rat is frightened and freezes. It has become conditioned to fear a previously innocuous stimulus. If the tone is repeated many times in a row, eventually the rat learns that the tone and shock are not paired and stops freezing to the tone alone. The conditioned fear is thus extinguished.
Illustration by Catherine DiDesidero.

for a while, a period of time that varies among species and conditioning methods. The second form of reactivation is "reinstatement," in which the UCS is presented again. If you put the rat back in the conditioning chamber and give it an UCS—the electric shock—it will start freezing to tones without shocks again. The third is called "renewal," in which the CS, the tone, is presented outside of the extinction context. To do this, one constructs a new conditioning chamber that does not resemble the original one in which fear conditioning and extinction were accomplished. The new chamber, or context, is painted a different color and has a different odor. The rat will freeze immediately to unpaired tones presented in this new context.

The return of fear after extinction may be related to stress-induced weaknesses in dendrites that carry signals between neurons. In Chapter 4, we showed that stress causes a retraction of dendrites, effectively disconnecting parts of the brain. VEGFD is a protein that is required for the maintenance of dendritic integrity. Interfering with VEGFD by blocking the flow of calcium ions into neurons weakens the retention of fear extinction memory in mice.[28] The scientists who made this discovery noted that new stress is a cause of relapse for patients with conditions like PTSD and speculated that "a stress-dependent reduction of dendritic complexity may render the neuronal network less permissive to long-term persistence of new memories such as those acquired during extinction-based therapies" (p. 6954). We know that stress in humans decreases brain volume in specific regions such as the anterior cingulate cortex and hippocampus. This happens in mice as well, and it turns out that the decrease in brain volume in the stressed mouse is almost entirely due to loss of dendrites.[29] We can thus propose that when a patient like Sam gets stressed and his fear returns, it is because what he learned from his exposure treatment is disrupted by a retraction of dendrites and decrease in connections within parts of the brain key to memory, like the hippocampus.

Spontaneous recovery, reinstatement, and renewal all demonstrate that an extinguished memory is never destroyed but rather exists side by side with the more recent extinction memory. In Sam's case, his fear of heights had been extinguished by behavioral exposure therapy, but we can view the sale of his company and its attendant stress as a kind of new context. In this way, his fear of heights was subject to renewal. In general, people who have had successful behavioral therapy may relapse spontaneously or if new life stresses present themselves.

Kim Nader, now at McGill University, did a postdoc with Joe LeDoux at New York University. There, he and his colleagues discovered an intriguing aspect of reactivated fear memories—they are labile and can be disrupted using the same methods that block the acquisition of fear memory in the first place (Figure 8.4). If, for example,

[28] Hemstedt TJ, Bengtson CP, Ramirez O, Oliveira AMM, Bading H: Reciprocal interaction of dendrite geometry and nuclear calcium-VEGFD signaling gates memory consolidation and extinction. *J Neurosci* 2017;37:6946–6955.

[29] Kassem MS, Lagopoulos J, Stait-Garnder T, et al.: Stress-induced grey matter loss determined by MRI is primarily due to loss of dendrites and their synapses. *Mol Neurobiol* 2013;47:645–661.

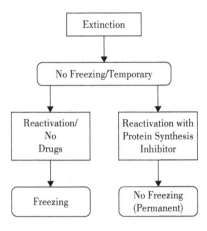

**Figure 8.4** At the top of this figure, the conditioned fear has been extinguished and the rat no longer freezes when it hears the tone. Next, the conditioned fear memory is reactivated. The conditioned fear memory is now briefly labile. If nothing further is done, it is reconsolidated into long-term memory (left side) and the rat once again freezes whenever it hears the tone. If, on the other hand, drugs that block reconsolidation are administered while the conditioned fear memory is labile, it will not be reconsolidated and the conditioned fear memory is permanently abolished (right side). Illustration by Catherine DiDesidero.

you renew a previously extinguished fear memory like freezing to a tone, the animal ordinarily resumes freezing whenever the tone is sounded, as if extinction had never been done. In this case, the reactivated fear memory has been reconsolidated into permanent memory in exactly the form in which it was originally acquired during conditioning. But reconsolidation requires many of the same molecular processes as the original consolidation of a conditioned fear memory does, including activation of several genes and synthesis of new proteins. If, immediately after renewing the fear memory, you give the animal a drug that blocks DNA transcription, protein synthesis, or glutamate binding to its receptors, the renewed fear memory is not reconsolidated (see Figure 8.4). The animal continues not to freeze, as if the extinguished fear memory had never been reactivated and therefore remains extinguished. Even more important, blocking reconsolidation of an unstable, reactivated fear memory appears to eliminate it completely—it is no longer subject to reactivation. The fear memory trace is permanently abolished.

## PSYCHOANALYSIS AND RECONSOLIDATION

As Steve and I pointed out in our 2011 paper, the first I had ever published in a psychoanalytic journal, there are many similarities, but also key differences, on a molecular and cellular level between the fresh consolidation of a conditioned fear memory and its reconsolidation back into permanent memory after it is reactivated. Hence, reconsolidation of a memory after reactivation is a unique biological process that calls on some specific biological processes to occur. There is a very short period of time after a "forgotten" memory is reactivated when it is labile and unstable. Blocking the reconsolidation process within that "reconsolidation window" of time makes it impossible for the labile, reactivated memory to be returned to permanent memory, and it is thereby lost forever. Moreover, studies in laboratory animals show that it is even possible to manipulate and reconfigure reactivated memories while they are labile and not just destroy them. Is it possible, then, that psychoanalytic therapies reactivate unconscious memories and reconfigure them before they are reconsolidated into the unconscious? If so, does that mean that whereas exposure therapy leads to successful outcomes that are nevertheless susceptible to relapse, a successful psychoanalytic treatment can produce more permanent change?

One of the statements that used to infuriate me is the claim that psychiatric medications and cognitive and behavioral therapies provide only superficial, temporary relief of symptoms but psychoanalytic psychotherapy "gets to the root of the problem" and establishes a more permanent cure. Where is the evidence for that, I would demand to know? In fact, I am not aware of any long-term studies that document that psychoanalytic therapies offer a more complete recovery than other approaches. In fact, short-term studies show that the effects of psychoanalytic and cognitive behavioral therapies yield approximately equal outcomes for conditions like panic disorder. And given that we don't really know for sure what the "roots" are of any psychiatric illness, it is hard to see how any school of therapy could claim to get to those putative roots.

What we do know, however, is that cognitive behavioral therapies are highly effective for depression, anxiety disorders, eating disorders, obsessive compulsive disorder, and PTSD and even offer help for patients with schizophrenia and bipolar disorder. We also know that CBT doesn't work equally well for all patients and that responders often relapse months or years later. In fact, it has recently been pointed out that there may more be more shortcomings and unknowns about CBT than we, in our enthusiasm for it, sometimes want to admit.[30] So, perhaps we need to be a bit more open-minded about different types of psychotherapy. After all, a more permanent response to treatment would surely be welcome.

The reconsolidation phenomenon suggests a biological mechanism whereby psychoanalytic therapy might accomplish just that. The hypothesis goes as follows: in the course of a psychoanalytic therapy, patients uncover unconscious, repressed memories and attitudes. These might be memories of early life traumas or of distant, unapproachable parents. They might be a tendency to attach anger to anyone giving them a compliment or to automatically feel inferior when a potential competitor appears. It is often hard, intensive work to get at these kinds of unconscious memories and attitudes. At certain, carefully chosen points in the course of treatment when the patient is reliving these memories, the analyst makes interpretations about their significance and meaning, thus manipulating the memories when they are in a labile state.

---

[30] Leichsenring F, Steinert C: Is cognitive behavioral therapy the gold standard for psychotherapy? The need for plurality in treatment and research. *JAMA* September 21, 2017.

When these memories are then returned to the unconscious, they are no longer as harmful because they have been reframed.

For example, when Sam was late to one of his sessions he practically fell all over himself apologizing to his therapist. He also seemed defensive about his lateness, pointing out over and over again that he got caught in a traffic jam that was beyond his control. In fact, his therapist had noted a long time ago that Sam was a rare patient who, over the course of a whole year, had never been even a minute late. His penchant for being on time seemed almost neurotic.

The therapist made an observation: "You seem to feel as if I am going to be angry at you for being late." Sam pauses, and then recognizes that there is some truth to this. The analyst then continues, "and you seem to feel you need to defend yourself by repeating multiple times that being late wasn't your fault." This leads to a discussion of Sam's tendency to always assume that authority figures are angry at him, including the therapist. Sam lives in a state of near constant terror, in fact, that he is breaking a rule or performing incompetently and will be severely chastised, if not ridiculed.

Now the therapist asks Sam if his fear of reprisal from the therapist reminds him of anything else in his life, and Sam summons up recollections of his hypercritical father that had been gradually coming to light during the previous months of his therapy. After discussing these memories, the therapist is able to make an interpretation: "You mean that your childhood fear of your father's criticism is transferred onto me and many other similar figures in your life, regardless of whether you have really done anything wrong or they are really angry at you. You feel and behave as if everyone in your life is just like your father, critical and punishing. In fact, not everyone is like your father. Some people actually want you to succeed and may even think you are smart and talented. But it is hard for you to see that."[31]

If we adopt the reconsolidation model to this exchange between Sam and his therapist, we might say that Sam has reactivated in this session memories of his harsh, critical father. These memories are now labile. His analyst reformulates them in a new way: these memories pertain only to your father; other people are not necessarily critical of you the way he was. The memories are then reconsolidated, but now they are reformulated and less harmful.

What is going on in Sam's brain when all of this happens in therapy? Remember that whatever happens in therapy is subject to the same biology as any other life experience. Sam's summoning of distant, unconscious memories requires the sprouting of dendrites within and between the brain's memory centers, allowing him to articulate what for so long has been out of his awareness. To accomplish this, genes in Sam's amygdala and hippocampus (the two brain regions most critical for reconsolidation of memory) are activated, and new proteins are synthesized as he remembers distant

[31] I fully recognize that this is not precisely what an experienced analyst would do or say. First of all, the process of going from the memories of a critical father to such an interpretation might occur over several sessions. Second, this interpretation is quite a mouthful and the analyst probably would not be quite as direct. Nevertheless, I believe it captures a fair representation of a likely part of an analytic process.

events in his life. Among these are the proteins that serve as receptors for the neurotransmitter glutamate. But the memories of early life events that Sam is recalling in therapy are labile when they are summoned, so that when the analyst makes interpretations about them they are reframed and reformulated in a way that is analogous to giving a rat protein synthesis inhibitors or glutamate receptor blockers when a conditioned fear memory is reactivated. For Sam, our hypothesis goes, similar biological processes now alter the reactivated, labile memories and beliefs as they are reconsolidated into permanent memory. To the extent that this process actually replaces the original memories with altered ones that are less harmful, it is conceivable that psychoanalysis offers a patient a form of permanent relief.

There is good evidence that the reconsolidation phenomenon occurs in humans[32] and that it involves the same brain regions in humans as it does in nonhuman animals, especially the amygdala.[33] In one fascinating study done by Elizabeth Phelps and her colleagues at New York University,[34] human volunteers underwent classical, Pavlovian fear conditioning. This is done by first pairing a neutral stimulus, blue squares projected on a screen for example, with a mild electric shock. Yellow squares are also shown, but these are not paired with shocks. The experimenters then measure the subjects' skin conductance reaction—a measure of arousal akin to a lie detector test—each time blue squares appear, but this time without any shocks, and red squares are projected on the screen. Skin conductance goes up each time the blue squares, but not the red squares, are shown, demonstrating that fear conditioning has occurred and been consolidated into memory. The blue squares are now a CS.

The next day (day 2), the subjects returned to the laboratory. Half of them underwent a regular extinction procedure in which they were shown repeated images of blue squares without any shocks. As expected, they first showed the same elevated skin conductance reaction as they had the day before, but this diminished back to baseline after seeing the blue squares multiple times without receiving any shocks. The other half of the group received a CS reminder—a single presentation of the blue square—and then waited 10 minutes before beginning the extinction protocol. Their skin conductance response went down to baseline just as it had in the group that did not receive a CS reminder. So extinction worked in both groups.

One more day later (day 3), the subjects all returned to the laboratory and were given a single CS—blue square—presentation. The group that had not received the CS reminder before extinction the day before showed robust return of conditioned fear, with increased skin conductance. But the group that had received the CS reminder before extinction the day before did not. It was as if this group had never undergone fear conditioning in the first place. One year later, the experimenters were

[32] Schwabe L, Nader K, Pruessner JC: Reconsolidation of human memory: brain mechanisms and clinical relevance. *Biol Psychiatry* 2014;76:274–280.

[33] Agren T, Engman J, Frick A, Bjorkstrand J, Larsson E-M, Furmark T, Fredrikson M: Disruption of reconsolidation erases a fear memory trace in the human amygdala. *Science* 2012;337:1550–1552.

[34] Schiller D, Monfils M-H, Raio CM, Johnson DC, LeDoux JE, Phelps EA: Preventing the return of fear in humans using consolidation update mechanisms. *Nature* 2010;463:49–53.

able to get some of the original subjects to return to their laboratory. The same finding prevailed—a CS reminder 10 minutes before extinction blocked any response to seeing blue squares.

What happened in this experiment is that conditioned fear that has been suppressed by ordinary extinction in human subjects can be easily restored by presenting the CS again. So, showing the first group blue squares a day after extinction simply reactivated the fear response. In the second group, however, presenting the blue square right before extinction on day 2 meant that extinction was accomplished while the fear memory was reactivated and labile. When extinction is performed on a labile memory, that memory cannot be reconsolidated and is thus lost forever, just like administering protein synthesis inhibitors does to an animal's fear-conditioned memory if given right after the memory is renewed. Thus, when the second group came back a day later on day 3, unlike the first group, there was no fear memory to be reactivated because in the second group's case extinction had completely obliterated it on day 2.

This exciting study showed not only that reconsolidation of a fear memory can be permanently blocked in humans, but that the blockade can be accomplished using purely psychological means, in this case an extinction protocol, and not only with drugs. At the same time, drugs, like the beta-blocker propranolol can block reconsolidation in both humans and laboratory animals as well.[35] The reconsolidation process seems capable of updating memories, and a lot has been written since our paper in 2011 suggesting that this is one process that occurs during psychoanalytic psychotherapy.

The reconsolidation phenomenon is also the basis for attempts to wipe out cues for drug use among addicts.[36] Reminders of the contexts in which an addict took drugs are major contributors to relapse. Treatment of addiction to drugs and alcohol is often accomplished by removing the addict from his or her environment and placing him in a rehabilitation setting where there are by design no drug cues. But once the addict returns home, cues of drug-taking are all around—even just being in the room of the house where the addict drank or took drugs can be enough to stimulate craving for the abused substance. One group of researchers deliberately evoked memories of drug taking and, as in the Phelps experiment described, performed an extinction trial for them during the reconsolidation window. This led to a reduction in craving every time the addicts were subsequently shown drug cues as long as 6 months later.[37]

If the reconsolidation hypothesis is correct for psychoanalysis, then the timing of interpretations made by the therapist should be critical. In animals, there is a reconsolidation window of time beyond which a reactivated memory is no longer labile and subject to modification or erasure. If a drug that blocks glutamate's ability to bind to

[35] Kindt M, Soeter M, Vervliet B: Beyond extinction: erasing human fear responses and preventing the return of fear. *Nat Neurosci* 2009;12:256–258.

[36] Milton AL, Everitt BJ: Wiping drug memories. *Science* 2012;336:167–168.

[37] Xue YX, Luo YX, Wu P, et al.: A memory retrieval-extinction procedure to prevent drug craving and relapse. *Science* 2012;336:241–245.

its receptors in the brain is given right after reactivation of a fear memory, the memory cannot be reconsolidated and is lost forever. But if the same glutamate blocking drug is given 6 hours after memory reactivation, reconsolidation will already have taken place. It would be interesting to learn if interpretations must be given within a similar reconsolidation window during psychoanalytic psychotherapy. Does a traumatic memory have to be fresh in the patient's mind for an interpretation to work?

Another interesting thing to consider is whether the experience of being in psychoanalytic psychotherapy should be an emotionally charged or emotionally neutral one. In classic psychoanalysis, the analyst maintains a neutral posture, revealing no personal details and making no direct, practical suggestions. The analyst is there to guide the patient through his or her free associations, making interpretations when they are most likely to have an impact. But studies with both rodents and humans demonstrate that memories are more strongly reconsolidated if their reactivation is accompanied by a strong emotional experience.[38] This implies that an emotionally neutral therapy experience might be less effective than one in which the patient feels emotionally aroused. This, again, is an eminently testable hypothesis. Psychoanalysts who are interested in studying the fundamental basis of their craft might be guided by neuroscience in designing meaningful experiments.

Cristina Alberini is one of the basic scientists whose outstanding work elucidated the biology of memory reconsolidation. In the last chapter of her book *Memory Reconsolidation*, she does what all top scientists do and considers objections to the psychoanalytic reconsolidation hypothesis.[39] She points out that it might be that psychoanalysis does not modify old, harmful memories that are then reconsolidated but rather creates new, more adaptive memories that exist side by side with old ones. She also reminds us that reconsolidation is subject to time effects. Old memories are less susceptible to the modification and reconsolidation process. Psychoanalysis deals with very old memories, of course, so this is a reason to pause in our quest to link reconsolidation blockade to the psychoanalytic process. Finally, Alberini notes that reactivating a previously consolidated memory does not always weaken it. Sometimes the old memory is strengthened. An interpretation of a reactivated memory could theoretically make the patient feel worse!

Alberini's reservations have very interesting implications for an emerging biology of psychoanalysis. Given that I have reframed all psychotherapy as types of experience, it is totally plausible that psychoanalytic psychotherapy involves the creation of new memories that inhibit, rather than replace, old ones. This might mean that psychoanalysis does not produce permanent relief after all because the old, toxic memories would

[38] Dunsmoor JE, Murty VP, Davachi L, Phelps EA: Emotional learning selectively and retroactively strengthens memories for related events *Nature* 2015;520:345–348.

[39] Alberini CM, Ansermet F, Magistretti P: Memory reconsolidation, trace reassociation and the Freudian unconscious. In Cristina M. Alberini ed. *Memory Reconsolidation*. Amsterdam: Academic Press, 2017, pp. 293–312.

still be there, capable of reactivation. One can easily imagine experiments designed to tease apart these possibilities.

The time effects are also concerning. I believe, however, that psychoanalysts could easily counter that reservation because psychoanalysis isn't simply about dredging up memories of distant events, like a beating from a parent at age 4. Although the reactivated memories may be of things that occurred long ago, they are still eminently present in the patient's brain and disrupting her emotional life and behavior in the present. The transference phenomenon, whereby the patient reenacts these memories in the present by attaching them to the analyst is very much a current event. What is recalled in psychoanalysis is the present representation of the past and therefore may still be amenable to updating and reconsolidation.

Could psychoanalysis actually make someone worse? That is the implication that follows the laboratory evidence that reactivation of memories sometimes makes them stronger. Stress clearly strengthens the reconsolidation of a reactivated memory.[40] If the psychoanalytic process results in conscious awareness of troubling memories and beliefs, and these are not updated by careful interpretation, theoretically, these adverse memories might actually be made stronger and reconsolidated in an even more destructive form. Psychoanalytic theorists and practitioners should take this possibility seriously. Medications used to treat psychiatric illnesses all have adverse side effects, some of which are very serious. It may be that effective nonmedication treatments also have adverse side effects. Medications intended to make patients feel better can clearly make a minority of them feel worse; perhaps that is true for psychotherapy as well. In my psychopharmacology-obsessed days, I used to say that "the only effective treatments that don't cause bad side effects are placebos."[41] Maybe that is true for psychotherapy as well. We will only know things like this when the psychoanalytic community undertakes some rigorous experimental tests of their theories and methods.

Despite her reservations, Alberini herself concludes that "the new perceptions present in the psychoanalytic treatment, and importantly, the new affect and emotional state of the present while recalling the past, do indeed provide an opportunity for changing consolidated memories via new memory traces (updating) or even, in certain conditions, weakening recent memory traces by interfering with their reconsolidation (extinction or new learning during reconsolidation)" (p. 303).[42] Hopefully, the psychoanalytic community will take advantage of insights from neuroscientists

---

[40] Bos MG, Schuijer J, Lodestijn F, Beckersw T, Kindt M: Stress enhanced reconsolidation of declarative memory. *Psychoneuroendocrinology* 2014;46:102–113.

[41] Even this statement is not entirely correct. The "nocebo" effect occurs when patients in a clinical trial get adverse side effects while on placebo. It turns out that even this phenomenon is subject to interesting psychological manipulation. See for example, Tinnermann A, Geuter S, Sprenger C, Finsterbusch C, Buchel C: Interactions between brain and spinal cord mediate value effects in nocebo hyperalgesia. *Science* 2017;358:105–108.

[42] Alberini CM, Ansermet F, Magistretti P: Memory reconsolidation, trace reassociation and the Freudian unconscious. In Alberini CM, ed. *Memory Reconsolidation.* London, Academic Press, 2013, pp. 293–312.

like this one and pursue rigorous research into memory reconsolidation and the psychoanalytic process.

## TO SLEEP, TO DREAM

I will touch on a few more areas in which recent neuroscience may have relevance to psychoanalytic theory and practice. Interpreting dreams was, of course, one of the most important parts of the Freudian version of psychoanalysis. In Freud's seminal book, *The Interpretation of Dreams* (1899), he calls dreams "the royal road to the unconscious." The back and forth between neuroscientists and psychoanalysts about dreaming is a good example of how antagonism can slow progress. It was believed for many years that dreams only occur during a specific stage of sleep, called rapid eye movement (REM) sleep. In 1977, Harvard psychiatrists Allan Hobson and Robert McCarley proposed that dreams have no meaning. Rather, they argued that the brain stem randomly fires during REM sleep and other parts of the brain put these randomly generated signals into arbitrary images and stories.[43] Psychoanalysts shot back that it seems impossible to believe that the detailed narratives people remember from their dreams could possibly be arbitrary. Then it was discovered that dreams are not, in fact, limited to the REM period of sleep, calling into question the entire Hobson and McCarley hypothesis. Most recently, scientists showed that dreaming, whether it occurs in REM or non-REM sleep, activates a "hot zone" in the back of the brain that is linked to consciousness.[44] This finding means that all of the rancor between neurobiologists and psychoanalysts based on REM sleep theories of dreaming was basically a waste of time. The science moved on while they were arguing.

Dreaming is clearly an experience that we all have. There will likely be a great deal more learned about its brain biology. Whether this will synchronize with psychoanalytic dream theory is a question we simply do not have enough information yet to address. Rather, psychoanalysts and neurobiologists should be working together to ask what kind of experiments and findings would push the field of dream neurobiology toward or away from a link to psychoanalytic ideas. If it turns out that the brain works in ways that seem completely unrelated to the idea that dreams reveal things about our unconscious minds that are useful in treating psychiatric illness, then that will be an important advance. If, on the other hand, experimental findings do not support that view, then psychoanalysts will need to accept the data and move on. The results of one recent study found that the content of dreams was associated with conscious, daytime feelings. Study participants who felt their psychological needs were not being met reported more negative dreams, including frightening dreams and dreams with sad or

---

[43] Hobson JA, McCarley RW: The brain as a dream state generator: an activation-synthesis hypothesis of the dream process. *Am J Psychiatry* 1977;134:1335–1348.

[44] Siclari F, Baird B, Perogamvros L, et al.: The neural correlates of dreaming. *Nat Neurosci* 2017;20:872–878.

angry emotions, than participants who felt less psychological frustration.[45] More work like this is clearly needed to convince us of the utility of dreams in understanding unconscious mental life.

One thing we know for certain about sleep is that it is a period of reactivation and reconsolidation of memories, a process that occurs mainly during deep (non-REM) sleep. It is the case that taking a nap after learning something increases the chances that you will remember it because what you have learned while awake is rehearsed while you sleep and laid down in increasingly more secure memory banks. It is also the case that memories and beliefs can be manipulated during sleep, just as reactivated memories can be modified before reconsolidation while we are awake. In a fascinating experiment, the level of prejudicial beliefs was assessed in a group of people using the Implicit Association Test (IAT).[46] Then, the subjects underwent "counterbias" training, in which they were shown pictures of faces paired with words that counteract common biases, for example, a female face with words associated with science and math. During this training, the subjects also heard a sound that was unique for each type of bias (that is, one sound for gender bias training and a different one for racial bias training). Then, while they slept in the laboratory, the sounds were presented. When awake after the 90-minute nap, the subjects again completed the IAT. In trials when the sounds were presented, the subjects who were given the sound associated with gender counterbias training while they slept had reduced gender bias immediately after waking and 1 week later, but not reduced racial bias. Conversely, subjects who heard the sound associated with racial counterbias training while they slept had reduced racial bias. The sounds served as cues that reminded the sleeping subjects of what they had learned while awake, and these new beliefs were then reconsolidated into permanent memory. Commentators noted that this study "is the first to demonstrate that this method can be used to break long-lived, highly pervasive response habits deeply rooted in memory and thereby influence behavior at an entirely unconscious level" (p. 971).[47] This seminal experiment demonstrates three things we have been stressing in this chapter: (1) the unconscious exists as a dynamic entity; (2) the unconscious is subject to neurobiological processes, like reconsolidation of memory; and (3) unconscious memories can be manipulated.

## PATHWAYS FOR SUPPRESSING DISTRESSING THOUGHTS

Emphasizing the role of unconscious mental processes might create the impression that psychoanalytic therapy relies solely on memories that are completely out of awareness. Of course, people who seek therapy often do so because of very conscious and very

[45] Weinstein N, Campbell R, Vansteenkiste M: Linking psychological need experiences to daily and recurring dreams. *Memory and Emotion* 2018;42:50–63.

[46] Hu XS, Antony JW, Creery JD, Vargas IM, Bodenhausen GV, Paller KA: Unlearning implicit social biases during sleep. *Science* 2015;348:1013–1015.

[47] Feld GB, Born J: Exploiting sleep to modify bad attitudes. *Science* 2015;348:971–972.

distressing thoughts and memories. For example, Angie is a college student who visited the student health facility at her school because she cannot stop obsessing about a break-up. The important thing, however, is that this break-up occurred a year ago, when Angie was a sophomore. It was traumatic—she thought she was in love and then found out her boyfriend was cheating—but after a few months of crying she seemed to be getting over it. But for the past month, Angie told the counsellor at student health, she had started thinking about the boyfriend again, feeling nearly murderous rage at his betrayal. She could not get these angry thoughts off her mind; they kept her up at night and disturbed her ability to concentrate in class. She also started isolating herself, refusing to attend social events or even go out to dinner with friends. She knew something serious was wrong, but also felt as if her intrusive thoughts were totally justified. After all, the boyfriend was a total creep who got away with hurting her without any consequences.

Obviously, Angie's most immediate symptom is not unconscious; she is all too conscious of her feelings. She wants her ex-boyfriend to suffer, but will settle for the vengeful thoughts to just go away. We know that conscious distressing thoughts like Angie's are an important part of many emotional disorders. How might a person deal with such distressing thoughts? A collaboration among three scientists from the United Kingdom, the United States, and France used fMRI to show that we are capable, to varying degrees, of suppressing unwanted thoughts by activating a pathway that starts in the most sophisticated part of the human brain, the dlPFC and runs to a major center for emotional memory, the hippocampus.[48] The more able our dlPFC is at inhibiting the hippocampus, the better we are at suppressing distressing memories. But suppressing such memories may not make them any less painful. It turns out that a parallel circuit runs from the dlPFC to the amygdala, that source of so much pain and fear. When the dlPFC suppresses the hippocampus, it also tries to suppress the emotion behind a painful memory by inhibiting the amygdala as well. Practice makes people better able to suppress unwanted thoughts and the feelings associated with them, "decreasing the likelihood of those traces reentering consciousness and triggering upsetting thoughts" (p. 6434). Further research using an imaging technique called magnetic resonance spectroscopy (MRS), described in Chapter 5, revealed that the concentration of the brain's main inhibitory neurotransmitter, GABA, in the hippocampus correlates with how successful we are at suppressing unwanted thoughts.[49]

These fascinating studies presents a perfect opportunity for psychoanalytical research. The study's implication could be that training a person like Angie to suppress her intrusive thoughts would lead to symptomatic improvement. There may be risks to thought suppression as a therapeutic approach, however. "Unfortunately," wrote a trio of neuroscientists, "it seems that thought suppression can lead to paradoxical

[48] Gagnepain P, Hulbert J, Anderson MC: Parallel regulation of memory and emotion support the suppression of intrusive memories. J Neurosci 2017;37:6423–6441.
[49] Schmitz TW, Correia MM, Ferreira CS, Prescott AP, Anderson MC: Hippocampal GABA enables inhibitor control over unwanted thoughts. Nat Commun 2017;8:1311. doi:10.1038/s41467-017-00956-z.

increases in the frequency of intrusions and the intensity of associated distress, a phenomenon known as the rebound effect that is observed across a variety of clinical conditions" (p. 11295).[50]

A psychoanalyst might wonder instead why, after so many months, Angie's unwanted thoughts cropped up again. The psychoanalyst's inquiry turns up that, shortly before Angie started thinking about her boyfriend again, she had spent a 1-week school break at home with her parents. As usual, her mother criticized Angie's hairstyle, clothing, and shoes on several occasions. More exploration revealed that Angie's mother had been criticizing her appearance since she was a young girl. Angie had actually internalized a belief that she is unattractive and that boys would not be interested in her. Angie's anger at her mother for criticizing her is largely unconscious, however, and if asked she will say that her mother was a generally supportive, loving parent. Young children may figure out that being angry at their parents is perilous given their dependency on them. The anger at a parent is repressed into unconscious memory, but it is there. When her boyfriend rejected her, Angie's anger at her mother was transformed into rage at him that clearly outlived its usefulness. By working through her relationship with her mother, the psychoanalyst might argue that an enduring solution to Angie's problems, not only helping her overcome her anger at her ex-boyfriend but also leading her to understand that she is neither unattractive nor uninteresting to men, could be achieved.

A cognitive behavioral approach to Angie's situation would focus on her angry thoughts, trying to put them into a realistic framework and challenging her negative ideas about herself. A psychoanalytic approach would be to understand how her relationships with her critical mother had caused her to harbor unconscious rage and distorted self-image. A neuroscientist hearing this might ask "which approach gives the most enduring increase in dlPFC suppression of both the hippocampus and the amygdala whenever Angie is presented with cues relevant to these ways of thinking and seeing herself?" Comparing outcomes for the two approaches in terms of which makes the patient feel better is certainly of paramount interest. Showing that improvement is accompanied by strengthening of a relevant brain pathway would make the finding that much more powerful. I can imagine many objections to this suggestion, but those often come from people who are afraid of the answer. My own prediction is that the psychoanalytic approach would provide a more enduring strengthening of the dlPFC-to-hippocampus/amygdala pathway and therefore be a better intervention in the long run. But perhaps it is time to let the chips fall where they may. How about a study in which the relationship between clinical outcome and the strength of the dlPFC-to-hippocampus/amygdala pathway is compared among various treatment approaches?

[50]  Cowan CSM, Wong SF, Le L: Rethinking the role of thought suppression in psychological models and treatment. *J Neurosci* 2017;37:11293–11295.

Transference is another key concept in psychoanalytic theory and central to psycho-analytic therapies. It fits in nicely with my idea of psychotherapy as a kind of experience that changes the brain, but is it real? Through the course of psychoanalytic therapy, the patient begins to redirect feelings and behaviors once directed to a significant person in his life onto the therapist. We saw this with Sam, who feared that his therapist would be mad at him for being late to a session. In another example, after a year of a psychoanalytic therapy, a therapist notices that her patient, Emily, is constantly demeaning the things she tells the therapist during the sessions as "unimportant." "I know I am boring you," Emily often says during sessions. In fact, the therapist does not find what Emily is talking about to be unimportant and is not at all bored. Careful dissection of this behavior reveals that Emily's father is a professor who only listened to his children when they discussed great books or important political trends. He would quickly change the subject if they brought up ordinary events of childhood, like friendships, plans for the weekend, or television shows they liked. By denigrating the importance of what she says in treatment sessions, Emily is "transferring" onto the therapist a feeling she had derived from her father: that nothing she talks about could possibly be interesting. Harboring this notion led to Emily's chronic feelings that she is stupid, uninteresting, and unimportant, leading in turn to anxiety in social situations and depression. "Working through" the transference reaction helped her realize that it was her father's cold, distant personality that was abnormal; Emily herself is not remotely close to a stupid or boring person at all.

Susan Andersen of New York University has conducted many experiments showing that transference is indeed a common, unconscious mental process.[51] Her psychological experiments allow measurement of the degree to which we apply attitudes we have to our significant others—attitudes often developed during childhood with respect to our parents—to people we encounter in our daily lives. Her group has shown that we are attracted to people who have characteristics of the significant others in our lives and that this kind of transference reaction occurs outside of conscious awareness. She and her colleague Serena Chen wrote that this work "may have implications for the long-standing clinical assumption that human suffering may result from inappropriately superimposed maladaptive responses learned in previous relationships onto new relations" (p. 627).[52]

Andrew Gerber and Bradley Peterson proposed to use Andersen's work to design brain imaging studies that would define how the brain works when we perform this transference operation.[53] So far, they have identified three brain regions that seem

[51] Przbylinski E, Andersen SM: Systems of meaning and transference: Implicit significant-other activation evokes shared reality. *J Pers Soc Psychol* 2015;109:636–661.

[52] Anderson SM, Chen S: The relational self: an interpersonal social-cognitive theory. *Psychological Rev* 2002;109:619–645.

[53] Gerber AJ, Peterson BS: Measuring transference phenomena with fMRI. *J Am Psychoanal Assoc* 2006;54:1319–1325.

associated with the propensity to transfer the attitudes we develop to early authority figures in our lives onto new people we meet: the insula, the caudate, and the motor cortex.[54] This work does not mean that Freud was "right" or "wrong" about transference. It signifies that a psychoanalytic concept can be identified and measured in the laboratory and that it has a potentially identifiable representation in specific brain circuits. After all, we psychiatrists get very excited when we can show that a drug we prescribe has an actual effect on brain function, even though it may not explain why the drug works. We have every reason to be similarly excited—and cautious—when we find a similar relationship between a psychoanalytic concept and brain function.

An imaging study of transference tell us that it is a phenomenon linked to psychotherapy that affects the brain. This opens the possibility that we might be able to tell if the effect on brain function is associated with a therapeutic benefit. For instance, researchers might develop a rating scale for the strength of transference. Is it correlated with a patient's perceived benefit from the treatment? Does stronger transference exert a stronger effect on the caudate, insula, or motor cortex, and is this correlated with improvement in treatment? Having this kind of information, which is definitely possible to obtain, would surely go a long way to telling us if transference is actually an important component of a psychoanalytic therapy.

## ENTER NEUROPSYCHOANALYSIS

The newly kindled interest in neuroscience among psychoanalysts has led to the creation of a field called "neuropsychoanalysis." Founded in 2000 by South African neuropsychologist and psychoanalyst Mark Solms, the International Neuropsychoanalytic Association aims "to promote interdisciplinary work between the fields of psychoanalysis and neuroscience" (https://npsa-association.org/who-we-are/the-international-neuropsychoanalysis-society/). Solms and his followers often cite the work of some of the most eminent modern neuroscientists, including Eric Kandel, who did psychoanalytic training early in his career; Antonio Dimascio; the late Jaak Panksepp; and Joe LeDoux. Solms began his work conducting psychoanalytic treatments on people who had sustained severe brain trauma, such as strokes that resulted in a loss of function of large swaths of brain tissue. He and his colleague Oliver Turnbull describe why they chose this approach:

> In sum, having researched small populations of such patients . . . we have developed a method that offers a respectable degree of experimental control, a reasonable degree of neuroanatomical localization, excellent construct validity, and a direct observational window into the subjective life of the brain in a reasonably naturalistic setting. (p. 7)[55]

[54] Schwartz C: Tell it about your mother: can brain-scanning help save Freudian psychoanalysis? *New York Times,* June 24, 2015.
[55] Solms M, Turnbull OH: What is neuropsychoanalysis? *Neuropsychoanalysis* 2011;13:1–13.

But not everyone is happy with the approach that neuropsychoanalysis is taking. In the opinion of French cognitive neuroscientist Franck Ramus, neuropsychoanalysis is "just an attempt to rehabilitate psychoanalysis by giving it a fashionable prefix and by attributing it the merits of other disciplines?"[56] Ramus fears that by attaching neuroscience to psychoanalysis we will give the latter a false veneer of scientific validity. Unless psychoanalysis itself can be shown to have valid capabilities to explain psychiatric illness or to offer an empirically proven treatment that is effective for patients with those illnesses, no attempt to find a biological basis for psychoanalysis is useful, according to Ramus. He concludes his scathing reappraisal of neuropsychoanalysis by stating "Merely finding inspiration in Freud's writings and making vague analogies between psychoanalytical concepts and neuroscientific findings will not do" (p. 171).

Ramus has a point, of course. Right now, neuroscience has great luster among scientists and science journalists, and deservedly so. There have been many impressive breakthroughs in our understanding of how the brain works in recent years, all nicely replicated by multiple laboratories. Psychoanalysis, on the other hand, has been around for more than a century but still has very little evidence supporting either that its theories are correct or its treatments effective. I often have a feeling, although I cannot prove this, that when eminent neuroscientists like Kandel, LeDoux, and DiMascio talk about a unification of neuroscience and psychoanalysis, they are engaging in wishful thinking. One cannot imagine any of these people actually engaging in psychoanalytic research.

Sometimes, proponents of neuropsychoanalysis seem to be pushing psychoanalysis in exactly the wrong direction. In her book about neuropsychoanalysis,[57] journalist Casey Schwartz describes her growing fascination with the field and with Mark Solms. But she writes things like "what I thought about was how dramatically the richness of Freud's ideas crashed and burned at the doors to the fMRI lab" (p. 42) and, in considering neuroscientific studies, "Nowhere did I find an acknowledgement that these [neuroscience] formulations did not actually resemble human experience; that they were at best, radically impoverished sketches of inner life" (p. 42). Rather than encouraging an application of science to psychoanalysis, she seems to be warning us that the former intends to destroy the latter:

> Yet I was troubled by how many people appeared to be participating in the reducing down of the brain's most complicated questions with little apparent regard for the long history of clinical insight established by psychoanalysis and psychiatry. The rush of findings about the brain that was permeating our current moment seemed to me like a new reality we would define ourselves by, and then wouldn't be able to turn back from. And I didn't want to subscribe to

[56] Ramus R: What is the point of neuropsychoanalysis? *Br J Psychiatry* 2013;203:170–171.
[57] Schwartz C: *In the Mind Fields: Exploring the New Science of Neuropsychoanalysis*. New York, Pantheon, 2015.

a version of life where creativity is explained as patterns of electrical waves, sadness as the number you circle between one and nine, and love confused with the mating habits of prairie voles. (p. 72)

Although her book verges on Mark Solms hagiography, I do not know whether these ideas would be embraced by him or any other members of the International Neuropsychoanalysis Association. But Schwartz's statements are troubling because they fly in the face of the kind of thinking that will be needed to locate any biology of psychotherapy. Schwartz again falls into the trap of believing that neuroscience is a mindless enterprise devoted to reducing the wonderful creative spirit of our species to mechanical trivialities. Imagine wondering if we can learn anything about the biology of love and affiliation by studying prairie voles! No doubt, Schwartz will not like this book, but her ideas strengthen the hand of those who believe science has passed psychoanalysis by, a contention she paradoxically seems intent on fighting against.

The charges against psychoanalytic psychotherapy are, of course, valid. And yet, no current theoretical system of psychiatric illness is satisfactory, and we have very little idea why any of our treatments work. We do not know why antidepressants relieve depression nor what causes schizophrenia. Has psychoanalysis survived this long out of pure nostalgia? There is no question that the psychoanalytic community has mostly failed to conduct the kind of clinical trials that would be necessary to decide once and for all if psychoanalytic therapies work. Hopefully, they will start doing that, although, as I noted earlier, such studies are methodologically very difficult to design or implement. In the meantime, it is now possible for us to isolate aspects of psychotherapy—including CBT and psychoanalysis—and use neuroscientific methods to see if there is any biology that might be explanatory. If the models of extinction and reconsolidation help us to find ways to improve psychotherapy and find biological markers that correlate with efficacy, then this search for a biology of psychotherapy will surely have merit.

# 9

# Conclusion

... and the whole plasticity of the brain sums itself up in two words when we call it an organ in which currents pouring in from the sense-organs make with extreme facility paths which do not easily disappear.
—William James, *Psychology: Briefer Course* (1892)[1]

I have emphasized throughout this book that experience changes the brain. Those changes can be seen and quantified on a molecular and cellular basis in animals and in the activity patterns of brain regions and connections among them in animals and humans. I have taken a position on three current controversies in neuroscience, psychiatry, and psychology. First, I asserted that the human brain is unique even when compared to our nearest genetic neighbors, chimpanzees and other great apes. Second, I sided with the mantra that the mind is the organ of the brain and that all functions of the human mind can ultimately be explained by the physical activities of molecules within the brain. Finally, I claimed that psychotherapy is an experience that changes the physical brain and that there may therefore be a neuroscience that is applicable even to the "pariah" among psychotherapies, psychoanalysis.

If these ideas are correct, then no doubt writing a book is itself an experience that has changed my brain. Certainly, I have learned many new things in researching what is in this book, and that has resulted in the creation of new synaptic connections in my brain. I didn't feel this as it happened, of course, but surely some dendrites in my hippocampus and prefrontal cortex extended their branches and sprouted new spines on their surfaces, permitting new connections with axons on receiving neurons. I also recognize that areas of my brain associated with the experience of fear and anxiety were undoubtedly stimulated because, at many junctures, I ran into new research that contradicted something I believed or thought I knew. The sense that I was probably wrong about some things made me feel frightened, and that perhaps caused new synaptic connections to arise in my amygdala and anterior insula. Finally, writing about the brain is fun for me and undoubtedly stimulated the reward pathway from my VTA to my nucleus accumbens.

Does this mean that writing a book is a mere matter of neurons firing away? Would I be satisfied if my head were in a magnetic resonance imaging (MRI) scanner as I write

[1] Reprinted in Robert Richardson, ed. *The Heart of William James.* Cambridge, MA, Harvard University Press, 2012, p. 104.

to learn that writing increases activity in my dorsolateral prefrontal cortex? What if I were a creative writer (I've tried that and failed)? Wouldn't I believe that an ethereal muse inspired me, something that no electrophysiology, optogenetic imaging, or brain scanning can capture? Is it really all just genes, cells, and neurons?

## IS NEUROSCIENCE SUPERFICIAL?

In February 2017, after I had already begun writing this book, I came across two blogs from the magazine *Psychology Today*, to which my daughter Sara Gorman and I also contribute a monthly blog on science denial. The articles voice a very common sentiment in the worlds of psychiatry and psychology. In one of those articles, David Ludden, a professor of psychology at Georgia Gwinnett College, wrote "there is a big difference between stating that the mind is a product of the brain and claiming that the mind is nothing more than brain activity. This second position is called *eliminative reductionism* [italics in original]. Neuroscientists who take this stance believe that eventually our understanding of the brain will so complete that all other psychological theories will become superfluous."[2]

Then, a few days later, Gregg Henriques, professor of psychology at James Madison University, wrote "Neuroscience deals with a fundamentally different subject matter than psychology. Neuroscience is about neurons and brains. Psychology is a science about conscious experiences, the behaviors of animals and persons as whole entities, and the application of psychological assessment and interventions to foster human well-being. These subjects are simply not the same entities."[3]

The arguments in these blogs are very well crafted and seemingly convincing. And when I read them, I am sure that my amygdala went wild; perhaps, I thought, I am wrong about everything. I am sure that from now on whenever I see an article by Drs. Ludden or Henriques I will have an increase in skin conductance, signaling an uncomfortable arousal.

Yet, I am going to stand my ground here. Let's take Ludden first. He says that neuroscientists think the mind is "nothing more than brain activity." But I really don't know any neuroscientists who would put it in such a dismissive way. What does Ludden mean by "nothing more than?" My hope is that you who have trudged through this whole book are now thoroughly convinced of at least one thing: there is nothing "nothing more than" about the human (or any other) brain. Brain function is based on a beautiful and intricate system of genes, proteins, transmitters, cellular components, and electrical signaling that rivals anything in the universe for complexity and intrigue. Just look at Figure 9.1. For years, neuroscientists at the University of Pennsylvania collected data from patients with epilepsy undergoing clinical monitoring and

---

[2] Ludden D: Is neuroscience the future or the end of psychology? *Psychology Today* February 2, 2017; https://www.psychologytoday.com/blog/talking-apes/201702/is-neuroscience-the-future-or-the-end-psychology

[3] Henriques G: Psychology's grand unified theory. *Psychology Today* February 5, 2017; https://www.psychologytoday.com/blog/theory-knowledge/201702/psychologys-grand-unified-theory

constructed this image of the electrical network activity of a small area of human brain tissue during a memory task. Does this look simple? To me, and I bet to most neuroscientists, it is actually quite beautiful. I have no trouble accepting that human cognition, emotion, and behavior is encoded in electrical activity like that shown in Figure 9.1. This is our complicated, beautiful mind at work.

Ludden's blog was the first time I had encountered the phrase "eliminative reductionism." It seems to signify the process by which nefarious neuroscientists will render everything in psychology obsolete. That, too, seems to me not just an exaggerated fear but really a basic misunderstanding. Neuroscientists are not motivated by any desire to replace psychological theories, but instead work to find support for them in brain function. Knowing the basis for a theory doesn't necessarily supplant it but rather makes the theory more secure. For example, neuroscientists now understand a lot about the fundamental physical processes required for Pavlovian or classical fear conditioning, but this does not degrade psychological theories about conditioned and unconditioned stimuli or stop psychology professors from teaching students about Pavlov's dogs. Instead, they can now add to their description powerful molecular and cellular neurobiology that gives these behavioral theories another level of firm foundation.

What about Henriques? Notice how many more words there are in the sentence that describes what psychology is compared to the sentence that describes what neuroscience is. Talk about "reductionism"; neuroscience is reduced to just two things, "neurons and brains!" [exclamation point mine]. Psychology, on the other hand, is described as a rich discipline devoted to nothing less grand than

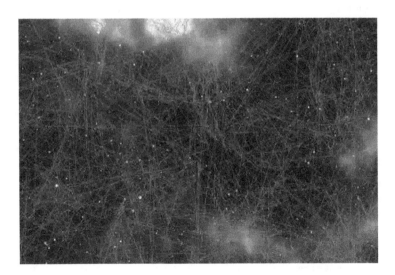

**Figure 9.1** An image of the electrical activity of networks in a small slice of the human brain while patients with epilepsy performed a memory recall task.

This work by neuroscientists at the University of Pennsylvania can be found at NeuroscienceNews.com; image in public domain.

the betterment of humankind. At this point, I decided that perhaps a psychoanalytic term was appropriate in understanding these blogs: defense mechanism. And it brought me back to an incident in my own career many years ago that perhaps evoked similar dynamics.

When I was at Columbia University, our psychiatry department chairman decided to recruit a wonderful psychiatrist and neuroscientist to our faculty. I was asked to interview the candidate and give him the pep talk to encourage him to make the move to us. In the course of the conversation, he said to me "Jack, everything is going to be brain imaging. Whatever you are doing now is going to be replaced by brain imaging." I was quite taken aback, but kept my composure (at least that is my recollection) and did everything I could to encourage him to join us at Columbia. He did and has had a wonderful career there.

I went home, however, in a disheartened and angry mood. How dare he denigrate my life's work. I was also in a panic because I had never done a brain imaging study and had no idea at the time how to go about one. My response was to be depressed for a while and consider going to law school. Ultimately, however, I developed relationships with brain imaging experts, began doing studies using imaging technologies in humans and animals, and was even given a joint appointment at Columbia in the Department of Radiology in order to help integrate neuroimaging into psychiatry.

But if I hearken back to my angry and depressed state, I think I understand how Ludden and Henriques must feel. Neuroscience is getting a lot of attention these days. Perhaps psychology is getting less notice, although I have no data to support that idea. Still, I imagine that neuroscience must seem like a threat to those not directly engaged in it, and the response, therefore, is to attack it as superficial and even a distraction from what is really important, an inchoate entity called "the mind." Psychology, not neuroscience according to these naysayers, stands to save our "humanness."

I would argue, however, that all good science serves the interests of human well-being. When psychologists and psychiatrists understand that the technologies and approaches used in the neurosciences may help us take psychology to the next level, there will be, I believe, an important burst in clinically meaningful progress. Think of the steps science took in understanding the basis for the earth's movement through space. At first, it was thought that the earth was the center of the universe and everything, including the sun, revolved around it. Then, scientific observation reversed this idea, and the modern notion that the earth and planets of the solar system revolve around the sun was born. Next, Newton showed us that it is a force called gravity that keeps the earth in its path around the sun, and then Einstein demonstrated that gravity is really a deformation in space-time that causes two objects to be "attracted" to each other. Today, physicists are trying to learn more about gravity, a relatively weak force that does not fit in with the other three forces of nature. We now have an amazing amount of very basic knowledge about what our earth is doing in space and lots of ideas about what the next set of observations and experiments must be. Has any of this work demeaned our appreciation of the beauties of the forests, mountains, and rivers of the earth? Has knowing the fundamental equations that govern the earth's movements dissuaded biologists and geologists from continuing their scientific explorations into things that are right in front of us on the earth on which we live? Of course not. The advance of physics has enriched all these other disciplines as they enrich physics.

The human mind should be proud to be associated with the human brain.

The point I made earlier about the physics of the gravitational attraction among planets also gives us reason for pause because those developments occurred over a span of nearly 400 years (from about the time of Copernicus to Einstein). The developments in neuroscience that I have been discussing in this book, by comparison, have mostly occurred in the past 50 years. One could easily argue that the brain is even more complex than the solar system, hence we have every reason to expect that we now stand at the very beginning of our inquiry into the brain.

## SCIENCE RAPIDLY CHANGES

Even within the past year, as I've worked on this book, I have been struck by how many things I had to rethink or change because of newly reported research findings. Here are a few of them:

- In a study published in *Science* in 2003 that dazzled me and many of my colleagues, Avshalom Caspi, now at Duke University, and colleagues produced one of the first pieces of evidence of a gene–environment interaction for a psychiatric illness. In a study involving 1,037 people from New Zealand followed from birth through adulthood, Caspi et al.[4] found that those with a particular form of a gene had increased risk for depression, but only if those people with the gene variant had also been exposed to significant stressful life events. To make the study even more remarkable, the particular gene involved happens to encode the protein directly involved in the mechanism of action of the selective serotonin reuptake inhibitor (SSRI) antidepressants (the serotonin transporter protein). I cited this study often in papers and talks in which I promoted the idea that psychiatric illness must be caused by a combination of heredity (i.e., nature) and adverse life experiences (i.e., nurture). The study itself seemed methodologically impeccable and indeed was published in one of the two most prestigious scientific journals in the world. And yet, in April 2017, a group from Washington University, St. Louis, published a study in which they analyzed data from 31 studies involving 38,802 people and could not replicate the association between the serotonin gene variant, stressful life experiences, and risk for depression.[5] Some newspapers picked up the story, declaring that this association, long touted by many to be definitive, simply isn't

---

[4] Caspi A, Sugden K, Mofitt TE, et al.: Influence of life stress on depression: moderation by a polymorphism in the 5-HTT gene. *Science* 2003;301:386–399.

[5] Culverhouse RC, Saccone NL, Horton AC, et al.: Collaborative meta-analysis finds no evidence of a strong interaction between stress and 5-HTTLPR genotype contributing to the development of depression. *Mol Psychiatry* 2017; Epub ahead of print.

true. While I still insist that gene–environment interactions must be at the root of most illness, including psychiatric ones, it seems that I must stop using the 2003 study to prove that point.

- I opened this book by trying to make the case that the human brain is unique. Although the main ideas of this book would not be overturned if in fact our brains are not that different from other species, including our nearest genetic neighbors the chimpanzee and bonobo, in trying to explain how life experiences change the physical structure of the human brain it is useful to recognize that we have specialized brain structures, especially the prefrontal cortex, that mediate the things only humans can do. As one writer put it when contemplating the great apes he saw at the zoo "these creatures are so clearly *not* us. Our upright walking, capacious and clever brains, and a list of other traits sharply set us apart."[6] My contention is that if humans are unique in developing many psychiatric and neurological illness, these must then necessarily involve parts of our brains that are different from all other species. Those brain regions, I have tried to show, are in the prefrontal cortex. I claimed, for example, that only humans have a deep knowledge that we have a future, making us uniquely prone to anxiety and despair, and that only humans get Alzheimer's disease. Once again, I may not be entirely correct on either point. It turns out that some other species, even including ravens, plan for the future "at least as well as 4-year-old children."[7] And elderly chimpanzees indeed have the characteristic neuropathological changes seen in humans with Alzheimer's disease, neurofibrillary tangles and amyloid plaques.[8] Dolphins may also, it turns out, develop something like Alzheimer's disease.[9] I still believe we can make a clear case that human brains are different—not better—than all other species, but I may not be on such solid ground making that case on the basis of knowing the future or developing dementia with aging.

- Remember how I said in Chapter 4 that the brains of adult mammals can only create new neurons in two areas, the hippocampus and the olfactory bulb? I've been saying that for quite some time now based on what is written in many papers and textbooks. Then, I suddenly came across a paper in August 2017 whose authors claim that they found evidence for new neuron creation—or neurogenesis—in a completely distinct part of the mouse brain, the amygdala.[10] I cannot tell you why this is only

[6] Reno, PL: Missing links: Our big human brains, upright gait, and style of love may exist because we shed key pieces of DNA. *Sci Am* May 2017, 43–47 (quote on p. 44, italics in the original).

[7] Boeckle M, Clayton NS: A raven's memories are for the future. *Science* 2017;357:126–127 (quote on p. 126).

[8] Edler MK, Sherwood CC, Meindl RS, et al.: Aged chimpanzees exhibit pathologic hallmarks of Alzheimer's disease. *Neurobiol Aging* 2017;59:107–120. doi:10.1016/j.neurobiolaging.2017.07.006.

[9] Gunn-Moore D, Kaidanovich-Beilin O, Iradi MCG, Gunn-Moore F, Lovestone S: Alzheimer's disease in humans and other animals: A consequence of postreproductive life span and longevity rather than aging. *Alzheimers Dement* 2018;14:195–204. doi:10.1016/j.jalz.2017.08.014.

[10] Jhaveri DJ, Tedoldi A, Hunt S, et al.: Evidence of newly generated interneurons in the basolateral amygdala of adult mice. *Mol Psychiatry* 2018;23:521–532.

being discovered now, and, of course, it is in mice, not humans. This is the first such report, so it needs to be replicated. But it reminds me that neuroscience is a rapidly moving field and that things we firmly believe can be overturned rather quickly as new research emerges. In fact, in 2016, neuroscience was abuzz at the finding that the human brain is even more complex than previously believed—more than 100 new brain regions were discovered using newly developed technologies.[11]

• I make a big case for a role for epigenetics in mediating the effects of life stress on the human brain. Although the genes we inherit at birth, with a few exceptions, cannot be changed during our lifetime, how extensively our genes are expressed is modified on a minute-by-minute basis by a process called epigenetics. Moreover, some animal studies have shown that epigenetic changes can be passed on from one generation to the next. One recent study even showed that epigenetic changes in gene expression were passed on for 14 generations.[12] Of course, that was in a species of worm. Still, recent studies in humans show that epigenetic changes present at birth, some influenced by prenatal exposure to alcohol and nicotine, influence conduct disorders in children[13] And another recent study showed epigenetic differences at age 4 ½ between children who had been held more as infants by their mothers and those who had had less physical contact.[14] But I know that I have to temper my enthusiasm for this phenomenon, especially after reading a more recent article by two criminologists.[15] They point out that most of the data supporting the interactions between life events, epigenetic control of gene expression, and brain function come from rodents, and we don't know for sure yet how well epigenetic changes can be passed from one generation to the next in the much more slowly reproducing and neurobiologically complex human.

Why in the world would I bring up things that seem to undermine what I have written and you have, perhaps, labored to read in this book? Because that is how science works, especially a rapidly evolving field like neuroscience. I am prepared for many of the things that I have said here to be proved incorrect because I know that hard-working, sometimes brilliant women and men working in laboratories and clinical centers around the world will find out many new things about the human brain. They are undoubtedly doing so right now as I write, but I am going to have to stop

[11] Glasser MF, Coalson TS, Robinson EC, et al.: A multi-modal parcellation of human cerebral cortex. *Nature* 2016;536:171–178.

[12] Klosin A, Casas E, Hidalgo-Carcedo C, Vavouri T, Lehner B: Transgenerational transmission of environmental information in *C. elegans. Science* 2017;356:320–323.

[13] Cecil CAM, Walton E, Jaffe SR, et al.: Neonatal DNA methylation and early-onset conduct problems: A genome-wide prospective study. *Dev Psychopathol* 2017;9:1–15. doi:10.1017/S095457941700092X.

[14] Moore SR, McEwen LM, Quirt J, et al.: Epigenetic correlates of neonatal contact in humans. *Dev Psychopathol* 2017;29:1517–1538. doi:10.1017/S0954579417001213.

[15] Boutwell B, Barnes JC: Epigenetics has become dangerously fashionable. *Quillette* April 7, 2017; http://quillette.com/2017/04/07/epigenetics-become-dangerously-fashionable/

adding new studies sometime soon! In fact, I decided not to go back and add the four new things I just described to the preceding chapters because to do so would begin an endless process, albeit one that I find totally exciting—the march of science toward better and better evidence about how the brain works.

Despite this acknowledgment that progress in neuroscience research will undoubtedly change many of our current ideas, there are a number of things I believe we can rely on that we have touched on in this book.

## A FEW THINGS I BELIEVE WILL HOLD

I am convinced that no matter how much progress we make in understanding the neurobiology and behavior of other species, we will nevertheless still conclude that the human brain is unique. That is not because it is bigger than all other brains or because we are better than all other species. Neither is true. It will always be the case, however, that the part of the brain in the front, the prefrontal cortex, has developed a complexity and sophistication that is unmatched in any other species. We must be humble about this. For every poem that gets written, a horrible new weapon is also created. For every medical advance developed that saves lives, our technologies release more toxic substances into the atmosphere to hasten our collective and individual demise. Chimpanzees are capable of great intellectual sophistication and social organization, and although they can be very violent creatures they will never devise methods capable of exterminating their or any other species. Only humans do that. Hence, we pay a very heavy price for our neurobiological uniqueness. Among those burdens are things like depression, schizophrenia, and bipolar disorder. The more complex anything becomes, the more room there is for error. Psychiatric illness is, in my opinion, the inevitable result of having such a complicated brain.

That unique status does set the stage for the intuition that our brains are especially flexible in the face of environmental stimuli. What we see, hear, and feel from the moment we are born and throughout our lives set in motion an incredibly complex system of genes, proteins, cells, and networks in our rather small brains. This gives us unprecedented abilities to manipulate and remember what we learn. So, there is no question in my mind that a another basic tenet of this book—that all experiences produce physical changes in our brains—is the case.

It is true that we can only see such changes in humans when they occur at the systems level, using brain imaging techniques, or at the molecular and cellular level after death at autopsy. Our ability to examine changes in gene expression, protein synthesis, and dendrite expansion in living brains is restricted to laboratory animals. But it would be a big surprise to learn that these processes are substantially different in animals than in humans in those areas of the brain that are similar among species. A gene that gets turned on by a frightening stimulus in a rat amygdala is very likely also going to be activated in a human amygdala. It is when we get to the prefrontal cortex that extrapolations like that become strained. The rat prefrontal cortex is just not that sophisticated.

And that is what, I believe, some people are referring to when they talk about the human "mind"—the mind, I firmly believe, is really the sum of things about which we do not yet have enough information. All of the epigenetic effects on gene expression, the differences in protein synthesis, the expansion and retraction of dendrites, and the strengthening and weakening of connections among brain regions are undoubtedly the basis for mind and consciousness. That is what we mean when we declare that the "brain is the organ of the mind." The word "mind" is a metaphor for all the cognitive and emotional functions of the brain, and when people complain that "brain" does not include all the glorious things of which humans are capable, I think they are simply referring to those things about the brain about which we are still in the dark. As we learn more about the brain, there will be less and less of an unknown entity called "mind" about which to be concerned.

That's right. I unabashedly join those who think that the mind is indeed "brains and neurons." Just like a beautiful forest is composed of trees that are made of tiny cells, minds are composed of brains that are made out of neurons and other cell types. Knowing that the forest is really a collection of cells does not impede our ability to appreciate beautiful, variegated leaves on a bright New England fall morning. But if a virus or fungus begins to attack those trees, it is only armed with our knowledge of the basic biology of plants and microorganisms that we will have a chance of saving what we so cherish.

Similarly, asserting that the mind is made of neurons does not stop us in any way from seeing every person as a unique and wonderful individual. Psychologists who deal with these people need not deny that neurons are ultimately involved when they attempt to "treat the whole person." Indeed, when a mind becomes sick with depression, anxiety, or psychosis, it is ultimately going to be our understanding of how its neurons work that will give us the best chance to cure it. And by that I do not mean by medication only.

## NEUROSCIENCE IS NOT JUST ABOUT DRUGS

Somehow, many of us, myself included, were led to believe that the process of using neuroscientific knowledge to treat psychiatric illness only means prescribing medications. In this book, I have argued strongly that this is not the case and that neuroscience today gives us as much if not more reason to seek solutions in psychotherapy as in medication. That does not mean that I am turning my back on my years of work in psychopharmacology, of course.

Medications are essential for some of the most severe mental illnesses. These are some of the areas in which our use of psychopharmacology is essential to ensure positive outcomes:

- *Schizophrenia*: Most patients with schizophrenia require antipsychotic medication to achieve any form of symptomatic improvement and functional capacity. It is true that these medications have adverse side effects that can sometimes be severe. But without them most patients with schizophrenia are forced to live their lives in institutions, including prison, and often to die violent deaths at a young age. Two forms of antipsychotic medication—long-acting injectable (LAI) antipsychotics and a specific drug, clozapine—are actually seriously underutilized and could reverse a great deal of misery for patients, their families, and society. At the same time, however, psychosocial interventions are also crucial for patients with schizophrenia, including family therapy, vocational assistance, and cognitive behavioral therapy (CBT).

- *Bipolar disorder (formerly known as manic-depressive illness)*: Lithium, the first drug approved for bipolar disorder, is truly a miracle drug, and, once again, most patients with bipolar disorder need to take one of the mood-stabilizing medications now available. But it is also the case that psychotherapy is a critical component in achieving the best outcomes for bipolar patients.

- *Depression*: Although psychotherapy should be considered the first-line approach for patients with depression in my opinion, there are patients whose depression is so severe that they cannot meaningfully participate in psychotherapy or for whom psychotherapy does not work. These patients should be put on antidepressant medications, which clearly work. But we need to stop giving them to patients with mild and even moderately severe depression without first at least considering a trial of psychotherapy. And, in many cases, patients who do not fully respond to antidepressant medication will get better if the treatment is supplemented with cognitive behavioral psychotherapy.[16]

- *Attention deficit hyperactivity disorder (ADHD)*: Psychostimulant medications like methylphenidate—the most familiar form of which is sold under the brand name Ritalin—have been studied as well or better than almost any drugs in all of modern medicine. They work for children with ADHD and are remarkably safe. For a child with ADHD, withholding methylphenidate can have tragic consequences: poor school performance, low self-esteem, increased risk for accidents and drug abuse, and poor long-term vocational and social prospects. But we have to be much more careful that we give psychostimulant medication only to children who really have carefully diagnosed ADHD; that we stop falling for misleading drug company hype that amphetamines are equally safe as methylphenidate and reserve the mixed amphetamine salts like Adderall only for children who do not respond to methylphenidate; that we work harder to stop college students from buying, selling, and abusing amphetamine psychostimulants like Adderall; and that we remember that there are nonmedication treatments for ADHD that work.

My point here is to be very clear that I am far from anti–psychiatric medication. Having spent a career studying them, I have seen both the strong scientific evidence for their efficacy and the help they have afforded many patients.

[16] Nakagawa A, Mitsuda D, Sado M, et al.: Effectiveness of supplementary cognitive-behavioral therapy for pharmacotherapy-resistant depression: a randomized controlled trial. *J Clin Psychiatry* 2017;78:1126–1135.

But there is actually surprisingly little neuroscientific sophistication surrounding our current psychiatric drugs. For instance, all the antidepressants manipulate one or both of two neurotransmitter systems (serotonin and norepinephrine), and this mechanism of action hasn't changed since they were first introduced in the 1960s. Newer drugs like the SSRIs (which aren't really that new anymore) may have fewer adverse side effects than the first generation of antidepressants, but they don't work any better. Most striking is the fact that we have been unsuccessful in connecting what we know the drugs do—increase levels of serotonin and/or norepinephrine— and exactly how they work to treat depression. We just keep developing variations on the same theme, allowing drug companies to claim that each new drug is a major advance over the old ones when in fact there haven't been any major advances in 50 years. Antidepressants work, but not nearly as well as we would like. And neuroscience has not revealed much yet that has guided the development of anything radically different. We have a similar situation with antipsychotic medications, all of which operate to reduce dopamine transmission in the brain. As psychiatrist, molecular neurobiologist, and former director of the National Institute of Mental Health Steven Human wrote "The molecular actions of all widely used antidepressants, antianxiety drugs, and antipsychotic drugs are relatively unchanged from their 1950s prototypes."[17]

And that may be the case for quite some time to come. A psychiatrist and researcher I respect a great deal, University of Oxford's Guy Goodwin, was recently quoted as saying "I'd be very surprised if we were to see any new drugs for depression in the next decade. The pharmaceutical industry is simply not investing in the research because it can't make money from these drugs."[18]

To be sure, there are some novel ideas for new psychiatric drugs that have grown out of neuroscience research. Ketamine, for example, is an anesthetic agent—and street drug—that blocks the ability of an excitatory neurotransmitter, glutamate, to bind to one of its receptors in the brain. Preclinical research suggested that excessive glutamate signaling might be involved in depression, and so ketamine has been tested as a potential antidepressant. Clinical trials of ketamine and drugs that have a similar mechanism of action look very promising. Similarly, basic science studies showing a relationship between inflammation and depression-like behavior in laboratory animals have led to studies of anti-inflammatory drugs as a treatment for depression.

Yet I am dismayed that right now a lot of the excitement in psychopharmacology for depressions seems to be focusing on very old compounds that are currently drugs of abuse. Studies are querying whether opioids and cannabinoids (marijuana) have antidepressant qualities. Much is now being made of research that suggests that

---

[17] Hyman SE: Psychiatric drug development: diagnosing a crisis. *Cerebrum* April 2, 2013. https://www.ncbi.nlm.nih.gov/pmc/articles/PMC3662213/

[18] Kelland K: No new antidepressants in sight despite growing need, experts warn. *Reuters* June 11, 2017; http://www.reuters.com/article/us-health-antidepressants/no-new-antidepressants-in-sight-despite-growing-need-experts-warn-idUSKBN14V2AQ

psychedelic mushrooms (psilocybin) and ecstasy (MDMA) may work to treat depression. I am not suggesting that developing these medications is a bad idea. Our current antidepressant drugs leave much to be desired. Only about one-third of people with depression get a complete response with the first antidepressant drug they take, and those who do respond to medications often relapse as soon as they are discontinued.[19] We clearly need more effective medications for serious depression. We should develop whatever works. But opioids, marijuana, psilocybin, and ecstasy do not represent scientific breakthroughs. There is no connection between anything we know about the causes of depression and the way these drugs work.[20] We are purely operating on observation here: people who take these drugs, sometimes illegally, claim that they relieve depression, and so we put them into formal clinical trials to see if that is true and if they can be delivered safely. US Food and Drug Administration (FDA) approval for any of these drugs as an antidepressant means that they will become widely available. That is already the case for opioids and marijuana, but do we really want doctors prescribing mushrooms and ecstasy?

It is important, then, to focus attention on what neuroscience has told us may be one of the causes of psychiatric illnesses. I have stressed throughout this book that we do know quite a bit about a major contributor to depression, anxiety disorders, and other psychiatric illness—adverse life experiences. We understand many of the specific ways that stress changes the brain on a molecular and cellular level from laboratory studies with animals. Epidemiologists repeatedly confirm that early childhood adversity and later stressful life events are linked to psychiatric illness, in most cases preceding its onset. We can use brain imaging to see the changes adversity makes in the human brain.

As neuroscientists push along making these connections between adverse life experiences and mental illness, psychiatrists and psychologists have often resisted them. It is difficult for those of us who grew up in the world of "biological psychiatry" to grasp the idea that what happens in life may cause depression and schizophrenia. That sounds "Freudian," and we were taught from the '70s on to oppose Freudian ideas as unscientific and clinically unproven. So, we persist in trying to prove that mental illness is solely caused by inherited factors that are completely unrelated to our lived experiences. In such a misguided view, we "catch" depression and bipolar disorder as if it were pneumonia.

[19] Batelaan NM, Bosman RX, Muntingh A, Scholten WD, Huijbregts KM, van Balkom AJM: Risk of relapse after antidepressant discontinuation in anxiety disorders, obsessive-compulsive disorder, and post-traumatic stress disorder: systematic review and meta-analysis of relapse prevention Trials. *BMJ* 2017;358:j3927.

[20] A recent study did show that psilocybin decreased activity in the amygdala and increased activity in the prefrontal cortex in patients with treatment resistant depression. But this seems to be a characteristic finding of all treatments research for depression, including psychotherapy. Carhart-Harris RL, Roseman L, Bolstridge M, et al.: Psilocybin for treatment-resistant depression: fMRI-measured brain mechanisms. *Sci Rep* 2017;13:13187.

# THE PRICE OF IGNORING ENVIRONMENTAL INFLUENCES

In a piercing and eye-opening article in *Scientific American* in 2017, Michael Balter reviewed one such example of ignoring the role of environment in favor of searching for the gene that causes a psychiatric illness.[21] He begins with a finding that was hailed as a landmark by top-level media, the isolation of a gene mutation that appears to increase the risk for schizophrenia.[22] I will explain a bit about this finding in order to make the controversy surrounding it clear.

Schizophrenia occurs in approximately 1% of the world's population. It has been known for many years that it must in part be an inherited disorder. Whenever the risk of a disease is higher in first-degree relatives of someone with that disease than in first-degree relatives of someone without the disease, inheritance is obviously suspected. For nonpsychiatric diseases, this kind of familial risk usually means there is a mutation in one or more genes causing the illness. But for psychiatric illnesses there looms the possibility that living with someone with an illness, rather than inheriting an abnormal gene, is the reason a person gets the disorder. For most purely physical diseases, we do not think that a parent can influence a child to get the disease. You don't get breast cancer because your mother had it, and you are somehow copying her example. Any link between a parent and child both having breast cancer is purely genetic,[23] but the experience of living with a parent with depression might be the reason someone develops depression himself. Growing up in a home with depression could affect brain development so that the environment, not just genes, is responsible. So, for psychiatric illnesses, a different kind of test is needed to determine if there is any genetic basis.

Twin studies are the gold standard for deciding if a psychiatric illness is passed on from parent to child via abnormal genes. Remember that identical (also called monozygotic) twins share all the same genes, whereas fraternal (or dizygotic) twins have only 50% of the same genes, just like ordinary brothers and sisters. If one identical twin has a purely genetic disease, the other should have it 100% of the time as well, whereas if one fraternal twin has a purely genetic disease, the chance the other fraternal twin has it should be only 50%. If a disorder is partly genetic and partly caused by environmental factors (as is the case, for example, with type 2 diabetes, which is partly caused by obesity), then those rates will be lower than 100% and 50%, respectively, depending on how strong the environmental factor is and how similar or dissimilar the childhood environments were of the twins. We call the number of times the two members of a twinship have a disease the *concordance rate*. Even when an

[21] Balter M: Schizophrenia's unyielding mysteries. *Sci Am* May 1, 2017; https://www.scientificamerican.com/article/schizophrenia-rsquo-s-unyielding-mysteries/

[22] Sekar A, Bialas AR, de Rivera H, et al.: Schizophrenia risk from complex variation of complement component 4. *Nature* 2016;530:177–183.

[23] Even this statement is a bit glib. Excessive alcohol intake is a risk factor for breast cancer, and alcoholism is familial. Hence, one can construct a plausible scenario whereby a daughter getting breast cancer is partially the result of a genetic link (for alcoholism) with her mother.

illness is partly genetic and partly environmental, the concordance rate for identical twins should be higher than for fraternal twins.

And that is exactly what is found in people with schizophrenia. The concordance rate for schizophrenia among identical twins is about 50%, whereas the concordance rate for schizophrenia among fraternal twins is only about 15%, a very statistically significant difference. Hence, it is clear that some part of schizophrenia is genetic.

But it is also unlikely that a single mutation in a single gene is involved. It is probably the case that we know all the diseases that are caused by a single gene mutation already. These are illnesses like sickle cell anemia and Huntington's disease. If an identical twin has Huntington's disease, the other identical twin always has it. Most diseases, however, are the result of mutations in several genes that work together to cause the illness. This makes it very difficult to find them, especially since different sets of genes may be causative in different people with the same disease.

One way to search for abnormal genes in this multigene scenario is to gather thousands of people with the disease and thousands of people without it and compare their DNA, base pair by base pair, through all their chromosomes. Once a daunting task, modern technology makes the genome-wide association study (GWAS) possible. In 2014, a huge GWAS study involving 36,989 people with schizophrenia and 113,075 control subjects without schizophrenia identified 128 differences in base pairs between patients and controls on 108 genes.[24] These 108 genes, therefore, may be involved in why some people develop schizophrenia. One of the genes codes for a protein called C4, and that attracted particular attention.

The immune system uses a group of about 30 small protein molecules, called the *complement system*, to enhance the ability of antibodies and immune cells to neutralize pathogens like bacteria and viruses. C4 is one of these complement proteins, and the gene that codes for it was also one of the 108 genes found to have a mutation in patients with schizophrenia in the 2014 study. This led to the study that got Michael Balter so exercised. In that study,[25] a group of scientists did three things. First, they used GWAS techniques to confirm the finding that the C4 gene is strongly associated with schizophrenia. Second, they examined 700 postmortem brains and found that the C4 protein is more abundant in schizophrenia brains, that a particular variant of the C4 gene that they called C4A was elevated in brains of people with schizophrenia compared to controls, and that the C4 gene is located in neurons in places involved with making synaptic connections. Third, they looked at what C4 does in mouse brain and found it is necessary for "pruning" or eliminating unnecessary connections between neurons during brain development. This process occurs in humans, too, mostly during adolescence, and some postmortem studies of human brains show a deficiency in synaptic connections in people with schizophrenia.

[24] Schizophrenia Working Group of the Psychiatric Genomics Consortium: Biological insights from 108 schizophrenia-associated genetic loci. *Nature* 2014;511:421–427.
[25] Sekar A, Bialas AR, de Rivera H, et al.: Schizophrenia risk from complex variation of complement component 4. *Nature* 2016;530:177–183.

The National Institutes of Health (NIH), which funded the study, issued a press release in which the then acting director of the NIH is quoted as calling the finding "a breakthrough."[26] Media emphasized that the link to the C4 gene is the strongest for schizophrenia yet reported and that because it has plausible biological significance—the possibility of abnormal synaptic pruning in schizophrenia—it should encourage the search for new and specific treatments.

But Balter points out some clear reasons to be circumspect about the finding. First, he points out, about 22% of the healthy controls in the study also had the C4A form of the gene. This means that even though the C4 gene association is the strongest yet discovered for schizophrenia, it turns out that, by itself, it explains only a very, very small part of the risk to get the illness.

A second issue is that it is a big leap from showing that C4 is involved in pruning synapses in developing mouse brain to knowing if it is involved in this process in developing human brains. Remember that the evidence for a reduced number of synaptic connections between neurons in schizophrenia comes from examination of postmortem brain samples. By the time they die, people with schizophrenia have been exposed to many things that might eliminate synapses, including poor nutrition, stress, cigarette smoking, alcohol use, and antipsychotic medications.

Finally, Balter points out that GWAS studies require very large numbers of subjects, mandating that diagnoses of the patient participants have to be done with relatively brief screens. These are generally accurate, but it is likely that some people get into these studies who do not really have the illness in question. This will introduce error into the findings.

But the biggest reason that Balter balks at the genetic findings is that they systematically ignore the strong evidence that environmental factors also contribute to schizophrenia. Many studies, for example, have shown that growing up in a city increases the risk for schizophrenia compared to growing up in a rural area. Whereas the high-risk form of the C4 gene increases the risk for schizophrenia by about 27%, growing up in an urban neighborhood increased the risk by 80% in one study.[27] Now some of that city risk could itself be partially explained by genetics if people who harbor the high-risk genes for schizophrenia are more likely to move to urban areas than people without these genes, but not all of it. My friend and former colleague, Columbia University psychiatrist and epidemiologist Ezra Susser, told an audience in 2004 that "It's not clear if it is birth in cities, or upbringing in cities, but there is something about city living that increases risk." Susser is reported to have gone "on to explain that where you are born and brought up is a larger contributing factor to risk than genetic predisposition. Indeed, 34.6% of schizophrenia cases would be prevented if people were not

[26] National Institutes of Health: Schizophrenia's strongest known genetic risk deconstructed. January 27, 2016, https://www.nih.gov/news-events/news-releases/schizophrenias-strongest-known-genetic-risk-deconstructed

[27] Newbury J, Arseneault L, Caspi A, Moffitt TE, Odgers CL, Fisher HL: Why are children in urban neighborhoods at increased risk for psychotic symptoms? Findings from a UK longitudinal cohort study. *Schizophr Bull* 2016;42:1372–1383.

born and brought up in cities, compared to 5.4% of cases that would be prevented if people did not have parents or siblings who suffered from the illness."[28]

None of this should be taken as eschewing the importance of searching for genes for schizophrenia or any other illness. Even finding a gene with a small effect on disease causality could point scientists toward an intervention. The C4 finding tells us that genes involved in the body's immunological system are somehow tied into a brain disorder and opens up a whole area of research. Perhaps this will lead to new treatments that are more securely based on the actual cause of schizophrenia.

It might seem easier to find a medication to treat an overabundance of C4 in the brain of people with schizophrenia than to do something about the effects of growing up in a city. What aspects of living in a city are linked to schizophrenia? Crowding, poverty, pollution, crime? People are already working on those issues, and it is not immediately obvious how learning that they affect the risk for schizophrenia will help us find a better treatment. Should we advise people to move out of the city if they are concerned that their children are demonstrating behaviors that have been shown to be precursors of schizophrenia, like social isolation, learning difficulties, or smoking marijuana? Doing so would entail a mass exodus from urban areas because the great majority of children who exhibit those behaviors will not in fact get schizophrenia.

But developing a new drug based on a genetic finding is hardly going to be easy either. Consider for a moment another attempt at basic science-guided drug discovery. It has been known for decades that a major pathological signature in the brains of people with Alzheimer's type dementia is something called an amyloid plaque. These are tiny plaques composed of an abnormal form of a protein that are found outside of neurons throughout the brains of Alzheimer's patients. For a variety of reasons, it seems logical to attempt to dissolve those plaques in order to improve memory loss and other impairments in Alzheimer's patients, so scientists developed an intriguing approach: injecting antibodies that see the amyloid plaques as foreign invaders and destroy them. In a mouse model of Alzheimer's disease, this approach not only reduces the number of plaques in the brains of aged mice, it also improves their memory. Some evidence even suggests that these medications reduce plaque burden in humans with Alzheimer's disease. Yet, despite numerous clinical trials, none of them has resulted in any meaningful clinical improvement.

The brain is such a tricky organ. It seems to defy logic and thwart our every attempt at intervention. Some medications are quite successful for brain diseases, like anticonvulsants for epilepsy. But most medications offer only symptomatic improvement without addressing underlying causes. Suppose that too much C4 protein is a problem that causes some cases of schizophrenia. We could conceivably develop a drug that specifically reduces the amount of the high-risk form of the protein, C4A. But if excess pruning of synapses is the problem with C4, this occurs mainly during adolescent years, before most patients can reliably be diagnosed with schizophrenia.

---

[28] Ezra Susser's comments at a 2004 conference are reported in http://www.schizophrenia.com/prevention/country.html

And remember that C4A was present in a lot of people without schizophrenia. We might not know to whom to give the drug because we wouldn't know exactly who is going to get schizophrenia.

Furthermore, the complement system is essential for the proper functioning of our immune systems. Although C4A may be associated with schizophrenia, it probably also plays a role in fighting infections. If we attack it, would we be increasing the risk for serious infectious diseases? Even if we could somehow restrict an "anti-C4A" drug to the brain—which would be very hard to do—it might still cause an increase in brain infections. It is true that scientists are making remarkable progress developing strategies to use the immune system to fight cancer and other diseases, and we have every right to hope that work like this might someday help with psychiatric illnesses. But that someday is not going to be soon. All indications are that we are going to be using the nonspecific antidepressants and antipsychotics, or variations on their basic themes, for the foreseeable future.

## PSYCHOTHERAPY CAN CHANGE THE BRAIN

We aren't going to eliminate child abuse, poverty, or homelessness in the near future either. So how can knowing that these things are linked to psychiatric disorders help us develop better interventions?

The path, I believe, lies in accepting two propositions of this book; first, that adverse life experiences alter brain function and structure, and, second, that psychotherapy is a form of life experience that can repair some of those changes. What we need is more psychotherapy studies that are linked with neurobiology. The critical questions to ask here are what forms of psychotherapy work for which disorders, when do those psychotherapies work better with the addition of medication, and what effect do successful psychotherapies have on the physical structure and function of the brain.

Hopefully, I have convinced you that neither of these propositions is at all far-fetched and that it is eminently possible to begin doing the kind of research I propose right now. It will have to be funded by the NIH; drug companies are not going to pay for psychotherapy studies. Nor will this work replace drugs and drug research. That absolutely must continue. Lithium is for a bipolar patient what insulin is for a person with diabetes, nothing short of life-saving. It would be nice, of course, to know what lithium actually does in the brain and to find something that is better tolerated. But we are not going to be able to help many people suffering from severe psychiatric illnesses without prescribing medications.

It is a rare patient, however, who won't benefit from psychotherapy, many without taking medications at all. Patients with some conditions, like depression and anxiety disorders, should be treated with psychotherapy before going to medication; patients with schizophrenia and bipolar disorder should get both medications and psychotherapy. A concerted effort at psychotherapy research combined with neurobiological studies using both animal models and brain imaging studies in humans will refine what types of therapy to use for which patients and develop more powerful psychotherapeutic approaches.

I envision that CBT and psychoanalytic therapies will both turn out to be effective and both have a neurobiological basis. We touched on some examples of this biology in Chapter 8, but there is much more interesting work that can already be pursued in this area. CBT, psychoanalytic therapy, and other types of psychotherapy will be useful in different situations and for different patients. A recent meta-analysis of 207 studies showed that both forms of therapy are capable of producing large and long-lasting changes in neurotic personality traits.[29] Research will undoubtedly show that modifications in how these therapies are conducted will have to be made, particularly for psychoanalytic therapies, to make them more effective and practical. But we already know that psychotherapy works and changes the brain; the scientific basis for these studies already exists.

What is needed as much as anything is a change of attitude from all camps involved in treating psychiatric illnesses. Those who regard neuroscience as the enemy and think it is only there to make reductive pronouncements and promote psychopharmacology will need to look harder at what neuroscience is really doing. Those who think that psychotherapy has no scientific basis need to examine the evidence. More than any other organ of the body, the brain works by assimilating experiences into its biological processes. Throughout life, what we see, hear, feel, and experience changes how our brains work and look in profound ways from the molecular level of gene expression to the cellular level of synaptic connections to the systems level of connections among brain regions. It should be no surprise, then, that an intervention in which a therapist and a patient embark on an intense process over time should not only work but also change the brain as well.

Yes, I still get excited every time a new genetic association for a psychiatric or neurological disease is announced or a potential new medication is characterized. Psychopharmacology is an indelible part of my background. But I have learned that our drugs are blunt instruments that work, but not well enough and not without consequences. I have seen both in studies and from personal experience how well psychotherapy can work. It needs more experimental validation and a firmer biological basis. I hope today's neuroscientists and clinical researchers will take up the challenge.

This book clearly represents not only what I have learned about the brain, but also the ways in which my own experience has changed my view of many aspects of psychiatry and psychiatric illness. Once, I was an avid biological psychiatrist and psychopharmacologist. Have I changed all that much? Perhaps; but, without meaning to be glib, I have started to think that psychotherapy is in every sense like a psychiatric medication. It is directed at damage done to the human brain by adverse life experiences, and it makes adjustments to limit the consequences of that damage by changing physiological processes put in motion by those experiences. Like a medication, psychotherapy affects the physical brain. It is a powerful tool and one that is based on as much basic neuroscience as is any medication we currently prescribe. But it needs

---

[29]  Roberts BW, Luo J, Briley DA, Chow PI, Su R, Hill PL: A systematic review of personality trait change through intervention, *Psychol Bull* 143:2017:117–141.

to be studied, refined, and harnessed to make it more acceptable and more effective. Right now, people with psychiatric problems should try their best to get evidence-based psychotherapy of some sort whether or not they take medications.

So, in the end, I do not think the basic premises upon which I have operated have changed all that much in the past 40 or so years. I still believe that the mind is driven by molecules and cells. I still believe that the brain is physically altered in people with emotional disorders. What I have done is to accede to the data, data which clearly show both that adverse life experiences are part of the reason people get ill and that psychotherapy works. From there, it has been a fascinating journey to figure out how neuroscience might connect them. Right now, it feels like being on the border between the mind and the brain. In the not too distant future, that border will be eliminated and progress toward helping more people more effectively will be made.

# Index

Figures are indicated by an italic *f* following the page number.